Textbook of
Inorganic Pharmaceutical and
Medicinal Chemistry

Textbook of
Inorganic Pharmaceutical and
Medicinal Chemistry

ELEVENTH EDITION

Professor J. S. Qadry

M. Pharm. (Pb.), D. Sc. (Germany),
MSEI, FGAG (Germany), MASP (USA)
Dean-Director, Shekhawati College of Pharmacy, Dundlod, Rajasthan

Formerly
Dean, Dubai Pharmacy College, Dubai, UAE
Founder Principal, Hamdard College of Pharmacy, University of Delhi
Founder Dean and Vice Chancellor, Hamdard University, New Delhi
Chairman, Board of Pharmaceutical Education and Research, AICTE, New Delhi
Advisor-Specialist, Ministry of Public Health, Kuwait
President, Pharmacy Council of India

S. Z. Qadry

M. Pharm.
Hamdard College of Pharmacy, New Delhi, India

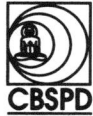

CBSPD

CBS Publishers & Distributors Pvt Ltd

New Delhi • Bengaluru • Chennai • Kochi • Kolkata • Lucknow • Mumbai
Hyderabad • Jharkhand • Nagpur • Patna • Pune • Uttarakhand

Textbook of Inorganic
Pharmaceutical Chemistry

ISBN: 978-81-239-1919-5

Eleventh Edition 2004
Reprint: 2012, 2017, 2018, 2019, 2020, 2024

Published by **Satish Kumar Jain** and produced by **Varun Jain** for

CBS Publishers & Distributors Pvt Ltd

4819/XI Prahlad Street, 24 Ansari Road, Daryaganj, New Delhi 110 002, India.

Ph: 011-23289259, 23266861

Website: www.cbspd.com
e-mail: delhi@cbspd.com

Corporate Office: 204 FIE, Industrial Area, Patparganj, Delhi 110 092

Ph: 011-4934 4934

Fax: 011-4934 4935 e-mail: publishing@cbspd.com;publicity@cbspd.com

Branches

- **Bengaluru:** Seema House 2975, 17th Cross, K.R. Road, Banasankari 2nd Stage, Bengaluru 560 070, Karnataka, India
  Ph: +91-80-26771679/79   Fax: +91-80-26771680   e-mail: bangalore@cbspd.com
- **Chennai:** 7, Subbaraya Street, Shenoy Nagar, Chennai 600 030, Tamil Nadu, India
  Ph: +91-44-26680620, 26681266   Fax: +91-44-42032115   e-mail: chennai@cbspd.com
- **Kochi:** 42/1325, 1326, Power House Road, Opp KSEB, Ernakulam 682 018, Kochi, Kerala, India
  Ph: +91-484-4059061-67   Fax: +91-484-4059065   e-mail: kochi@cbspd.com
- **Kolkata:** 147, Hind Ceramics Compound, 1st Floor, Nilgunj Road, Belghoria, Kolkata 700 056, West Bengal, India
  Ph: +91-33-25633055/56   e-mail: kolkata@cbspd.com
- **Lucknow:** Basement, Khushnuma Complex, 7-Meerabai Marg (Behind Jawahar Bhawan), Lucknow 226 001, UP, India
  Ph: +0552-4000032   e-mail:tiwari.lucknowl@cbspd.com
- **Mumbai:** PWD Shed. Gala no. 25/26, Ramchundra Bhatt Marg, Next to JJ Hospital Gate no. 2, Opp. Union Bank of India, Noorbaug, Mumbai 400 009, Maharashtra, India
  Ph: 022-66661880/89   e-mail: mumbai@cbspd.com

Representatives

• Hyderabad	0-9885175004	• Jharkhand	0-9811541605	• Nagpur	0-8692091830
• Patna	0-9334159340	• Pune	0-9664372571	• Uttarakhand	0-9716462459

Printed at: Sanjay Printers, Sahibabad, U.P, India

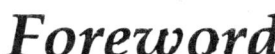

Foreword

I am happy that Prof. Qadry has undertaken the task of writing a textbook on inorganic pharmaceutical and medicinal chemistry. Although books on pharmaceutical chemistry by Indian authors have been published in the past, the publication of a book bringing the information up-to-date is to be welcomed. This book would be useful not only to students of pharmacy but also to teachers of inorganic pharmaceutical chemistry. The redeeming feature of this book is that the information has been presented in a simple manner and would therefore be easily understandable for diploma students.

The chapter on pharmaceutical methods of analysis and assay methods would be useful not only to students but also to pharmacists working in hospital pharmacies and in the industry. The alphabetical classification of official compounds and preparations that has been followed is more convenient, particularly since the Indian Pharmacopoeia, with which the students would have to remain acquainted, adopts such a classification.

The book contains information that is relevant to the syllabus prescribed by the Pharmacy Council of India for diploma students and books such as these could help in bringing about uniformity not only in the standard of education but also in the standards of teaching in pharmacy institutions.

Prof. Qadry, who is an eminent pharmaceutical educationist, has rendered valuable service to the profession of pharmacy by publishing this book which should find a place in all institutions imparting education in pharmacy.

Drugs Controller (India)   **Dr. D.S. Gotoskar**
New Delhi, December 1980

v

Preface to the Eleventh Edition

When I first started writing this book on Inorganic Pharmaceutical and Medicinal Chemistry way back in 1979, the existing syllabus of PCI at that point of time consisted of inorganic compounds and their preparations arranged on the basis of individual metals and compounds thereof. The pharmacists' bible at that time was the Indian Pharmacopoeia 1966. Having had long experience in teaching, I noticed that it was only at the end of the completion of a pharmaceutical agent's "monograph" that the uses were generally only cursorily mentioned. This made the subject not only a lot monotonous, but it did not even do justice with the medicinal and pharmaceutical values of the compounds and their preparations in so far as their usefulness and applicability in medicine and industry was concerned. By this time the students were also not exposed to pharmacological teaching, which could give them understanding about therapeutic and technical applications of the inorganic agents being taught in the classes.

There was, therefore, need to classify these inorganic compounds and their preparations on the basis of their medicinal and therapeutic usefulness and industrial utility. This, I thought, could make the teaching more explanatory and interesting to make the students understand the pharmacological/ therapeutic background of each of the compound and its preparations. Fortunately, I could put this idea into practice as the new Education Regulation 1992 started being framed with my full involvement as a member of EC and Vice President of PCI. I saw to it that ERC of PCI designed its courses, especially of pharmacognosy and chemistry in a more rational way. This I achieved through the ERC by seeing to it that the new syllabus of ER 1992 overhaul the content of both pharmacognosy and inorganic pharmaceutical chemistry on the basis of therapeutic classification and in a manner that did give the subjects the practical importance they deserve. Some time later, fortunately, I again had the occasion to involve myself in devising the degree courses by the AICTE, with me as the Chairman of All India Board of Pharmaceutical Education, AICTE, New Delhi and President, Pharmacy Council of India. At AICTE also we framed the courses on the same lines, making it rather look more meaningful under the clear cut therapeutic and technical headings, keeping in mind the fact that the Bachelor Course was being framed collectively for the whole of India (which in fact was supposed to be utilized by PCI, as it was popularly believed at that time that the PCI would soon switchover to the degree course, after doing away with the Diploma course). I, as usual, again revised the books keeping in view the AICTE syllabus in my mind. This also did not in any way undermine the requirements of the Diploma course. The newly designed and drafted degree course by the AICTE also fulfilled the desirability of colleges conducting the courses to give parity to almost all the courses conducted by them in different parts of India. This parity in the AICTE courses was but natural as the sword of AICTE was always hanging on the colleges, as it (AICTE) threatened them not to recognize the colleges, if they did not seek their permission and approval of conducting the courses in Pharmacy as per their directives. I recently came to know that the PCI has formed Pharm. D. Regulations, 2008 under Section 10 of the Pharmacy Act, 1948, and that it has already notified the regulation in the Gazette of India. I am more than satisfied to see the new shape of the courses and find Inorganic Pharmaceutical Chemistry course fall into the same pattern, covering essentially the same course contents as considered rational and desirable.

The present revised edition will thus continue to cater to the needs of all the courses, including the newly adopted Pharm. D. course. The changes made in the textual subject matter have been introduced in view of the latest I.P. 2007 requirements. The appendices, which had got deleted inadvertently by the publisher from the 7th edition onwards, have been reintroduced with modifications whenever necessary. When I first wrote the book, I had to lay hand on the official compound and their preparations that were included in the I.P. 1966. The fourth edition was revised by following the I.P. 1985. The fifth and subsequent editions were revised keeping in mind the latest I.P.s as and when they appeared. Ever since the I.P. 1966 to I.P. 2007 enormous changes and advances have taken place. I.P. 2007 increasing to three volumes and putting on about 10 kg weight. This also has resulted in quite a few compounds and/or their preparations having been deleted in subsequent I.P.s. However, the importance of medicinal/ pharmaceutical and industrial materials has not abated a bit. On the contrary they continue to have almost the same importance in practice. That is why the present edition has not excluded any compound and its preparations. I am sure the readers will agree with me in this respect. I may further add that the inorganic pharmaceutical and medicinal chemistry is just not a basic inorganic chemistry of the school level, but it deals with the special applied course. The basics of the subject in question have already been taken care of in the schools until the 12th Class. Hence, the subject matter of the course as given in the syllabus should be respected and followed in letter and spirit and dealt with as an applied course, covering the molecular structure, nomenclature, origin, preparation, properties, identification, tests for purity, detection of impurities, assay methods, knowledge of therapeutic and technical values, dosage forms, storage, posology, etc. of the official and other important inorganic compounds and their preparations. Although I have faithfully tried to refer to the I.P. 2007 during the revision of the book, I have not deleted the few compounds which have been official in earlier I.P.s most of which still find them included in other pharmacopoeias and other official books and formularies. I must stress here that I find all the inorganic compounds which have been officially recognised at a particular given time still as important as they have been through all these years and are in use and demand as usual.

Wherever I have used the term I.P., it means I.P. 2007 and its appendix. At places old I.P.s references have also been retained. Also since the original 1980s descriptive textual style has been liked and appreciated, it has been retained. A new feature of this edition is that I have myself taken the responsibility to publish the book in my personal care in Dubai and Delhi. I am happy that the book is going to be marketed by the distinguished All India fame Medical Books Distributors, the CBS Publishers & Distributors, Ansari Road, New Delhi. I thank Mr. Satish K. Jain, Managing Director and Mr. Vinod K. Jain, Production Director of CBS Publishers & Distributors for volunteering to market the book on my behalf. Let me take this opportunity to thank those of my friends, teachers and former students (now teachers) who have appreciated my student-friendly style in writing the book. Their appreciation will surely lead to my further motivation and encouragement.

J.S. Qadry

Contents

Introduction

Chemistry as a subject is as vast as the whole universe. Name anything, it is comprised of chemistry. The subject of chemistry now consists of many branches. Earlier when one talked about the branches of chemistry one just mentioned them as organic, inorganic, physical and analytical chemistry. Later on, and more so now, we have to know to name the other branches of chemistry, like biochemistry, polymer chemistry, material science chemistry, environmental chemistry, thermo chemistry, electro chemistry, nuclear chemistry, computational chemistry and of course dear to us the applied and important pharmaceutical/medicinal chemistry.

This book deals with the medicinal compounds of Inorganic Chemistry, a branch of chemistry which is concerned with the preparations, properties, reactions, analysis and utilisation of inorganic compounds. Even though these days most of the required pharmaceuticals belong to the organic chemical nature, yet a great number of inorganic medicinal compounds of exceptional importance are in great demand for therapeutic use. A single inorganic chemical compound contains fixed proportions of two or more elements. The compounds which are obtained from living organism - plants and animals - are called organic and all others are called inorganic. All the organic compounds contain carbon, while very few of the inorganic compounds do so. Accordingly any compound of carbon is an organic compound except carbon monoxide, carbonates, cyanides, cyanates, thiocyanates and some carbides. This book deals mainly with the inorganic pharmaceutical and medicinal compounds.

It is understood that by now the students, who are going to be exposed to the inorganic pharmaceutical chemistry course, have abreast themselves quite well with the general inorganic and physical chemistry in either the first year of the course in pharmacy or previously up to the 12th class of the 10 + 2 system of school education or in the pre-medical course or in intermediate or equivalent course, which made them eligible for admission to the Degree or Diploma Course in Pharmacy. Hence it is neither possible nor desirable to treat here basic general inorganic and physical chemistry in any detail.

This book will essentially deal with the study of inorganic substances and their preparations that are official in the Pharmacopoeia of India. The word official normally denotes a substance which is defined in the monograph and is official in I.P., B.P., and U.S.P. and in any other authoritative book of a country or a group of countries.

All the important inorganic compounds commonly used in pharmacy will be dealt with their origin (definition), chemical formula, preparation, description, solubility, tests for identity, tests for purity, method of assay, storage, pharmaceutical preparations, pharmaceutical/therapeutical uses and doses.

Since the compounds are mostly intended for their therapeutic action and uses, it is desired that they should conform to definite standards and be devoid of impurities. A student is thus supposed to have thorough practical knowledge about the identification and tests for purity, assay methods and limit tests for the presence of common impurities like arsenic (As); lead (Pb); iron (Fe); sulphate (SO_4); chloride (Cl), etc. As the determination of the purity of pharmaceutical substances is of significant importance, it is desired that certain general physical and chemical methods are outlined in the beginning itself in Part I to enable the students to know about their details in anticipation of their occurrence in the texts that will follow. The details of other particular methods relating to some special pharmaceutical compounds will be described under the individual compounds as and when they occur.

Special care has been taken and restraint exercised to limit the scope of this book to suit the requirement of pharmacy students. Even the Degree Courses all over India include the study of pharmacopoeial compounds and hence references to I.P. standards have been made in describing tests for identity, tests for purity, assay, etc.

I.P. requirements and methods, especially for testing the limits of impurities wherever described in this book, are indicated in the text. Tests for identity as applied to the inorganic compounds for qualitative reaction for some common substances and radicals, as given in I.P. Appendix, are also included in this book.

The beginning of the chapters and the compounds included in them are preceded by a fairly detailed introduction from all angles viz. therapeutic aspect of elements and the compounds, etc. Explanation of the procedures adopted for testing methods and for assay methods are given at proper places. References in the text to the I.P. appendices and other I.P. standards followed are also cited.

PART I

Methods of Pharmaceutical Analysis

Common Impurities in Official Compounds

An understanding of the nature and sources of impurities in pharmaceuticals is necessary to apply various tests for their detection and control. Impurities in chemical/pharmaceutical compounds are introduced from starting materials, intermediates, reagents, solvents, catalysts, etc., used in their manufacture and through the use of metallic plants (equipment, apparatus, reaction vessels, etc.). In these the solvents act on the metals like silver, copper, lead, cast iron, steel, iron, aluminium and other alloys of which the apparatus, vessels, pans, etc., are made. In order to find the nature and magnitude of impurities in a chemical/pharmaceutical compound, one has to have the knowledge of raw materials, intermediates, reagents, etc. and the process of manufacture involved in obtaining the compound. However, it is out of scope of this book to go into details about the occurrence, causes and sources of impurities in pharmaceutical compounds. In short it can be stated that the methods of manufacture of a pharmaceutical compound can always afford to point out the source and types of expected impurities.*

The most common qualitative official limit tests for impurities such as chloride, sulphate and iron and the quantitative tests for arsenic and lead are given below. There are general qualitative and quantitative limit tests which are applicable to almost all the pharmaceutical compounds, sometimes in special cases with little modification. Special data concerning description, solubility, identification, test for purity, and also other standards, such as melting point, distillation range, specific gravity and methods of assay of each pharmaceutical compound will be given under each compound, along with the method of preparation, storage, uses and doses.

Limit Tests for Chlorides, Sulphates and Iron

These tests are based on the production of an opalescence, turbidity or colour and comparing any of these with that obtained in standard solutions.

---

* Impurities in commercial products are common and vary much in their proportion. Sometimes being so small that for a layman they may not be of any significance. They are likely to be higher in commercial products compared with those which are produced on smaller scales in laboratories. The commonest source of impurities in pharmaceutical products is the material used for plant construction and decomposition of substances on storage. Sometimes imurities can creep in due to the nature and properties of substances, e.g. impurity of sodium carbonate in sodium hydroxide due to highly deliquescent nature of sodium hydroxide. Impurities may also occur due to the preecess of manufacture followed for obtaining a particular substance and due to adulteration with cheaper materials.

Limit Test for Chlorides

The test is performed by dissolving a specified quantity of the substance (to be tested for Cl ion) in water and transferring the solution to a Nessler glass.[*] To the solution in Nessler glass is added 1 ml of nitric acid (HNO_3) and sufficient water to make the volume up to 50 ml. 1 ml of a solution of silver nitrate is then added to the Nessler glass and the solution after stirring with a glass rod is set aside for five minutes. An opalescence, due to the formation of silver chloride, is produced which is compared with that produced by adding silver nitrate to a standard solution containing a specified quantity of hydrochloric acid.

Standard opalescence: This is produced by measuring 1 ml of 0.01 N (N/100) hydrochloric acid (HCl) and 1 ml of nitric acid (HNO_3) in a Nessler glass, adding sufficient water to make 50 ml. 1 ml of a solution of silver nitrate is then added and the solution is stirred with a glass rod and set aside for five minutes. The reaction involved is as follows:

$$NaCl + AgNO_3 \xrightarrow{\quad HNO_3 \quad} AgCl\downarrow + NaNO_3$$

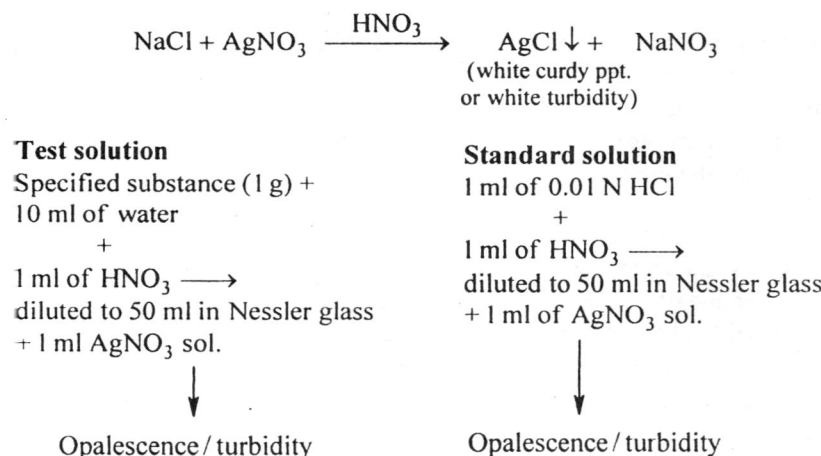

(white curdy ppt.
or white turbidity)

Test solution
Specified substance (1 g) +
10 ml of water
+
1 ml of $HNO_3 \longrightarrow$
diluted to 50 ml in Nessler glass
+ 1 ml AgNO₃ sol.

Opalescence / turbidity

Standard solution
1 ml of 0.01 N HCl
+
1 ml of $HNO_3 \longrightarrow$
diluted to 50 ml in Nessler glass
+ 1 ml of AgNO₃ sol.

Opalescence / turbidity

.If the turbidity appears to be greater in test solution than that in standard solution, the Cl impurity is greater and hence the substance does not pass the limit test for chloride.

Note: Sometimes the solution, to be tested, is to be prepared by special method and instruction to this effect, if given, should be followed for preparing the test solution.

Limit Test for Sulphates

In this case also the turbidity produced in the test solution is compared with that produced in standard solution.

Test solution: A specified quantity of the substance (to be tested for SO_4 ions) is dissolved in water and transferred to Nessler glass. To the Nessler glass is added 1 ml of hydrochloric acid (if HCl is not already used for preparing the test solution) and the volume is made up with water upto 50 ml. 1 ml of

---

[*] **Nessler glass/cylinder:** They are tubes of clear, colourless glass with uniform internal diameter and a flat, transparent base. They are made of transparent glass with a capacity of 50 ml. They measure $150 \times 124 \times 3.0$ mm. They are used for comparative tests.

a solution of barium chloride ($BaCl_2$) is added to the Nessler glass and the solution stirred immediately with glass rod and set aside for five minutes. The turbidity produced is compared with that produced by the standard solution simultaneously.

Standard solution: This solution for standard turbidity is prepared by taking 2.5 ml of N/100 H_2SO_4 and 1 ml of HCl into a Nessler glass and diluting the solution to 50 ml by adding sufficient water. To this standard solution is then added 1 ml of $BaCl_2$. The solution is immediately stirred with a glass rod and set aside for five minutes.

The reaction involved is as follows :

$$H_2SO_4 + BaCl_2 \xrightarrow{\text{HCl}} \downarrow BaSO_4 + 2HCl$$

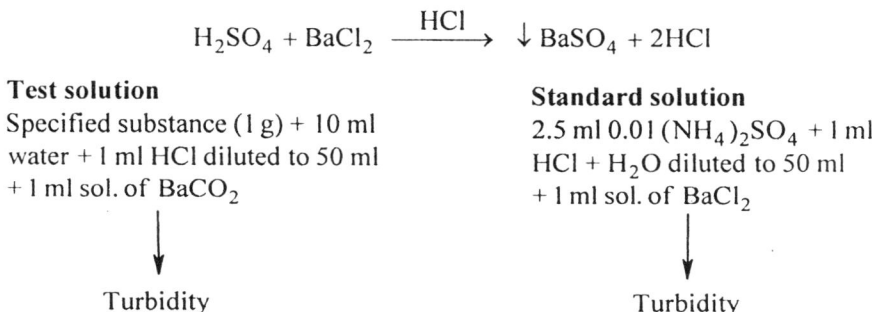

Test solution
Specified substance (1 g) + 10 ml water + 1 ml HCl diluted to 50 ml + 1 ml sol. of $BaCO_2$

Turbidity

Standard solution
2.5 ml 0.01 $(NH_4)_2SO_4$ + 1 ml HCl + H_2O diluted to 50 ml + 1 ml sol. of $BaCl_2$

Turbidity

The turbidity produced in the test solution should not be greater than that produced in the standard solution.

Limit Test for Iron

In this test, colour produced in the test solution is compared with that produced in the standard solution.

Test solution: A specified quantity of substance (to be tested for iron) is dissolved in 40 ml of water to which is added 2 ml of a 20% w/v solution of iron free citric acid in water and two drops of thioglycollic acid. The solution is mixed, made alkaline with (iron-free) solution of ammonia and diluted with water to make the volume up to 50 ml in Nessler glass. The solution is allowed to stand for 5 minutes and the colour developed in Nessler glass is compared by viewing vertically with that developed in the standard solution.

Standard solution: Two ml of standard solution of iron (prepared as follows) is diluted with 40 ml of water and to this 2 ml of a 20% w/v solution of iron-free citric acid in water and 2 drops of thioglycollic acid are added. The solution is mixed, made alkaline with (iron-free) solution of ammonia and diluted with sufficient amount of water to make the volume up to 50 ml in Nessler glass. The solution is allowed to stand for 5 minutes and the colour developed is compared with that developed in the test solution by viewing vertically.

The colour developed in test solution should not be deeper than that developed in the standard solution.

Preparation of standard solution of iron: It is prepared by adding 0.173 g of ferric ammonium sulphate ($NH_4Fe(SO_4)_2 \cdot 12H_2O$) to 1.5 ml of HCl and adding sufficient water to produce 1000 ml. Each ml of solution contains 0.02 mg of iron.

Test solution

Sample + 40 ml of water + 2 ml of 20% w/v (iron-free) citric acid + 2 drops of thioglycollic acid; solution mixed, made alkaline with ammonia and volume adjusted to 50 ml; allowed to stand. Colour developed is viewed vertically and compared with standard solution.

Standard solution

2 ml of standard sol. of iron + 40 ml of water + 2 ml of 20% w/v citric acid + 2 drops of thioglycollic acid; solution mixed, made alkaline with ammonia and volume adjusted to 50 ml; allowed to stand and develop colour.

In ammonical solution thioglycollic acid ($HS.CH_2CO_2H$) gives with iron salts a pale pink to deep reddish colour which is due to the formation of ferrous compound:

$$(HS.CH_2.COO)_2Fe$$

The citric acid is added to prevent the precipitation of iron by ammonia.

Note: All the reagents used in the limit test for iron should themselves be iron-free. Hence they themselves should conform to the limit tests for iron.

Quantitative test for arsenic

Arsenic impurity in a substance is expressed as parts per million and the principle involved in its detection and determination is based on the reduction of arsenic compound to gaseous arsenious hydride or arsine (AsH_3) by nascent hydrogen. The reduction is achieved by using zinc and dilute hydrochloric acid.

The substance to be tested is dissolved in acid (in case the substance is in the form of an extract or if it is to be dissolved in water, it is acidified) whereby the arsenic present in the sample is converted to arsenic acid. The solution, when treated with a reducing agent, converts arsenic acid to arsenious acid.

$$H_3AsO_4 \longrightarrow H_3AsO_3$$

Arsenic acid   Arsenious acid

The nascent hydrogen reduces arsenious acid to arsine.

$$H_3AsO_3 + 6[H] = AsH_3\uparrow + 3H_2O$$

Arsenious acid   Arsine

Arsine gas then comes into contact with mercuric chloride paper and stains it yellow. The depth of yellow stain on mercuric chloride paper will depend upon the quantity of arsenic present in the sample.

Apparatus: It consists of a wide mouth glass bottle of 120 ml capacity, fitted with a rubber bung through which passes a glass tube, 20 cm long, having an external diameter of about 0.8 cm and internal diameter of 0.65 cm. The upper end of the tube is rounded off, while the lower end of the tube, towards the bottom of the glass bottle, is drawn out to a diameter of about 1 mm and a hole, not less than 2 mm in diameter, is blown in the side near the lower end where the constriction begins.

The upper end of the glass tube is to be fitted with two rubber bungs, each with a hole bored centrally and exactly 6.5 mm in diameter. One of the bungs is fitted to the upper end of the tube, while the second bung is required to be fitted upon the first bung in such a way that the mercuric chloride paper is exactly sandwiched between the central perforation of the two. The bungs are then kept in close contact with the help of rubber band or spring clip in such a way that gas evolved from bottle must pass through the 0.65 mm internal circle of mercuric chloride paper.

The glass tube with the lower rubber bung should be so arranged that it, on being fitted to the glass bottle containing 70 ml of liquid, should in no case touch the liquid and its side hole should be below the bung (Fig. 1.1).

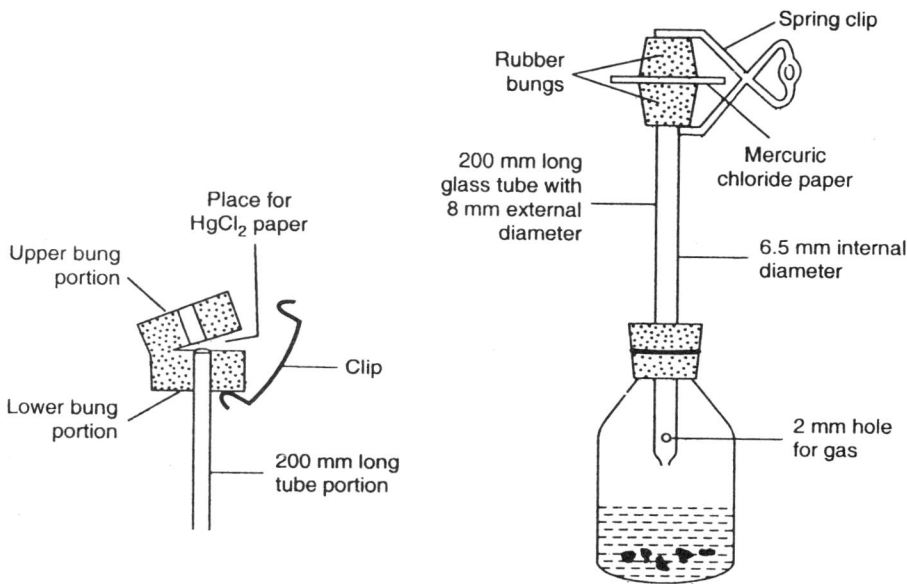

Fig. 1.1. Apparatus used for arsenic limit test; on the left is an alternative device for placing mercuric chloride paper.

Reagents: All the special reagents that are used in the limit test for arsenic are marked and distinguished by letter 'As T', meaning that they all should be arsenic free and should themselves conform to limit test for arsenic. Of course, dilute and strong arsenic solutions which are used for standard stains are exceptions.

Hydrochloric Acid 'As T'

HCl should comply with the following additional tests:

(i) Dilute 10 ml with sufficient water to produce 50 ml, add 5 ml of solution of ammonium thiocyanate and stir immediately. No colour is produced.

(ii) To 50 ml add 0.2 ml of bromine solution 'As T', evaporate on a water bath until reduced to 16 ml, adding more bromine solution 'As T', if necessary, in order that an excess, as indicated by the colour, may be present throughout the evaporation, add 50 ml of water and 5 drops of stannous chloride solution 'As T' and apply the general test. The stain produced is not deeper than 0.05 part per million.

Mercuric chloride paper: Smooth white filter paper, not less than 25 mm in width, soaked in a saturated solution of mercuric chloride, pressed to remove superfluous solution and dried at about 60° in the dark. The grade of the filter paper shall be such that the weight in g per sq. m. shall be between 65 and 120 g, the thickness in mm of 400 papers shall be approximately equal, numerically, to the weight in g per sq. m.

Note: Mercuric chloride paper should be stored in a stoppered bottle in the dark. Paper which has been exposed to sunlight or to the vapour of ammonia, affords a lighter coloured stain or no stain at all when employed in the quantitative test for arsenic.

Potassium Iodide 'As T'

Potassium iodide which complies with the following additional test:

Dissolve 10 g in 25 ml of hydrochloric acid 'As T' and 25 ml of water, add drops of stannous chloride solution 'As T' and apply the general test; no visible stain is produced.

Zinc 'As T'

Granulated zinc complies with the following additional test:

Add 10 ml of stannated hydrochloric acid 'As T' to 50 ml of water, and apply the general test using 10 g of the zinc, but allowing the action to continue for one hour; no visible stain is produced (limit of arsenic). Repeat the test with the addition of 0.1 ml of dilute arsenic solution As T; a faint but distinct yellow stain is produced (test for sensitivity).

Nitric Acid 'As T'

Nitric acid which complies with the following additional test:

Heat 20 ml in a procelain dish with 2 ml of sulphuric acid 'As T' until white fumes are given off. Cool, add 2 ml of water and again heat until white fumes are given off. Cool, add 50 ml of water and 10 ml of stannated hydrochloric acid 'As T' and apply the general test; no visible stain is produced.

Potassium Chlorate 'As T'

Potassium chlorate which complies with the following additional test:

Mix 5 g in the cold with 20 ml of water and 22 ml of hydrochloric acid 'As T'; when the first reaction has subsided, heat gently to expel chlorine, remove the last traces with a few drops of stannous chloride solution 'As T', add 20 ml of water, and apply the general test; no visible stain is produced.

Sodium Carbonate Anhydrous 'As T'

Anhydrous sodium carbonate which complies with the following additional test:

Dissolve 5 g in 50 ml of water, add 20 ml of brominated hydrochloric acid 'As T', remove the excess of bromine with a few drops of stannous chloride 'As T' and apply the general test; no visible stain is produced.

Stannated Hydrochloric Acid 'As T'

Prepared from solution of stannous chloride by adding an equal volume of hydrochloric acid, boiling down to the original volume and filtering through a fine-grained filter paper.

It complies with the following test:

To 10 ml add 6 ml of water and 10 ml of hydrochloric acid 'As T', distil, and collect 16 ml. To the distillate add 50 ml of water and a few drops of stannous chloride solution 'As T' and apply the general test; the stain produced is not deeper than a 1 ml standard stain showing that the proportion of arsenic present does not exceed 1 part per million.

Stannated Hydrochloric Acid 'As T'

Stannous chloride solution 'As T' .... 1 ml

Hydrochloric Acid 'As T' .... 100 ml

Sulphuric Acid 'As T'

Sulphuric acid which complies with following additional test:

Dilute 10 g with 50 ml of water, add 0.2 ml of stannous chloride solution 'As T' and apply the general test; no visible stain is produced.

Arsenic Solution Dilute 'As T'

Strong arsenic solution As T .... 1 ml

Water, sufficient to produce .... 100 ml

Dilute arsenic solution As T must be freshly prepared.

1 ml contains 0.01 mg of arsenic As T.

Arsenic Solution Strong 'As T'

Arsenic trioxide .... 0.132 g

Hydrochloric acid .... 50 ml

Water, sufficient to produce .... 100 ml

Brominated Hydrochloric Acid 'As T'

Bromine solution 'As T' .... 1 ml

Hydrochloric acid 'As T' .... 100 ml

Bromine Solution 'As T'

Bromine .... 30 g

Potassium bromide .... 30 g

Water, sufficient to produce .... 100 ml

METHODS FOR TESTING PURITY FOR ARSENIC

There are three methods which can be used for testing purity for arsenic:

1. Gutzeit Test; 2. Marsch Test; 3. Fileitmann Test.*

Note: For those substances which are soluble (simple organic compounds and large number of inorganic acids and salts) the solution under examination is prepared with water and stannated HCl

---

* In Gutzeit test arsine stains mercuric chloride paper yellow (as explained above). In Marsch test arsenic is decomposed to As mirror, while in Fileitmann test arsenic stains $AgNO_3$ paper greyish-black.

'As T'. But if the substances to be examined are insoluble, like $BaSO_4$, bentonite or kaolins, they are diffused in water.

The solution of substances, like metallic carbonates, etc., which effervesce with acids is obtained with brominated HCl As T. I.P. gives the methods of preparation of solutions of most of the substances which are required to be tested for arsenic impurity. Special reagents required for making solutions are given in I.P.

Procedure for Test for Arsenic

The glass tube (Fig. 1.1) is first lightly packed with cotton wool, which has been previously moistened with a solution of lead acetate and dried (because if impurity of H_2S is present, it will be trapped by lead acetate present in cotton, which otherwise itself would stain the mercuric chloride paper). The cotton is so arranged in the tube that the upper surface of the cotton is not less than 2.5 cm below the top of the tube and is lightly packed to allow the gas to quit efficiently.

The upper end of the tube is then inserted into the narrow end of one of the bungs and the two bungs secured by means of the rubber band after placing the mercuric chloride paper in between them as described above (Fig. 1.1).

The solution to be examined and prepared as specified is placed in the wide-mouthed bottle and to this is added 1 g of KI 'As T' and 10 g of Zinc 'As T'. The glass tube is placed in position quickly. The action is allowed to go on for 40 minutes. A yellow stain which is produced on the $HgCl_2$ paper, if arsenic is present, is compared in daylight with the standard stains which are produced by operating in a similar manner with known quantities of dil. arsenic sol. 'As T' (the action may be hastened by placing the glass bottle on warm surface).

The comparison of the stains is made immediately at the completion of the test and the standard stains used for comparison are prepared freshly as they fade on keeping. As a matter of fact both these tests should be performed simultaneously.

The proportion of arsenic in a substance can be determined by matching the intensity of colour with that of the standard stain.

A stain equivalent to 7 ml standard stain produced by operating on 10 g of a substance indicates that the proportion of arsenic is 1 part per million.

Standard Stains

Solutions are prepared by adding to 50 ml of water, 10 ml of stannated hydrochloric acid As T and quantities of dilute arsenic solution As T varying from 0.2 ml to 1 ml. The resulting solutions, when treated as described in the general test, yield stains on the mercuric chloride paper which are referred to as the standard stains.

Quantitative Test for Lead

The test is based on a reaction between lead and dithizone (diphenylthiocarbazone).

Dithizone in chloroform has the property of extracting lead (Pb) from alkaline aqueous solution as lead dithizonate, which is coloured red in chloroform solution. Since dithizone itself gives a green colour in chloroform, the resulting colour is a violet shade, which is compared with the standard colour.

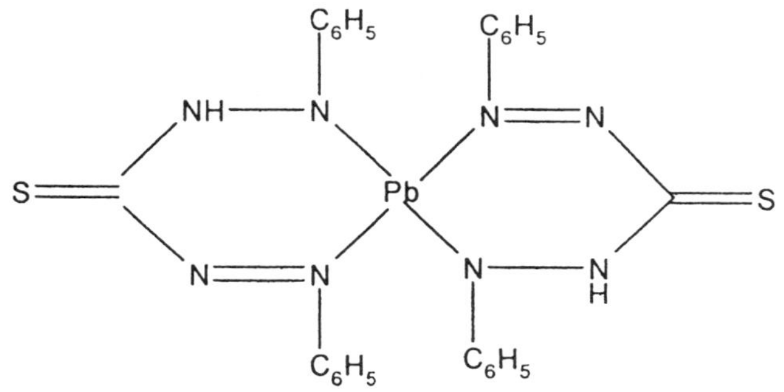

Diphenylthiocarbazone lead complex
(Lead dithizonate)

The test known as Diphenylthiocarbazone test for lead in I.P. involves the use of large number of reagents, which should be as lead-free as obtainable and are designated as Sp. The I.P. requires that all glasswares should be well rinsed with warm dilute nitric acid (1 in 2), followed by water before use.

Following are the reagents, which are prepared as follows:

Ammonia Solution Sp.

The heavy metals limit of solution of ammonia used in this test shall not exceed 1 part per million when determined as directed in the monograph for dilute ammonia solution.

Ammonium Citrate Solution Sp.

Dissolve 40 g of citric acid in 90 ml of water. Add 2 or 3 drops of a solution of phenol red, then cautiously add ammonia solution until the solution acquires a reddish colour. Remove any lead that may be present by extracting the solution with 20 ml portions of diphenylthiocarbazone extraction solution, until the diphenylthiocarbazone solution retains its orange-green colour.

Potassium Cyanide Solution Sp.

Dissolve 50 g of potassium cyanide (deadly poison, handle with care) in sufficient water to make 100 ml. Remove the lead from this solution by extraction with successive portions of Diphenylthiocarbazone Extraction Solution as described under ammonium citrate solution above. Then extract any diphenylthiocarbazone remaining in the cyanide solution by shaking with chloroform. Finally dilute the cyanide solution with sufficient water so that each 100 ml contains 10 g of potassium cyanide.

Ammonium Cyanide Solution Sp.

Dissolve 2 g of potassium cyanide in 15 ml of ammonia solution and dilute with water to 100 ml.

Hydroxylamine Hydrochloride Solution Sp.

Dissolve 20 g of hydroxylamine hydrochloride in sufficient water to make approximately 65 ml. Transfer to a separator, add a few drops of a solution of thymol blue; then add ammonia solution Sp., until the solution assumes a yellow colour. Add 2 ml of a 4 per cent solution of sodium diethyldithiocarbamate, mix well and allow to stand for 5 minutes. Extract this solution with two successive 10 to 15 ml portions of chloroform until a 5 ml portion of the chloroform extract does not assume a yellow colour when shaken with a dilute copper sulphate solution. Add dilute hydrochloric acid until the solution is pink, and then dilute with sufficient water to make 100 ml.

Nitric Acid 1 Per Cent

Dilute 10 ml of nitric acid with sufficient water to make 1000 ml.

Diphenylthiocarbazone Extraction Solution

Dissolve 30 mg of diphenylthiocarbazone in 1000 ml of chloroform and add 5 ml of alcohol. Store the solution in a refrigerator.

Before use shake a suitable volume of the diphenylthiocarbazone extraction solution with about half its volume of 1 per cent nitric acid.

Standard Diphenylthiocarbazone Solution

Dissolve 10 mg diphenylthiocarbazone in 1000 ml of chloroform. Keep the solution in a glass-stoppered, lead-free bottle, suitably wrapped to protect it from light and store in a refrigerator.

Lead Solution

Dilute 10 ml of standard lead solution (containing 10 micrograms of lead per ml) with sufficient 1 per cent nitric acid, make to 100 ml. This solution contains 1 microgram of lead per ml (1 part per million).

Sodium Diethyldithiocarbamate $(C_2H_5)_2N.CS.SNa.3H_2O$

Description: White or colourless crystals.

Sensitivity: Add 10 ml of 0.1 per cent w/v solution to 50 ml of water containing 0.002 g of copper, previously made alkaline with dilute ammonia solution. A yellow-brown colour should be apparent in the solution when compared with a blank containing no copper.

Procedure for Test for Lead

Transfer the volume of the prepared sample directed in the monograph to a separator and unless otherwise directed in monograph, add 6 ml of ammonium citrate solution Sp., 2 ml of potassium cyanide solution Sp. and 2 ml of hydroxylamine hydrochloride solution Sp. (for the determination of lead in iron salts use 10 ml of the ammonium citrate solution Sp.). Add 2 drops of a solution of phenol red and make the solution just alkaline (red colour) by the addition of ammonia solution Sp. Immediately extract the solution with 5 ml portions of diphenylthiocarbazone extraction solution, draining off each extract into another separating funnel, until the diphenylthiocarbazone extraction solution retains its green colour. Shake the combined diphenylthiocarbazone solution for 30 seconds with 30 ml of a 1 per cent nitric acid solution and discard the chloroform layer. Add to the acid solution exactly 5 ml of standard diphenylthiocarbazone solution and 4 ml of ammonium cyanide solution Sp., and shake for 30 seconds, the colour of the chloroform layer is of no deeper violet shade than that of a control made with a volume of lead solution equivalent to the amount of lead permitted in the sample under examination.

Test for Heavy Metals

This test is performed to detect the amount of all those metallic impurities which get coloured by hydrogen sulphide under the condition of the test. The Indian Pharmacopoeia includes a limit test for many official substances. The Heavy Metals' limit is also expressed as parts of lead per million parts of the substance by weight. The proportion of such impurities is expressed as the quantity required to produce a colour of equal depth as in a standard comparison solution.

The test is based on the reaction between hydrogen sulphide and certain heavy metals, like lead, iron, copper, nickel, cobalt and bismuth, the reaction products being the sulphides of the respective metals. The sulphides so formed are distributed in colloidal state and produce brownish solutions with soluble sulphides. The usual limit for heavy metals prescribed in I.P. is 20 parts per million. It is also indicated in the individual monographs in terms of ppm i.e. the parts of lead, Pb, per million parts (by weight) of the substance under examination.

The test requires the use of a large number of reagents which are designated as Sp. The reagents and their methods of preparation are given below:

Dilute Acetic Acid Sp.

Dilute acetic acid which complies with the following additional test:

Evaporate 20 ml in a porcelain dish nearly to dryness on a water bath. Add to the residue 2 ml of the acid and dilute with water to make 25 ml, then add 10 ml of a solution of hydrogen sulphide. Any dark colour produced is not darker than a control made with 0.04 mg of Pb and 5 ml of the dilute acetic acid.

Hydrochloric Acid Sp.

Hydrochloric acid which complies with the following additional test:

Evaporate 17 ml of the acid in a beaker to dryness on a water bath. Dissolve the residue in 2 ml of dilute acetic acid Sp., dilute to make 40 ml with water and add 10 ml of a solution of hydrogen sulphide till any darkening produced is not darker than that in a blank to which 0.02 mg of Pb has been added (1 part per million).

Acetic Acid Sp.

Acetic acid which complies with the following additional test:

Make 25 ml alkaline with dilute ammonia solution Sp., add 1 ml of solution of potassium cyanide Sp., dilute to make 60 ml with water and add two drops of solution of sodium sulphide; no darkening is produced.

Dilute Ammonia Solution Sp.

Dilute ammonia solution which complies with the following additional test: To 20 ml add 1 ml of a solution of potassium cyanide Sp. dilute to make 50 ml with water and add two drops of solution of sodium sulphide, no darkening is produced.

Stock Solution of Lead Nitrate

Dissolve 159.8 mg of lead nitrate in 100 ml of water, to which has been added 1 ml of nitric acid, then dilute to make 1000 ml with water. This solution must be prepared and stored in glass containers free from soluble lead salts.

Standard Lead Solution

Dilute 10 ml of the stock solution of lead nitrate, accurately measured, to 100 ml with water.

This solution must be freshly prepared. Each ml of this standard lead solution contains the equivalent of 0.01 mg of lead. When 0.1 ml of standard lead solution is employed to prepare the solution to be compared with a solution of 1 g of the substance being tested, the comparison solution thus prepared contains the equivalent of 1 part of lead per million parts of the substance being tested:

Bromine Solution Sp.

Bromine	30 g
Potassium bromide	30 g
Water, sufficient to produce	100 ml

Dissolve and mix. Evaporate 10 g in a porcelain dish to dryness on a water bath. Add 10 ml of water and again evaporate to dryness.

Repeat the process till all the bromine is driven off. Add 10 ml of water and 2 ml of dilute acetic acid Sp. and make up to 25 ml with water. Add 10 ml of a solution of hydrogen sulphide, the resulting solution is not darker than a blank to which 0.01 mg of lead has been added.

PROCEDURE FOR TESTING CHEMICALS

Solution A: Introduce into a 50 ml Nessler tube, 2 ml of dilute acetic acid Sp. and exactly the same quantity of standard lead solution containing the lead equivalent to heavy metals limit specified for the substance to be tested and make up to 25 ml with water.

Solution B: This consists of 25 ml of solution prepared for this test according to specific directions given in each monograph.

Transfer solutions A and B to matching 50 ml Nessler tubes and add 10 ml of solution of hydrogen sulphide to each tube; allow to stand for ten minutes; then view downwards over a white surface, the column of Solution B will be darker than that of Solution A.

The latest I.P. 2007 has described the limit test for heavy metals by use of four methods: methods (i) A, (ii) B, (iii) C and (iv) D. Different methods are used for different kinds of substances, e.g.

(i)   this method for one which affords clear and colourless solutions during a particular test condition;

(ii) this method is utilized for such substances which fail to give clear and colourless solutions as per the conditions similar to the first one;

(iii) this method is used for substances which due to their complex nature interfere with the precipitation of substance's metals by sulphide ion;

(iv) this method is used for those substances which impart clear colourless solutions with sodium hydroxide solution.

CHAPTER

2

Principles of Volumetric and Gravimetric Analysis

Volumetric or titrimetric analysis and gravimetric analysis are among the most widely used and accurate methods of quantitative analysis applied to the assay of a large number of pharmaceutical compounds. A brief description of these methods is given below.

Volumetric Analysis

It involves the measurement of the volume of a **standard solution** of known concentration. The standard solution is called the **titrant** and the process is known as **titration.** During titration, the titrant reacts with a quantity of the substance in the solution being titrated till the reaction is complete as indicated by the end point of titration.

A standard solution is a solution of known normality, N (concentration in equivalent/L or milli-equivalent/ml) or molarity, M (concentration in moles/L or millimoles/ml). It is prepared by dissolving an accurately weighed quantity of a highly pure substance, called a **primary standard,** and diluting it to an accurately known volume in a volumetic flask. A solution standardised by titrating with a primary standard is called a **secondary standard.** It is less accurate than a primary standard solution due to the titration errors involved. The determination of normality or molarity of a reagent by titration with a known quantity of a second reagent is known as standardisation.

Generally potassium hydrogen phthalate (AR), succinic acid (AR) and benzoic acid are recommended as primary standards for the standardisation of alkalis and anhydrous sodium carbonate for acids. These compounds occur in a highly pure form, are stable at drying temperature, and are readily available.

Normal solution for volumetric analysis is considered too concentrated for use, and hence dilutions are made, e.g. N/2, N/5, N/100. Such dilutions are amply indicated in assay methods followed under individual substances. In volumetric titrations the choice of an indicator for acid-alkali titrations is of great importance. At least two and preferably three titrations should be done to calculate the result from average litre.

Equivalent of various substances are the quantities that are equivalent in a chemical sense. In general, an equivalent is the quantity of the substance that is chemically equivalent to 1.008 g of hydrogen ion. For example, one mole or 36.46 g of HCl and 0.5 mole or 49.04 g of H_2SO_4 contains one equivalent of

1.008 g of H_2. A milliequivalent is one thousand of an equivalent, e.g. for HCl it may be expressed that 0.001 mole is equivalent to 0.0365 g of HCl.

Volumetric analysis embraces the following types of reactions :
   (i) Neutralization
  (ii) Reaction in non-aqueous media
 (iii) Precipitation
 (iv) Oxidation and reduction
  (v) Complexation

Neutralization: The titration can be conducted directly or by residual type reaction (back titration). Whenever the rate of reaction is slow or there is no sharp end point, the excess acid is titrated with another reactant. Examples are:

Direct titration: Assay of NaOH, HCl, citric acid

Residual titration: Lactic acid, aspirin, formaldehyde solution

Examples:
   1. 1.75 g of a tribasic organic acid was dissolved in water and diluted to 250 ml. 25.1 ml of this acid solution required on titration 25 ml of 0.1 N NaOH. Find out the equivalent and molecular weights of the acid.
   2. 25 ml of an approximately decinormal solution of caustic soda was neutralized by 23.5 ml of 0.1 N oxalic acid. How much volume of this solution is required for obtaining 250 ml of exactly 0.1 N NaOH?
   3. 6.3 g of borax sample was dissolved in water and diluted to 250 ml. 25 ml of this borax solution required 25.2 ml of 0.1 N HCl for complete neutralisation using methyl orange as indicator. Find the percentage purity of the borax sample.
   4. 25 ml of a solution containing a mixture of NaOH and Na_2CO_3 on/titration using phenol-phthalein as indicator consumed 18.7 ml 0.1 N HCl. On further titration of the same solution using methyl orange as indicator it required 6.3 ml of the acid for complete neutralisation. Calculate the percentage composition of the mixture.

Non-aqueous titration: Assay of many organic compounds which show poor solubility and are very weakly ionised in water can be carried out by using glacial acetic acid in place of water and carrying out the titration with perchloric acid, which acts as the strongest acid in this solvent and is very suitable for the titration of a weak base.

Non-aqueous titrimetry, now-a-days, has occupied an important place in quantitative pharmaceutical chemistry. Many of the organic medicinal agents which have been introduced recently are either poorly soluble in water or very weakly reactive in water. By the use of non-aqueous titrimetric methods, it is possible not only to perform titrations that cannot be carried out in an aqueous medium due to weak reactivity of the analyte, but also by the proper choice of solvent and titrant, the biologically active ingredient of a salt whether acidic or basic can be selectively titrated. Non-aqueous titrations are analogous to acid-base titrations in aqueous medium. In aqueous medium, acid-base neutralisation may be considered as a reaction between proton donors (acid) and proton acceptors (base). In non-aqueous medium, it can be regarded as a reaction between weakly protophilic substances which accept a pair of electrons and highly protophilic substances which tend to provide a pair of electrons in the formation of covalent bonds by co-ordination, i.e., a reaction between acids and bases.

Non-aqueous titrations are simple and accurate. The apparatus required are the same as that used in classical titrations except with some precautions that moisture and carbon dioxide are to be avoided. In presence of moisture, water being weakly basic would compete with the weak nitrogen base for $HClO_4$.

$$H_2O + HClO_4 \rightleftharpoons H_3O^+ + ClO_4^-$$

$$RNH_2 + HClO_4 \rightleftharpoons RN^+H_3 + ClO_4^-$$

Thus the sharpness of end point may be lost. Moisture contact in non-aqueous titrimetry should be less than 0.05%.

Organic acids or bases that are insoluble in water can be made to dissolve in non-aqueous solvents and then titrated.

The neutralization of a base with standard acid in non-aqueous titrimetry can be represented as:

$$BOH + CH_3ONa \longrightarrow BO^-Na^+ + CH_3OH$$

A greater difference in the protophilic properties of various substances occurs in non-aqueous solutions, such as acetonitrile, acetone and dimethylformamide, than in aqueous solutions, due to the "levelling effect" of water in the latter solutions. Though the following acids are of about equal strength in aqueous solution, in non-aqueous solvents, "acidity" decreases in the following order:

$$HClO_4 > HB_4 > H_2SO_4 > HCl > HNO_3$$

Classification of Solvents

(i) **Aprotic, neutral or inert solvents:** They have low dielectric constant and have no ionisable protons, e.g. benzene, chloroform, acetone. They have large potential ranges and do not increase dissociation of acids or bases. Therefore, they are not acting as levelling agents.

(ii) **Amphiprotic or amphoteric solvents:** They have high dielectric constant and are partially ionized, e.g. water, methanol, ethanol, isopropanol, etc.

They have reproducible limiting potentials both on acidic and basic sides. Often they are used in mixtures, e.g. benzene-alcohol, ethylene glycol-isopropanol.

(iii) **Protogenic (acidic) solvents:** They have high dielectric constants and are ionised. The ionic product of liberated anions and cations is greater than water. They exert a levelling effect in bases. They possess acidic properties, e.g. sulphuric acid.

(iv) **Protophilic (basic) solvents:** They possess basic properties. They are ionised and have high dielectric constant. Their ionic product is less than that of water, e.g. dimethylformamide (DMF), pyridine, ethylene diamine, etc.

Choice of Solvents

The selection of the solvents is based on the following considerations:

(1) Solubility and nature of the sample under investigation. If the sample is a weak acid, then the basic solvents like DMF or pyridine are used. If the sample is a weak base like ephedrine, then acidic solvents like glacial acetic acid are used.

(2) There should not be any side reaction between the sample or titrant and the solvent.

(3) The solvents chosen should not affect the sharpness of end point during titration.

Indicators commonly used in non-aqueous titration: End point in non-aqueous titrations can be located by the colour changes of the indicators or by potentiometric method. Commonly used indicators are of triphenylmethane group such as crystal violet or of azo group such as methyl yellow, methyl red or azo violet. For titration of basic substances, indicator solution is made in glacial acetic acid and for the titration of acidic substances, indicator solution is made in methanol.

Acidimetry in Non-Aqueous Medium

The titrant commonly employed in this titration is a standard acetous N/10 perchloric acid solution. Weakly basic substances (like alkali salts of organic acids, amines, amine salts, heterocyclic nitrogen compounds) are assayed by this method.

The **solvents** used in this case are either neutral or acidic solvents like alcohol, chloroform, benzene etc. or glacial acetic acid, acetic anhydride etc.

Reactions:

$$B + CH_3COOH \rightleftharpoons BH^+ + CH_2COO^-$$

$$\text{Base} \qquad\qquad\quad \underset{\text{acid of base}}{\text{Conjugate}} \quad \underset{\text{base}}{\text{Conjugate}}$$

Titrant reacts with the solvent and protonates it as follows:

$$HClO_4 + CH_3COOH \rightleftharpoons CH_3COO^+H_2 + ClO_4^-$$

Titration reaction with conjugate base anion is as follows:

$$CH_3COO^- + CH_3COOH_2^+ \rightleftharpoons 2CH_3COOH$$

So overall reaction can be written as

$$B + HClO_4 \longrightarrow BH^+ + HClO_4^-$$

Indicators: Crystal violet, methyl rosaniline chloride, quinaldine red or thymol blue (for relatively stronger base).

Preparation of N/10 Perchloric Acid

Perchloric acid occurs as a 70–72 per cent mixture with water. It has a sp. gr. of about 1.6. It must be handled with care as it is a strong acid.

8.5 ml of perchloric acid is mixed with 500 ml of glacial acetic acid and 30 ml of acetic anhydride. It is cooled and volume is made upto 1000 ml with glacial acetic acid. It is kept for a day for the excess acetic anhydride to combine with the water present. The molecular weight of perchloric acid is 100.46. So 1 litre of 0.1 N solution would contain one-tenth equivalent weight or 10.046 g.

Standardization of N/10 HClO$_4$

The solution prepared by the above procedure gives an approximately N/10 solution of perchloric acid. It can be standardized as follows:

About 700 mg of potassium hydrogen phthalate, previously dried at 105°C for 3 hours, is dissolved in 50 ml of glacial acetic acid in a 250 ml flask. Two drops of crystal violet are added and titrated with perchloric acid solution until the violet colour changes to emerald green. The volume of perchloric acid consumed by 50 ml of glacial acetic acid is deducted and the normality is then calculated.

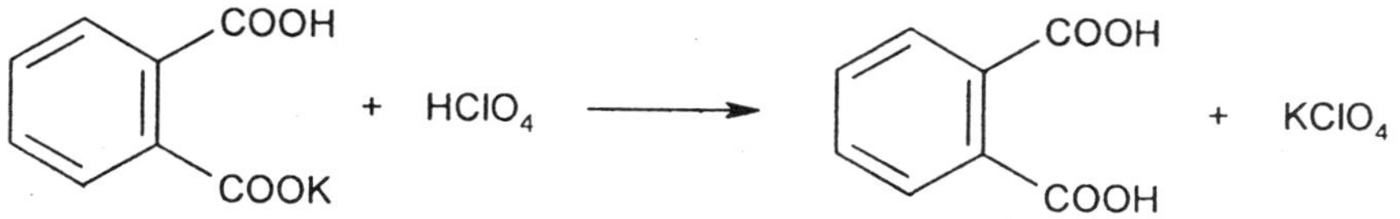

1 ml of 0.1 N HClO$_4$ ≡ 20.42 mg of C$_8$H$_5$KO$_4$

Assay of Ephedrine Hydrochloride

A weighed quantity of the sample is dissolved in sufficient amount of glacial acetic acid and to this is added a solution of mercuric acetate. It is then titrated with N/10 perchloric acid using crystal violet as indicator.

$$2C_{10}H_{15}NO \cdot HCl + (CH_3COO)_2 Hg + 2HClO_4 \longrightarrow 2C_{10}H_{16}NO + 2ClO_4^- + HgCl_2 + 2CH_3COOH$$

Mercuric acetate is added to provide sufficiently basic (acetate) ions as chloride ions are weakly basic.

Each ml of N/10 perchloric acid = 20.17 mg of C$_{10}$H$_{15}$NO.HCl.

Alkalimetry in Non-aqueous Medium

The titrant commonly used in this method is sodium methoxide or lithium methoxide. Potassium methoxide is not used as it produces gelatinous precipitate. Other titrants are sodium amino-methoxide which is the strongest base and sodium triphenylmethane which is used for weakly acidic compounds such as phenols and pyrroles.

The solvents employed in alkalimetry are dimethylformamide, pyridine, ethylenediamine, etc. Strong basic solvents like n-butylamine and morpholine are used for titration of weak acids such as enols. Sulfonamides, with N-alkyl substituents, are weakly acidic and hence strong solvent like ethylenediamine is used for their titration.

Indicators used are azo violet, o-nitroaniline and thymol blue.

For intermediate or weak acids azo violet is used and for strong acids thymol blue is the choice of indicator.

Preparation and Standardisation of 0.1 N Sodium Methoxide

One gram-atomic weight of Na (22.9) is equivalent to 1 gram-molecular weight of sodium methoxide (54.02 g). A 0.1 N solution contains 1/10 equivalent per litre. Therefore, 2.5 g of Na would produce 5.4 g or 1/10 equivalent of sodium methoxide.

Preparation: About 2.5 g of freshly cut sodium metal is added in small portions to 150 ml of ice cold methanol contained in a 1 L-volumetric flask. When the sodium metal has dissolved, sufficient quantity of benzene is added to make the volume to 1 L. It is mixed well.

Standardization: About 400 mg of benzoic acid is accurately weighed and dissolved in 80 ml of dimethylformamde (DMF) in a flask. To this are added 3 drops of a 1% w/v solution of thymol blue in DMF and titrated with sodium methoxide to a blue end point. The volume of sodium methoxide solution consumed by 80 ml of DMF is to be deducted and then the normality is calculated.

The correction to be applied for the volume of CH_3ONa consumed by DMF is to account for the reaction of water that may be present in the solvent and its reaction with the titrant.

Assay of Diphenylhydantoin

About 500 mg diphenylhydantoin is accurately weighed into a conical flask. It is dissolved in 50 ml of DMF and added to this are 3 drops of a saturated solution of azo violet in benzene. The solution is titrated with 0.1 N sodium methoxide to a blue end point. A blank experiment is carried out to make the necessary correction.

Diphenylhydantoin is an organic acid of weak strength and its acidity can be enhanced in DMF so that it can be titrated with sodium methoxide using azo violet as indicator.

Standardization Reaction:

$$C_6H_5COOH + CH_3ONa \longrightarrow C_6H_5COONa + CH_3OH$$

Reaction between the solvated proton and methylate ion is as follows:

$$C_6H_5COOH + HCON(CH_3)_2 \rightleftharpoons HCO^+NH(CH_3)_2 + C_6H_5COO^-$$

$$\underset{\text{Protonated DMF}}{HCON^+H(CH_3)_2} + CH_3O^- \longrightarrow \underset{\text{DMF}}{HCON(CH_3)_2} + CH_3OH$$

Precipitation: This type of reaction in volumetric analysis involves the interaction of silver nitrate with halogen acids or metallic halides, e.g. assay of NaCl :

$$AgNO_3 + NaCl = AgCl\downarrow + NaNO_3$$

Sometimes adsorption indicators, like fluorescein, phenosafranine are used. The AgCl, first precipitated, will adsorb Cl anions (before end point) and this in turn may cause secondary adsorption with Ag^+ cations. But at the end point where there is no more chloride, the AgCl will absorb Ag^+ first which in turn causes the secondary adsorption of the dye (fluorescein). This gives a sharp colour change in the nature of precipitate.

In the absence of interfering substance, silver salts are determined by direct titration with ammonium thiocyanate in presence of nitric acid. Assays for determination of mercury in some compounds are also carried out by use of ammonium thiocyanate.

Precipitation Method

It involves the formation of an insoluble substance or precipitate. The formation of precipitate is quantitative in nature. The end point in precipitation method is detected by cessation of precipitation or by use of indicator or by some instrumental method.

Precipitation methods can be divided into two categories:

(A) Mohr's Method or Direct Titration Method.

(B) Volhard's Method or Residual Titration Method.

Mohr's method: This method is based on quantitative precipitation into some definite compound, e.g. halides of sodium or potassium are directly estimated by titration with silver nitrate solution. When all the halides have been precipitated as silver halides, the silver nitrate reacts with the indicator, potassium chromate solution (5% w/v) to give a red to brown precipitate of silver chromate.

$$NaCl + AgNO_3 \longrightarrow NaNO_3 + AgCl\downarrow$$
$$KCl + AgNO_3 \longrightarrow KNO_3 + AgCl\downarrow$$
$$2AgNO_3 + K_2CrO_4 \longrightarrow Ag_2CrO_4\downarrow + 2KNO_3$$

Preparation and Standardization of 0.1 N AgNO$_3$ Solution

It is prepared by dissolving 17.5 g of silver nitrate in 1000 ml of distilled water and standardising it by titration with sodium chloride solution (0.1 N).

Similarly, compounds of silver and mercury are estimated by direct titration with standard ammonium thiocyanate solution. Ammonium thiocyanate precipitates mercury and silver salts as thiocyanate.

$$AgNO_3 + NH_4SCN \longrightarrow AgSCN\downarrow + NH_4NO_3$$
$$Hg(NO_3)_2 + 2NH_4SCN \longrightarrow Hg(SCN)_2 + 2NH_4NO_3$$

At the end point, ammonium thiocyanate reacts with ferric alum indicator to give red-coloured ferric thiocyanate:

$$Fe(NH_4)(SO_4)_2 + 3NH_4SCN \longrightarrow Fe(SCN)_3 + 2(NH_4)_2SO_4$$

The solutions of silver and mercury salts are acidified with nitric acid to avoid the hydrolysis of ferric. salts in neutral solution before titration with ammonium thiocyanate.

Preparation and Standardisation of 0.1 N Ammonium Thiocyanate Solution

It is prepared by dissolving 8 g of ammonium thiocyanate in 1000 ml of distilled water. For standardisation, 20 ml of 0.1 N AgNO$_3$ solution is acidified with nitric acid and titrated with an approximately prepared 0.1 N ammonium thiocyanate solution by using ferric alum as indicator. The normality of NH$_4$SCN is calculated.

Volhard's Method: In this method halides are completely precipitated as silver halides by silver nitrate solution. The precipitate is separated by filtration or coated by some organic solvent, e.g. nitrobenzene. The excess of N/10 silver nitrate is determined by standard ammonium thiocyanate solution.

Assay of NH₄Cl

An accurately weighed amount of ammonium chloride is dissolved in water, acidified with nitric acid and to it an excess of 0.1 N AgNO₃ solution is added in the presence of nitrobenzene. The excess of silver nitrate is titrated with 0.1 N NH₄SCN solution, using ferric ammonium sulphate as indicator (also see under Ammonium Chloride).

$$NH_4Cl + AgNO_3 \longrightarrow NH_4NO_3 + AgCl\downarrow$$

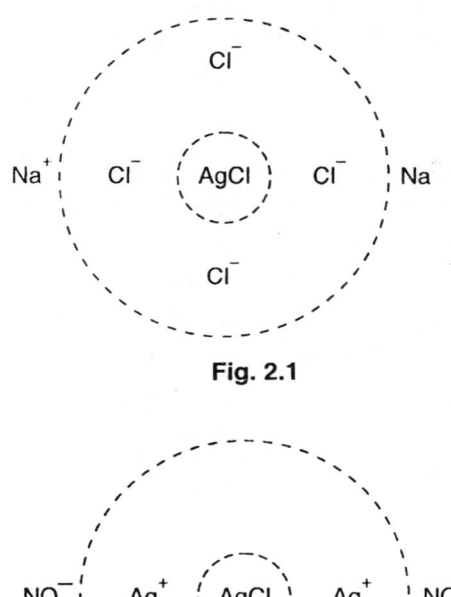

Fig. 2.1

Adsorption indicators: Besides potassium chromate and ferric alum, adsorption indicators, e.g. fluorescein and eosin dyes, are also used in the estimation of halides. The theory of the action of these indicators is based upon the properties of colloids. When a chloride solution is titrated with a solution of silver nitrate, the precipitated silver chloride forms an adsorbed layer of anions which is held by secondary adsorption by oppositely charged ions present in solution (Fig. 2.1).

As soon as the end point is reached, silver ions, present in excess, will be primarily adsorbed, while nitrate ions will be held by secondary adsorption (Fig. 2.2). If adsorption indicator, e.g. fluorescein, is present in solution, the negative fluorescein ions are more strongly adsorbed than nitrate ions and give their own colour (Fig. 2.3).

Fig. 2.2

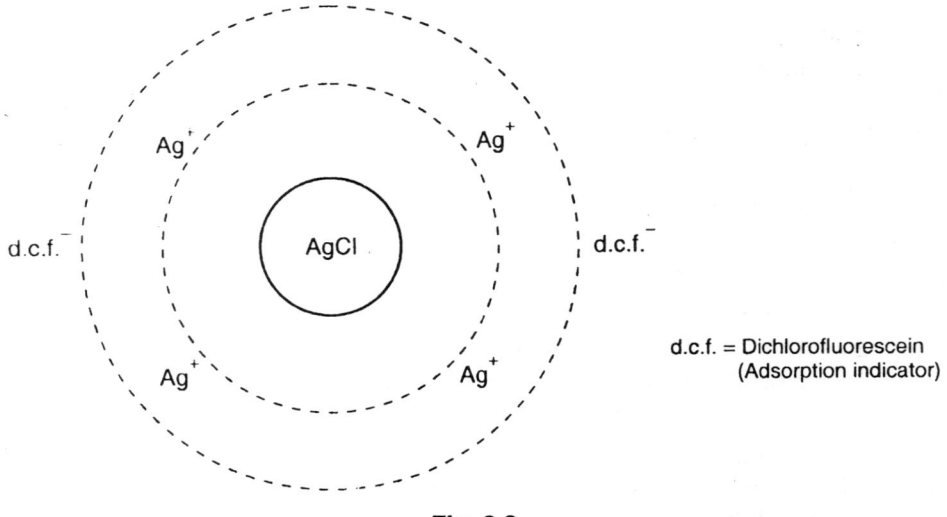

d.c.f. = Dichlorofluorescein
(Adsorption indicator)

Fig. 2.3

A few examples of precipitation method are given below:

Precipitation Problems

(1) A 0.219 g of sample of sodium chloride was assayed by the Volhard method using 50 ml of 0.0985 N silver nitrate and 11.75 ml of 0.134 N ammonium thiocyanate. Calculate the per cent of NaCl in the sample.

Hint:

$$NaCl\ per\ cent = \frac{(ml\ Ag^+ \times N) - (ml\ SCN^- \times N) \times 0.05844 \times 100}{Sample\ weight}$$

(2) A 250 mg sample of ammonium bromide was found to be equivalent to 25 ml of 0.1 N $AgNO_3$ in a Volhard determination. What volume of 0.0962 N sulphuric acid would be required to neutralize the ammonia produced from 0.4689 g sample of same material?

(3) If 25 ml of hydroiodic acid syrup (1.4% w/v) was treated with 45.0 ml of 0.102 N silver nitrate, what volume of 0.097 N NH_4SCN would be required in back titration?

Complexometric Titrations

A complexing agent mostly includes any electron donating system which may form bond or bonds with a metal ion and produce a complex. If the complexing agent contains two or more groups that donate electrons, then the complex formed is called a **Chelate**. Aminopolycarboxylic acids are excellent complex forming agents. The most important of such agents being ethylenediaminetetraacetic acid (EDTA), as it chelates with many metals.

This method of volumetric analysis was developed after the introduction of the analytical reagent commonly known as EDTA disodium salt. The metal-ion detectors are used in the similar way as that of pH indicators are used in acid-base titrations.

The reaction between a metal ion and the molecule which can donate electrons is referred to as **complexation** reaction. The resulting compound is known as a "complex". The EDTA-metal complex is water-soluble. The reaction is rapid and quantitative with polyvalent metal ions. Monovalent metal ions yield relatively weak or unstable complexes.

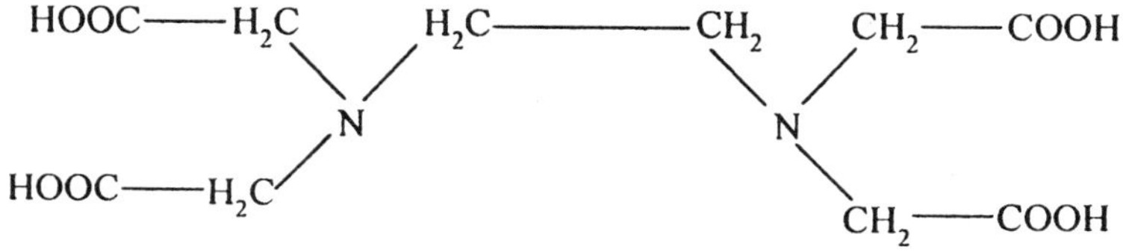

The ionisation of EDTA (ethylenediaminetetraacetic acid), represented by H_4Y, occurs as:

$$
\begin{aligned}
H_4Y &\rightleftharpoons H^+ + H_3Y^- & pK_1 &= 2.07 \\
H_3Y^- &\rightleftharpoons H^+ + H_2Y^{2-} & pK_2 &= 2.75 \\
H_2Y^{2-} &\rightleftharpoons H^+ + HY^{3-} & pK_3 &= 6.24 \\
HY^{3-} &\rightleftharpoons H^+ + Y^{4-} & pK_4 &= 10.34
\end{aligned}
$$

The predominant form of the dissociated forms of EDTA depends on pH at which the reaction is carried out.

In complexation, the ratio of EDTA to metal ion is 1 : 1.

$$Y^{4-} + M^{n+} \rightleftharpoons MY^{n-4}$$

Pharmacopoeia of India follows this method for the assay of calcium salts. With bivalent metals such as Ca^{++} there are six points of attachment or bonds between the metal ion and EDTA of which two are ionic, two are ordinate bonds involving oxygen atoms and two are co-ordinate bonds formed by unshared pair of electrons of nitrogen atoms which are donated to the metal. With Al^{3+} or trivalent metal one of ordinate bonds becomes ionic in character. The four oxygen and two nitrogen atoms of EDTA molecule are capable of entering complexation and make the molecule hexadentate. EDTA molecule which provides groups for attachment to metal ions is called a ligand. The stability of the complex varies with the number of rings that can be formed. The EDTA metal complexes are very stable, since the five-membered rings formed in the complex are strain-free and most stable.

The driving force in a complexometric reaction is the formation of a stable, soluble complex. When the law of mass action is applied to the reaction equilibrium, the stability constant is expressed as :

$$Ks = \frac{CaY^{2-}}{[Ca]^{2+} [Y]^{4-}} = 2.5 \times 10"$$

The value of the stability constant is large as the complex formed is very slightly ionized and the concentration of Ca-EDTA complex is greater than that of its constituent ions. The stability constants are valid only for that pH at which they are determined because concentration of Y^{4-} is a function of the pH at which the reaction is carried out.

Stability constants of some metals which are complexed and determined by EDTA titration are:

$$AlY^- = 16.1 \qquad BiY^- = 8.6 \qquad HgY^{2-} = 21.8 \qquad ZnY^{2-} = 16.5$$

$$CaY^{2-} = 10.7 \qquad CaY^{2-} = 18.8 \qquad MgY^{2-} = 8.7$$

If the stability constants are greater than 8, the titration will prove to be successful. Sodium and lithium form very weak complexes. Metal ions such as Fe^{3+} and Cu^{2+} yield highly coloured complexes and cannot be titrated visually.

Factors Influencing EDTA Reaction

The following factors influence the complexation of the metal ion with EDTA:

(1) Activity of metal ion.

(2) The pH at which reaction is carried out.

(3) Presence of interfering ions such as cyanide, citrate, tartrate, fluoride and other complex forming groups.

(4) Solvents in which reaction is carried out. Organic solvents influence the stability of complex.

Reagent (Titrant)

Disodium salt of ethylenediaminetetraacetic acid is the most commonly used titrant. Disodium salt is preferred to the free acid as the former is more water soluble, stable and non-hygroscopic. M/20 solution of disodium EDTA is normally employed. The molecular weight of disodium EDTA, $C_{10}H_{14}N_2Na_2O_8 \cdot 2H_2O$, is 372.24. So 1/20 M solution would contain 372.24/20 or 18.612 g dissolved in 1 litre of the solution. The solutions are made from metal-free glass distilled water and are stored in polyethylene containers or metal-free glass containers.

Indicators

They are organic compounds forming coloured complex with metal ion in high dilution. The stability constant of metal-indicator complex must be smaller than that of metal-EDTA complex. In other words, the indicator must release the metal ion to the titrant EDTA for complexing and not competing with it.

$$Mn^{2+} + HIn^{2-} \rightleftharpoons MIn^- + H^+$$
$$MIn^- + H_2Y^{2-} \rightleftharpoons MY^{2-} + HIn^{2-} + H^+$$

Red   Blue

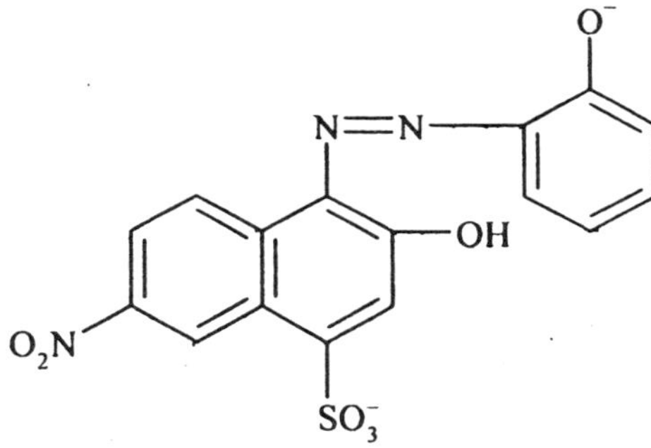

Blue HIn^{2-}

    The indicators used in complexometric titrations are Eriochrome Black T (Mordant Black) or murexide indicator (ammonium purpurate) preparation screened with the dye naphthol green. Hydroxynaphthol blue is also used as indicator.

    The Eriochrome Black T forms red complexes with:

$$Mg^{++}, \quad Zn^{++}, \quad Al^{+++}, \quad Ca^{++}, \quad etc.$$

Direct Titration Methods

Ca^{2+}, Mg^{2+} and Zn^{2+} are the metal ions determined by direct titration with EDTA. The method of standardization of EDTA (disodium salt) and the method of analysis of calcium compounds are similar in principle.

Preparation and Standardization of M/20 EDTA (Disodium Salt)

About 18.66 g of disodium EDTA is dissolved in sufficient water to make 1 L and the solution is standardized as follows:

    About 200 mg of calcium carbonate is accurately weighed, transferred to a suitable container and sufficient water and dilute hydrochloric acid are added to dissolve it. The solution is diluted with water to 150 ml. To this, 15 ml of NaOH T.S. and 300 mg of hydroxynaphthol blue as indicator are added and titrated with d'sodium EDTA solution until the solution is deep blue in colour. The molarity is calculated by the formula,

$$\frac{W}{100.1\,V}$$

where W is weight in mg of $CaCO_3$ in the sample of calcium carbonate and V is the volume in ml of disodium EDTA solution consumed.

In the above procedure, sodium hydroxide is added to make pH of about 13 at which **Ca-EDTA** complex is stable and any Mg^{++} ions present as impurity will not react.

The coloured Ca-indicator complex gives up metal ion, i.e. Ca^{++} to EDTA liberating free uncomplexed indicator which is blue.

Example: Assay of calcium gluconate I.P.

Masking: Masking refers to the determination of a particular metal ion in presence of another metal. The masking agent can also complex with metal ions. Masking can be done by adjusting pH of the titration media so that it will be favourable for complexation of a particular ion under investigation and not for another metal ion. For example, bismuth complexes at pH_2 in presence of other metals and without any interference of them. Zinc will not interfere with calcium titration at pH of 13.

Auxiliary complexing agents will also act as masking agents. **Triethanolamine** also suppresses Al-EDTA complexation in presence of Mg-EDTA reaction. Thioglycols inactivate metals such as Hg and Cu allowing the titration of Zn at pH 6. **Potassium cyanide** masks metals such as Co, Ni, Cu and zinc. **Ammonium fluoride** will inactivate Ca, Mg and Al permitting the titration of Zn. Ascorbic acid, citrates and tartrates are also used as masking agents.

Indirect or Residual Titrations

The indirect titration method is applied to the analysis of those compounds having Al or Bi because direct titration may cause errors by the precipitation of metals as hydroxides. In the residual titration method an excess of standard solution of EDTA is added to the sample, then pH is adjusted for back titration with metal-ion solution, zinc sulphate, using an indicator sensitive to titrant. The metal under analysis remains complexed with EDTA and does not interfere with Zn-EDTA complexation.

Assay of Aluminium Paste

About 2.5 g of the paste is accurately weighed into a 250 ml beaker and about 35 ml of dilute hydrochloric acid is added, it is heated gently first, then boiled until oil separates. It is chilled to solidify the oils, aqueous layer is decanted and filtered into a 250 ml volumetric flask. The same procedure is again followed with the residue in beaker. The filtrates and washings are collected and diluted to volume and mixed. By this procedure all aluminium and zinc oxide are converted into soluble chlorides.

From 250 ml, 25 ml of filtrate is pipetted in another beaker to which is added stronger ammonia water dropwise till a faint turbidity appears. The solution is cleared by the addition of HCl in drops followed by few drops in excess. To this is added with continuous stirring 50 ml of M/20 disodium EDTA, 20 ml of ammonium acetate buffer, 50 ml of alcohol and 2 ml of dithizone in order and the solution titrated with M/20 **Zinc sulfate** till colour changes from green violet to rose pink. The volume is recorded.

Zinc alone is determined by adding strong ammonia water and triethanolamine and ammonia-NH_4Cl buffer below 50°C. This is a masking technique by which only zinc complexes with EDTA and not aluminium. It is titrated with M/20 EDTA using mordant black as indicator. The difference between the volume of zinc sulphate consumed in first titration and volume of EDTA in 2nd titration gives the amount of aluminium present in 25 ml aliquot of paste.

$$\text{Each ml of M/20 solution} \equiv 1.349 \text{ mg of Al}$$

Oxidation Reduction Titrations (Redox Titrations)

It is well known that oxidation and reduction process occurs simultaneously. Oxidation-reduction concepts have recently been considerably broadened since they first came into use. Earlier oxidation meant the addition of oxygen to a substance; later it was used to include the removal of hydrogen. Reduction meant the opposite of oxidation.

During the last few decades, due to the importance of electron in chemical reactions, the terms oxidation and reduction, respectively, have been defined as the process in which there is loss of electrons (oxidation) and the process in which there is gain of electrons (reduction). Whenever there is a redox reaction, substance is oxidized and another substance is reduced.

Oxidizing agent is one which gains electrons and the reducing agent is one which loses electrons. A typical example of redox reaction is one in which a ferric salt is reduced by a titanous salt.

$$TiCl_3 + FeCl_3 \longrightarrow TiCl_4 + FeCl_2$$

In ionic form, the same equation can be written as :

$$Ti^{3+} + Fe^{3-} \longrightarrow Ti^{4+} + Fe^{2+}$$

In oxidation:

$$Ti^{3+} \longrightarrow Ti^{4+} + Fe^{2+}$$

whereas in reduction:

$$Fe^{3+} + e^- \longrightarrow Fe^{2+}$$

The gramme-equivalent of the reactant containing the element which is oxidized or reduced can be calculated on the basis of number of electrons transferred to or from one atom of the element.

For example, the half-equation describing the reduction of permanganate in acid solution is :

$$MnO_4^- + 8H^- + 5e^- = Mn^{2+} + 4H_2O$$

Here, for every atom of manganese taking part in the reaction, five electrons are transferred from the reducing agent. The gramme-equivalent of the molecule under these condition is thus:

$$\frac{KMnO_4}{5}$$

Some other common oxidizing and reducing agents and the half-equations are :

$$\text{Iodine} = I_2 + 2e^- = 2I^- \text{ (Iodide)}$$
$$\text{Ceric salt solutions} = Ce^{4+} + e^- = Ce^{3+} \text{ (Cerous)}$$
$$\text{Thiosulphate} = 2S_2O_3^{2-} = S_4O_6^{2-} + 2e^- \text{ (Tetrathionate)}$$
$$\text{Oxalic acid} = C_2O_4^{2-} = 2CO_2 + 2e^-$$

The following are the commonly used oxidising reagents:

I. N/10 Potassium Permanganate (KMnO₄)

In presence of excess dilute sulphuric acid and a reducing agent two moles of $KMnO_4$ provide **five** atoms of available oxygen :

$$2KMnO_4 + 3H_2SO_4 \longrightarrow K_2SO_4 + 2MnSO_4 + 3H_2O + 5(O)$$

Equivalent of $KMnO_4 = 31.6$

A solution of $KMnO_4$ containing 3.16 g of $KMnO_4$ in 1000 ml has approximately the normality, 0.1 N. Potassium permanganate is not a primary standard because it may be reduced by atmospheric organic matter or organic matter present in water. It is standardized by any of the methods described below:

A. Standardization with Oxalic Acid

In acidic medium oxalic acid is oxidized by $KMnO_4$ to water and CO_2.

$$2MnO_4^- + 5C_2O_4^{2-} + 16H^+ \longrightarrow 2Mn^{2+} + 10CO_2 + 8H_2O$$

This oxidation reaction takes place quantitatively only at a temperature of about 60°–70° C.

A solution containing 6.3 g of oxalic acid in 1,000 ml of water provides the normality of 0.1 N. A measured volume of this 0.1 N oxalic acid is treated with dilute sulphuric acid (about 2 N). It is then heated to about 70°C. While hot, the solution is titrated with approximately N/10 $KMnO_4$ till the solution becomes pink (end point).

B. Standardization with Sodium Oxalate

Sodium oxalate is a better standardizing agent than oxalic acid as sodium oxalate is available in a pure state and is free from water of crystallization.

$$\text{Equivalent wt. of sodium oxalate} = \frac{\text{Mol. wt.}}{2} = \frac{134}{2} = 67$$

The standardization procedure is same as described under standardization with oxalic acid. Reaction is expressed as:

$$2MnO_4^- + 5C_2O_4^{2-} + 16H^+ \longrightarrow 2Mn^{2+} + 10CO_2 + 8H_2O$$

C. Standardization with Ferrous Ammonium Sulphate

$FeSO_4 \cdot (NH_4)_2SO_4 \cdot 6H_2O$ (mol. wt. = 392) is a stable double salt which is oxidized in cold by $KMnO_4$ in presence of H_2SO_4 and is represented by the following equation:

$$2MnO_4^- + 16H^+ + 10Fe^{2+} \longrightarrow 2Mn^{2-} + 10Fe^{3+} + 8H_2O$$

No heating is to be done as Fe^{2+} gets oxidised on heating by air.

A known quantity of ferrous ammonium sulphate is dissolved in a measured volume of distilled water. Before making up the volume, a few drops of sulphuric acid are also added to avoid any oxidation by air. A measured volume of the solution is acidified and titrated with N/10 $KMnO_4$ solution.

Examples:

1. 25 ml of the solution containing oxalic acid and sodium oxalate required 12.5 ml of N/10 NaOH

for neutralization. 25 ml of solution mixture required 26 ml of 0.1 N $KMnO_4$. Calculate the strengths of oxalic acid and sodium oxalate in the given solution.

2. 25 ml of a solution containing Fe^{2+} and Fe^{3+} ions required 10 ml of N/10 $KMnO_4$ for titration. 25 ml of the solution mixture after reduction required 24 ml of N/10 $KMnO_4$ for titration. Calculate the strengths of ferrous and ferric iron in the solution.

II. N/10 Potassium Dichromate ($K_2Cr_2O_7$)

It is a salt of dichromic acid, $H_2Cr_2O_7$. In acid solution each mole of $K_2Cr_2O_7$ provides 3 atoms of oxygen available for oxidizing purposes.

$$K_2Cr_2O_7 + 5H_2SO_4 \longrightarrow 2KHSO_4 + Cr_2(SO_4)_3 + 4H_2O + 3[O]$$

$$Cr_2O_4^{2-} + 14H^+ + 6e^- \longrightarrow 2Cr^{3+} + 7H_2O$$

It is obtained in pure state and N/10 solution is prepared by dissolving one-sixtieth of the gramme molecular weight and diluting the solution to 1,000 ml. This reagent is useful in standardizing approximately 0.1 N iodine and also in ferrous iron titrations.

Iodimetry and Iodometry

Iodine is used as titrant because of its oxidising power:

$$I_2 + 2e \rightarrow 2I^-$$
$$I_2 \equiv 2e^-$$
$$126.90 \text{ g } I_2 \equiv 1000 \text{ ml N}$$
$$12.69 \text{ g } I_2 \equiv 1000 \text{ ml 0.1 N Iodine}$$

Iodine is insoluble in water and therefore potassium iodide is used to form KI_3, which behaves in solution as free iodine.

Iodometry: In this method of titration by selecting a suitable chemical reaction free iodine is liberated which is titrated with thiosulphate. A blank titration should be done on the same quantity of reagents, omitting the sample. Indicator is not needed and the end-point shows colourless solution, e.g.:

Determination of Phenols:

$$5KBr + KBrO_3 + 6HCl = 6KCl + 3Br_2 + 3H_2O$$
$$3Br_2 + Br_2 + C_6H_5OH = C_6H_2 \cdot Br_3OH + 3HBr$$
$$2KI + Br_2 = 2KBr + I_2$$
$$I_2 + 2Na_2S_2O_3 = Na_2S_4O_6 + 2NaI$$
$$\qquad\qquad \text{Sodium} \qquad \text{Sodium}$$
$$\qquad\qquad \text{thiosulphate} \quad \text{tetrathionate}$$

Iodimetry: It is a direct titration method with standard iodine.

The sample is titrated directly, using starch TS as indicator, e.g.:

Determination of Antimony Sodium Tartrate:

$$2C_4H_4O_7NaSb = Sb_2O_3$$

$$Sb_2O_3 + 2H_2O \rightarrow Sb_2O_5 + 4H^+ + 4e^-$$
$$2I_2 + 2e^- \rightarrow 2I^-$$
$$C_4H_4O_7NaSb \equiv Sb_2O_3 \equiv 4e^-$$
$$617.6 \text{ g } C_4H_4O_7NaSb \equiv 4000 \text{ ml N}$$
$$0.01544 \text{ g} \equiv 1 \text{ ml } 0.1 \text{ N}$$

Preparation of starch indicator: About 1 g of starch is ground with 5 ml of water to a thin paste in a mortar. This paste is poured into 100 ml of boiling water. The mixture is boiled for 2–3 minutes and is cooled for use.

N/10 Iodine Solution

An approximately N/10 iodine solution is made by transferring 12.7 g of iodine, 18 g of KI and 50 ml of water to a stoppered iodine flask, shaking the mixture until solution completes.

A decinormal solution therefore contains N/10 I_2.

$$I_2 + H_2O \longrightarrow 2HI + [O]$$

Iodine is quite volatile and very slightly soluble in water. It is, however, readily soluble in KI solution due to the polyiodine ion formation.

$$I + I_2 \longrightarrow [I^{3-}]$$
$$\text{Triiodide ion}$$

This ion liberates iodine so readily during the titration that the solution behaves as if dissolved iodine were all free iodine.

It is standardized with standard N/10 sodium thiosulphate solution which is in turn standardized using standard $KMnO_4$ solution or $K_2Cr_2O_7$ solution or KIO_3 solution as follows:

A. By using KMnO₄ solution*

It is based on the fact that $KMnO_4$ in acid solution liberates free iodine when treated with excess KI. The liberated iodine is titrated against the given sodium thiosulphate using starch as indicator.

$$2MnO_2^- + 10I^- + 16H^+ \longrightarrow 2Mn^{2+} + 8H_2O + 5I_2$$
$$I_2 + 2S_2O_3^{2-} \longrightarrow S_4O_6^{2-} + 2I^-$$

B. By using K₂Cr₂O₇ solution

It is also based on the fact that dichromate, like $KMnO_4$, liberates I_2 from KI in the presence of acid. The liberated iodine is titrated with N/10 $Na_2S_2O_3$ using starch as indicator.

$$Cr_2O_7^{2-} + 14H^+ + 6I^- \longrightarrow 2Cr^{3+} + 7H_2O + 3I_2$$

C. By using KIO₃ solution

In this case also the principle is the same as that of $K_2Cr_2O_7$ or $KMnO_4$.

---

* It is seldom, as in titrations with potassium permanganate, that an end point of a reaction is sharply visible. Thus an indicator is always required to be used to show a change in colour on precipitation at the end point. In volumetric determinations on an average three titrations should be done and the result calculated from the mean titre.

$$IO_3^{3-} + 6H^+ + 5I^- \longrightarrow 3H_2O + 3I_2$$

Equivalent weight of KIO_3 is $= \dfrac{\text{Mol. wt.}}{5} = \dfrac{214}{6} = 35.67$.

Example: A solution contains 25 g of hydrated copper sulphate ($CuSO_4 \cdot 5H_2O$) per litre. 25 ml of this solution on treatment with excess KI requires 25 ml of N/10 sodium thiosulphate solution for titration. Calculate the percentage of copper in the salt.

Gravimetric Analysis

It involves measurement of the weight of a substance in a sample or the calculation of the weight of a substance from the weight of chemically equivalent weight of some other substance. The substance to be determined can be converted into some other well-defined chemical compound which can be separated and purified, dried and weighed.

In general: $\qquad\qquad\qquad\qquad A + B \longrightarrow C + D.$

The weight of either reactant A or B can be calculated from the weight of either product, i.e. C or D.

Sometimes, depending upon the nature of the substance, volumetric and gravimetric methods can be applicable to one and the same substance. In practice, however, volumetric methods are preferred, as they are easy and rapid, compared to gravimetric methods, which are slow and tedious. Besides, they do not have any advantage as far as accuracy is concerned. That is why most of the determinations in I.P. are based on volumetric assays.

The gravimetric analysis involves the following steps:

1. Precipitation.
2. Filtration and washing of precipitate.
3. Drying and ignition.

Precipitation: It relies upon the production of a substance, the solubility of which is very negligible under the conditions employed, e.g. the solubility of AgCl is 1.4×10^{-5} g moles/litre.

In this operation, a solution of precipitating agent is usually added slowly to a suitably diluted solution of sample with stirring. Efficient stirring is essential to avoid contamination of the precipitate due to co-precipitation. Precipitation is usually done at elevated temperature to obtain an easily filterable precipitate. The formation of coarse particles is also enhanced by slow addition of precipitating agents with constant stirring at a slightly elevated temperature. Then the precipitate is allowed to settle down and slight amount of precipitating agent is added to check the completeness of precipitation. If further precipitation is obtained, then whole procedure is repeated with small quantities of precipitating agent until precipitation is complete. The precipitate is either left for some time or boiled to increase the coarseness of precipitate for easy filtration. This procedure is called "digestion" of the precipitate.

Filtration and Washing of Precipitate

The precipitate is separated by filtration either through a filter paper or through one of the varieties of filter crucible. 'Whatman' No. 40, 41 or 42 filter papers are generally used because they have very small ash values. The diameter of filter paper may vary according to the bulkiness of precipitate. Bulky precipitate such as aluminium hydroxide requires a large filter paper than dense precipitate, e.g. barium

sulphate. The folded filter paper is placed in a funnel moistened with
water and pressed to expel the air. Then the precipitate is transferred
in a usual way and separated.

Various other types of filtration units are also used in gravimetric
analysis which include:

    (A) Gooch crucible

    (B) Sintered glass crucible.

Both filtration units are used for quick filtration, washing and
drying of precipitate.

(A) Gooch Crucible

A Gooch crucible (A) is supported in glass adapter (B) which passes
through a rubber bug into a Buchner flask (C). Gooch crucibles have
perforated bottoms. The holes of the crucible are covered by a thin
layer of asbestos fibres.

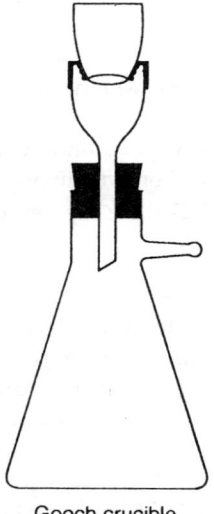

Gooch crucible

(B) Sintered Glass Crucible

Sintered glass crucibles have bases of sintered glass in various degrees
of porosity, numbered 1, 2, 3, 4, indicating decreasing pore size with
the increasing number. A number 3 crucible is suitable for coarse
precipitate and number 4 is usually employed for fine precipitate.
After filtration, precipitate is washed to remove unwanted anions like
Cl^- and/or SO_4^-.

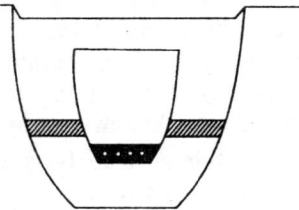

Sintered glass crucible

Drying and Ignition of Precipitate

The precipitate can be dried either in sintered glass crucibles or in porcelain crucibles depending on the
temperature. Sintered glass crucibles are used if temperature below 500°C is used because this is
susceptible to sudden change in temperature. If the precipitate must be ignited at a temperature above
500°C, it is collected on ash-less filter paper, transferred to a porcelain crucible and heated to the
required temperature. The charring of filter paper must be gradual and the paper should not catch fire.
Once charring is complete, the crucible is heated until no dark coloured material is left on the surface.

Sometimes, if there is a risk of reduction of precipitate by carbon, then special treatment is given,
e.g. $BaSO_4$ is cooled after ignition, treated with sulphuric acid and reignited to convert any sulphide
into sulphate.

$$BaSO_4 + 2C \longrightarrow BaS\downarrow + 2CO_2\uparrow$$
$$BaS + H_2SO_4 \longrightarrow BaSO_4\downarrow + H_2S\uparrow$$

The residue obtained after ignition of the precipitate along with the crucible is kept in a desiccator.
After cooling, the residue in the crucible is weighed until the weighings are concordant.

The calculations are made as follows :

$$\text{Percentage of the substance} = \frac{E \times S}{W} \times 100$$

where E = Wt. of the residue
      S = Gravimetric factor
      W = Weight of the sample taken

A few examples of gravimetric analysis are given below:

Problems of Gravimetric Analysis

(1) Estimate gravimetrically the percentage of lead in a lead alloy, 9 g of which is dissolved in dilute acetic acid and the solution is made to 1 L.

Hint: $Pb^{+2} + SO_4^{2-} \longrightarrow PbSO_4 \downarrow$

Let 25 ml of the solution = X g $PbSO_4\downarrow$

∴ Amount of $PbSO_4$ per litre = $40X$ g.

Now, $PbSO_4 = Pb$

$\quad\quad$ 303 = 207

∴ $40X$ g of $PbSO_4 = \dfrac{40X \times 207}{303}$ Pb

Hence, percentage of lead in the given alloy = $\dfrac{40X \times 207}{303 \times 9} \times 100$.

(2) Suppose a given solution contains 15.0 g/L of $Pb(CH_3COO)_2.nH_2O$. Find the value of n by gravimetric method.

Hint:

Let 25 ml of the solution = X g of $PbSO_4$

∴ Amount/litre of $PbSO_4 = 40X$ g

Now, $PbSO_4 = Pb(CH_3COO)_2.nH_2O$

$\quad\quad$ 303 = 325 + 18n

∴ $40X$ g of $PbSO_4 = \dfrac{40X \times (325 + 18n)}{303}$ g of $PbAc.nH_2O = 15$ g (Given)

So from the following equation, n can be calculated :

$$\dfrac{40X \times (324 + 18n)}{303} = 15$$

(3) A solution containing 0.375 g of $Pb(CH_3COO)_2.x\,H_2O$ gave 0.2997 g of dry $PbSO_4$ ppt. Evaluate x. **(Ans. 3.01)**

(4) In a phosphate determination, 0.6096 g of a mixture of Na_2HPO_4 and NH_4Cl gave 0.3270 g of $Mg_2P_2O_7$. Calculate the percentage composition of the mixture.

(Ans. Na_2HPO_4 = 68.61%, NH_4Cl = 31.39%)

Hint:

$$Mg^{2+} + PO_4^{3-} + NH_4^+ + 6H_2O \longrightarrow Mg(NH_4)PO_4, 6H_2O \downarrow$$

$$\text{white precipitate}$$

$$2MgNH_4PO_4.6H_2O \longrightarrow Mg_2P_2O_7 + 2NH_3 + 13H_2O$$

$$2NaHPO_4.7H_2O \equiv Mg_2P_2O_7$$

(5) An unknown sample of a soluble sulphate weighing 1.800 g yielded 0.900 g of $BaSO_4$. Calculate the percentage of sulphur in the unknown sample.

Hint:

$$\frac{S}{BaSO_4} = \frac{32.06}{233.40} = 0.1374$$

$$SO_4^{2-} + BaCl_2 \longrightarrow 2Cl^- + BaSO_4 \downarrow$$

(6) A 5.0 ml sample of sodium phosphate solution was diluted with water to a volume of 100 ml. A 10.0 ml sample of the resulting solution was treated with magnesia mixture TS (mixture containing magnesium ions in a buffered ammonium chloride-ammonium hydroxide solution). By ignition of the magnesium ammonium phosphate precipitate, 0.1515 g of pyrophosphate was obtained. Calculate the content of sodium phosphate solution in per cent W/V. If the sp. gr. was 1.39, what would be the Na_2HPO_4 content in per cent W/W?

(7) What weight of AgCl could be obtained from a sample of mercury bichloride capable of yielding 0.375 g of HgS?

(8) A sample consisting of only pure KCl and pure KI weighs 0.4811 g; it is quantitatively converted into KCl and then weighs 0.2982 g. Calculate how much KI is present in the original sample.

Methoxyl Determination : Methoxyl determination is carried out by following the Zeisel method. In this method the methoxyl groups of the sample are subjected to hydrolysis, which is brought about by boiling with hydroiodic acid. Carbon dioxide is passed through the apparatus to prevent oxidation of hydroiodic acid and to absorb the volatile methyl iodide in a bromine acetic acid (for potassium acetate in glacial acetic acid) solution, which liberates iodine monobromide as shown in the following reactions:

$$ROCH_3 + HI = ROH + CH_3I$$

$$CH_3I + Br_2 = CH_3Br + IBr$$

$$IBr + 2Br_2 + 3H_2O = HIO_3 + 5HBr$$

Formic acid is added to remove excess of bromine, followed by the addition of potassium iodide and dilute sulphuric acid. The reactions taking place are given below:

$$Br_3 + HCOOH = 2HBr + CO_2$$

$$HIO_3 + 5HI = 3I_2 + 3H_2O$$

The liberated iodine is titrated with sodium thiosulphate.

$$I_2 + 2Na_2S_2O_3 = Na_2S_4O_6 + 2NaI$$

Each ml of 0.1 N sodium thiosulphate is equivalent to 0.0005172 g of methoxyl (OCH_3).

Methoxyl determination is carried out in a specified apparatus.

Methoxyl can also be determined gravimetrically by passing methyl iodide into an alcoholic solution of silver nitrate and weighing the silver iodide.

PHYSICAL METHODS OF ANALYSIS

The official methods of analysis (I.P.) involve tests and procedures necessary to determine the identity, purity, quality and strength of pharmaceutical compounds and formulated products. These methods are based on chemical and physical principles and are applied to perform identification tests, limit tests and assays. The usual chemical tests are used to indicate development of colour, formation of turbidity, precipitate or characteristic stain, evolution of gas, etc. for identification and limit tests and volumetric and gravimetric methods for assay as described in the above sections.

In addition to the application of these methods, physical or instrumental methods (such as electrochemical, spectroscopic and chromatographic methods) are now extensively used for identification and limit tests and for assay of pharmaceutical substances. These methods are based on the measurement of a physical property such as refractive index, optical rotation, light absorption or emission, electrical current or potential and electrical or thermal conductivity, that is characteristically related to the particular substance. These methods have the advantage of being specific and more sensitive than the chemical methods.

Chromatographic methods (such as thin-layer chromatography, TLC, glass-liquid chromatography, GLC and high performance liquid chromatography, HPLC) are particularly useful for analysing complex mixtures or formulations. They perform the separation and measurement steps simultaneously and the analysis is conducted in a short time.

A few examples of the applications of these methods in I.P. are give below :

Substance	Identification	Limit test	Assay
Calcium folinate	Infrared absorption	–	HPLC
Calcium gluconate	TLC	–	–
Calcium pantothenate	TLC	–	Potentiometric titration
Activated charcoal	–	Atomic absorption (Cu, Pb, Zn)	–
Disodium edetate	Infrared absorption	–	–
Insulin zinc	HPLC	–	HPLC
Lithium carbonate	–	Atomic emission (K, Na)	
Magaldrate	–	–	Potentiometeric titration
Oral rehydration salts ORS powder (dextrose, NaCl, KCl)	–	Atomic absorption (Na, K)	Measurement of optical rotation (dextrose)
Potassium chloride	–	Fluorescence (Al) Atomic absorption (Na)	–
Sodium acetate	–	Fluorescence (Al)	–
Sodium chloride	–	Fluorescence (Al) Atomic emission (K)	–
Compound sodium chloride injection	–	–	Atomic absorption (NaCl, KCl)
Sodium phosphate	–	–	Potentiometric titration
Thiomersal	–	Light absorption at 323 nm (inorganic Hg compounds)	

CHAPTER

3

Radioactivity

RADIOACTIVE ISOTOPES AND THEIR APPLICATIONS IN PHARMACY

Before discussing the production, properties and applications of radioactive isotopes, it is desirable to define some of the units and terms that we often come across in the field of radioactivity.

Definitions

Curie is the unit representing the rate of decay and is equal to 3.7×10^{10} disintegrations per second. It refers to about the disintegration rate of 1 g radium.

Specific activity is the ratio of the number of radioactive atoms to total number of atoms or it is the disintegration rate per unit weight.

Roentgen (R) is the unit of exposure; $1 \text{ R} = 2.58 \times 10^{-4} \text{ C kg}^{-1}$ (C = coulomb).

Rad is the unit of absorbed dose; $1 \text{ rad} = 10^{-2} \text{ J kg}^{-1}$. The energy absorption equivalent of one roentgen in air is 0.87 rad and for water it is 0.97 rad. For tissue, the roentgen and rad are assumed to be numerically equivalent.

Rem refers to the unit of dose equivalent. The dose in rems is equal to the dose in rads multiplied by quality factor and the distribution factor.

Exposure rate constant (l) is the dose rate in roentgens per hour at 1 m distance from 1 curie. It is about one tenth the dose at a distance of 1 foot from 1 curie.

Electromagnetic radiation is a form of energy which consists of electric and magnetic fields vibrating at angles perpendicular to one another. Electromagnetic radiation is a wave particle. There are four main types of particulate radiation.

Alpha-particles: They possess positive charge (two units). The alpha-particles are similar to helium nuclei with a mass of 4 amu. These particles are produced by the disintegration of certain radioisotopes particularly those of heavy metals. All the alpha-particles have the same energy. These particles produce about 30,000 ion pairs per cm of path when they pass through the air. The thickness of a particular absorbing medium is expressed as mass per unit area. An aluminium foil of thickness (surface density) 1.62 g/cm^2 is able to slow down the alpha particles and this thickness is equivalent to 1 cm of air.

Beta-particles: These particles are negatively charged. Sometimes they are also positively charged with negligible mass, about 1/1836 that of the hydrogen ion. These particles are often accompanied by gamma radiation. They have less ionizing power than alpha particles, but have more penetrating power than alpha particles. Beta particles can pass through an aluminium foil of few millimetres.

Gamma rays: They have no mass or charge. There is not much difference between X-rays and gamma rays. Their distinction is based only on their origin. X-rays are produced by sudden stopping of the electrons by an anode or a target. Gamma rays are produced during disintegration of radioactive substances along with beta-radiation and during nuclear fission. The penetrating power of gamma radiation depends on atomic weight of absorber and wavelength of radiation.

Neutrons: They have no charge, but have a mass of 1 amu. Neutrons will be produced when alpha- or gamma-radiation interacts with a target element, generally beryllium, in which the neutrons are bound together with less energy than the bombarding radiation can impact.

Radioactive isotopes: Isotopes are classified into two types: (a) **stable isotopes** and (b) **radioactive isotopes**. The radioactive isotopes can undergo nuclear reactions producing alpha-, beta- and gamma-particles. The nucleus obtained after the nuclear changes or rearrangement may be that of a different element which may be stable. The original element is the **parent** and the product is called the **decay** or the **daughter product**. This phenomenon of nuclear changes is known as disintegration of radioactive decay.

Nuclear equations and reactions: The nuclear changes can be illustrated by equations. For example, the reaction in which a neutron is captured, producing an isotope of the target element and γ-radiation. This is (n, γ) reaction.

$$^{23}_{11}\text{Na} + {}^{1}_{0}\text{n} \longrightarrow {}^{24}_{11}\text{Na} + \text{r}$$

$$^{32}_{16}\text{S} + {}^{1}_{0}\text{n} \longrightarrow {}^{32}_{15}\text{P} + {}^{1}_{1}\text{P} \quad (n, p) \text{ reaction}$$

$$^{6}_{3}\text{Li} + {}^{1}_{0}\text{n} \longrightarrow {}^{3}_{1}\text{H} + {}^{4}_{2}\text{He} \quad (n, a) \text{ reaction}$$

The steps in a nuclear reaction involve the incident particle entering the nucleus with the formation of a **compound nucleus**, which ultimately decays to a product nucleus and to an emitted radiation. The probability that an incident particle strike a given type of nucleus is defined in terms of an effective cross-sectional area, referred to as (σ) cross-section. Its unit is 'barn' and barn is 10^{-28} m^2.

When once a particle has been captured by the nucleus to form an excited compound nucleus, the subsequent decay may occur in various fashions according to the amount of energy imparted to the nucleus by the initial step.

For example, let us see the bombardment of ^{35}Cl by neutrons:

$$^{35}_{17}\text{Cl} + \text{n} \longrightarrow {}^{36}_{17}\text{Cl}* \quad (\text{excited nucleus})$$

The excited nucleus may decompose in several fashions:

$$
^{36}_{17}\text{Cl}* \quad
\begin{cases}
\longrightarrow {}^{36}_{17}\text{Cl} + \text{r} \\
\longrightarrow {}^{35}_{17}\text{Cl} + \text{n} \\
\longrightarrow {}^{34}_{17}\text{Cl} + 2\text{n} \\
\longrightarrow {}^{35}_{16}\text{S} + \text{P} \\
\longrightarrow {}^{32}_{15}\text{P} + \alpha
\end{cases}
$$

Yield of a nuclear reaction: Let us consider a thin target of 1 cm^2 containing n nuclei which can undergo the given reaction. Suppose this is a flux of ϕ particles per cm^2 per second, and that the cross-section for the formation of a certain product is σ, then there will be $n\phi\sigma$-transformations per second.

If the product nuclei are radioactive, they will decay at a rate determined by the decay constant λ. Thus the radioactive nuclei being produced by one process are decaying by another. The rate of change of the number of radioactive nuclei (N) is given by following equation:

$$\frac{dN}{dt} = n\phi\sigma - \lambda N \quad (n = \text{number of atoms})$$

If irradiation continues for a finite time t sec, the number of resulting radioactive nuclei (N_t) is given by the following equation:

$$N_t = \frac{n\phi\sigma}{\lambda}(1 - e^{-\lambda t}) = \text{the activity after irradiation for } t \text{ seconds}$$

From this, we obtain a formula for calculating the yield in a practical case. If one introduces the Avogadro constant and the atomic weight, the result can be an expression of activity for a given mass. The above equation can thus be simplified by replacing the exponential as follows:

$$\text{Activity} = 6.02 \times 10^{23} \, \phi\sigma W(1 - t/2) \, t/t_{1/3} \text{ dis}^{-1} \text{ for W g}$$

Cross-section, σ, is measured in barn units.

Flux, ϕ, is expressed as bombarding particles per square metre. The two times, t and $t_{1/3}$ must be in the same units like seconds, hours, days, etc.

Half-life: The decay of individual atoms of a radioactive substance is irregular. If a certain amount of radionuclide is taken and the number of disintegrations per second is measured, we observe that, after certain time, half of the original atoms would have disintegrated and only half of the original active atoms would be present. The number of disintegrations per second will also now be half of the original value. The decay time of radionuclide to half is constant irrespective of the quantity present. This time is known as half-life of the radionuclide.

$$\text{Half-life } t_{1/2} = \frac{0.693}{\lambda}$$

where λ is disintegration constant in units of sec^{-1}.

Production of Radioisotopes

(a) **Reactor irradiation:** A reactor consists of an arrangement of fissionable material in a moderator, which slows down the fast neutrons to thermal energies. The fissionable material like uranium is in the form of rods arranged in a lattice pattern and hence the neutron flux is maximum in the centre where there is most uranium. A heavy water moderated reactor using enriched uranium (Harwell reactor DIDO) has a maximum flux of 10^{14} neutrons $cm^{-2} s^{-1}$.

(b) **Cyclotron irradiation:** While the reactor can only give a flux of neutrons and gamma-rays, accelerating machines can employ many other types of bombarding particles which are charged particles. They have to be accelerated to high velocities in order to overcome the repulsive forces of the nucleus. The beam of energetic particles is small and targets for irradiation have to be put in this beam. The number of samples that can be irradiated at a time is limited and the yields are low. But on the other hand many isotopes which otherwise cannot be produced in a reactor could be generated in a cyclotron.

Particle Detectors (Measurement of Radioactivity)

To measure the radiations of alpha, beta and gamma particles, several techniques involving detection and counting of individual particles or photons are commonly employed. The gas ionisation devices are Pulse Ionisation Chamber, Proportional Counter and Geiger-Muller Counter. Scintillation methods are available especially for counting gamma radiations.

I. Geiger-Muller Counter

It is still the most popular radiation detector. It does not need the use of a high-gain amplifier and it can detect alpha, beta and gamma-radiations.

G-M counter has the ionising gas and also contains a quenching vapour whose functions are (1) to prevent the spurious pulses that may be produced due to the positive ions reaching the cathode and (2) to absorb the photons emitted by excited atoms and molecules returning to their ground state. Both chlorine and bromine are used as quenching agents. Ethyl alcohol and ethyl formate have been used as organic-quenching agents. The filling gas pressure is much below the atmospheric pressure to avoid the use of high operating voltages.

Construction: The Geiger-Muller counter has a cylindrical cathode, usually 1–2 cm in diameter, along the centre of which is a wire anode. The space is filled with a gas which is readily ionised together with a small proportion of quenching vapour.

The design and construction of G-M counters entirely depend on the purpose for which they are needed. For counting the radioactive solid sources, the end window type G-M counter is the most popular which is shown in Fig. 3.1. The window is made of an aluminium alloy (7 mg cm^{-2}), mica or may be a thin glass bubble (about 15 mg cm^{-2}).

For counting the medium and high energy beta-particles (above 0.5 MeV) and for gamma counting thin glass-walled counters may be used. These are normally about 1 cm in diameter with a glass wall of 20–40 mg cm^{-2} thickness, the actual thickness depending on the length of the counter. The tube is coated on the inside with graphite to form the cathode. A counter of this type is shown in Fig. 3.2.

For counting the radioactive liquids, the counter takes the form shown in Fig. 3.3. It has the capacity of 10 cm^3 in annular space. In such a counter, 10 cm^3 of 3% solution of a uranium salt gives approximately 10,000 counts per minute. The type shown in Fig. 3.4 has a capacity of approximately 5 cm^3 and is connected by a plug and a socket. There are other types of G-M counters containing a thin-walled tube or spiral through which radioactive liquids can be drawn.

For counting the radioactive gases, the type shown in Fig. 3.5 is used. In this counter radioactive gas is introduced together with the counting gas. For the more efficient gamma-counting, counters with lead or copper cathode are used.

Operation of Geiger-Muller Counters

A Geiger-Muller probe unit is considered as an electrical switch, in which each pulse causes current to pass to scaler or counting unit to record the number of pulses. For the operation of Geiger-Muller

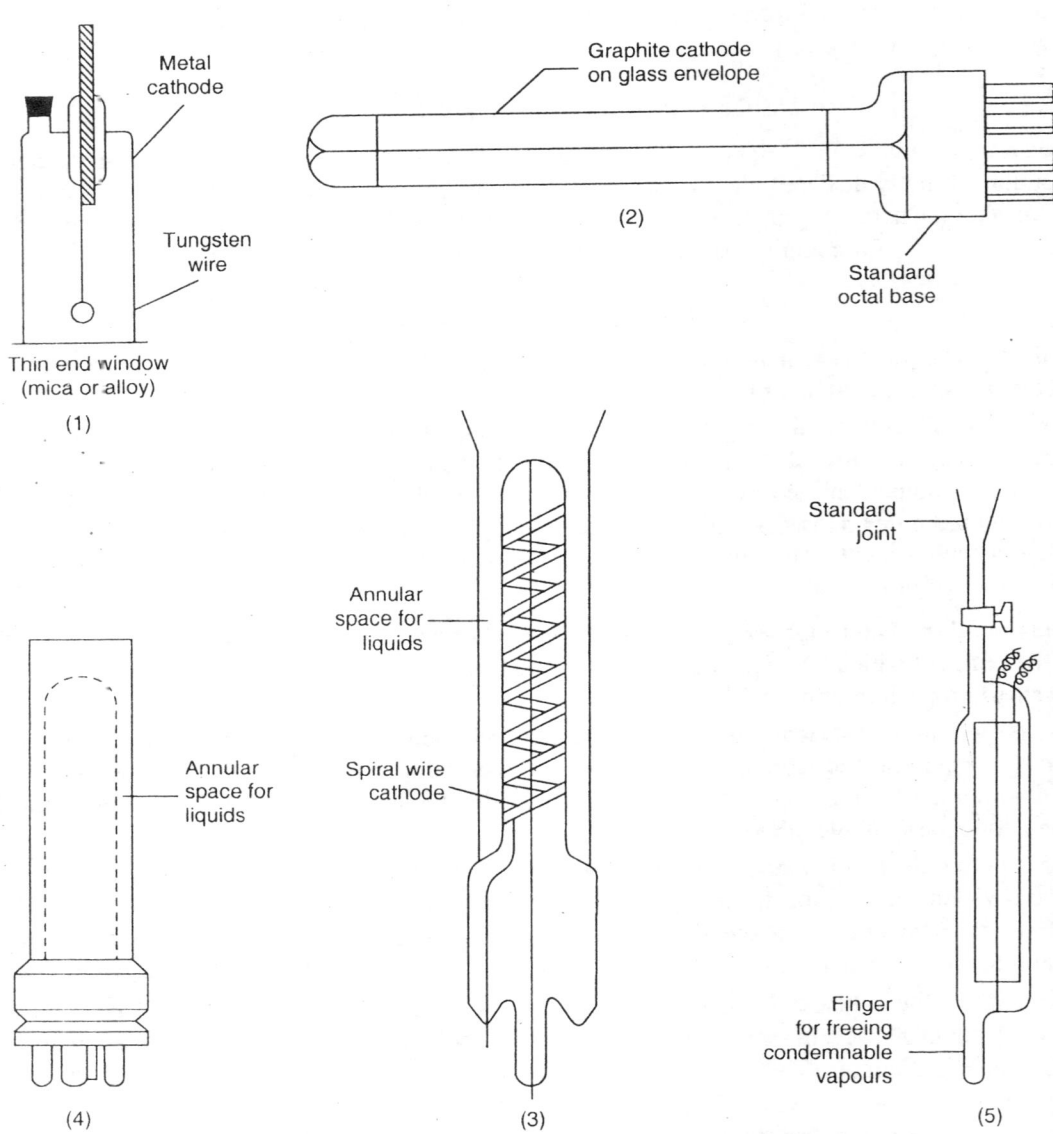

Figs. 3.1–3.5. Geiger-Muller counters. 3.1 & 3.2. for radioactive solids: 3.3 & 3.4 for liquids and 3.5 for gases.

counters, a source of high voltage, together with a low-gain amplifier and sealing unit for registering the pulses are required. To reduce the counting rate without any source in position, i.e. 'background' counting rate, the Geiger/counter is mounted in a lead shield. It has shelves for holding a source in one or more positions and for holding absorbers between the counter and the sourse. The reduction of the active length of an end window tube reduces the background, but it has little effect on counting rate.

The high voltage is adjusted so that the counter is operating on the plateau of its characteristic curve as shown in Fig. 3.6.

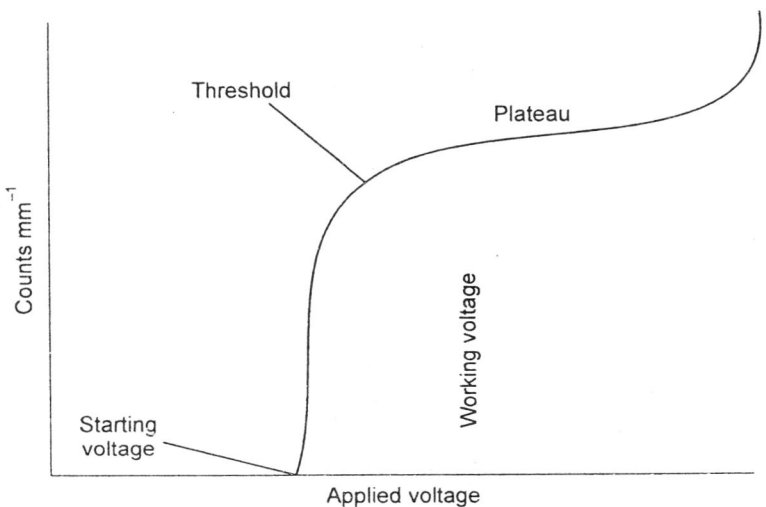

Fig.3.6. Plateau of Geiger-Muller counter.

As the voltage on the counter is raised, no registration of pulses will be observed till a certain voltage is reached (starting voltage). The counting rate rises rapidly to the threshold and at 150–200 volts or more, the counting rate is sensibly constant. At the same time size of individual pulses increases with voltage, so that at higher voltages there is a tendency for spurious discharges to be initiated. It is one of the causes for slope of plateau. The other reason may be variation in sensitivity.

The usual voltage selected for operating point is 100 volts above the threshold voltage.

II. Scintillation Counters

This method has gained popularity in the recent past. It is mainly useful in the counting of gamma emitters. In earlier devices, counting of scintillations was done visually. This method was obviously tedious, slow and not sensitive.

The development of photomultiplier tubes, consisting of photoelectric cells directly linked to electron multipliers have led to sensitive detection devices, which together with solid-state detectors are now-a-days enjoying a supremacy over other methods of counting. Fluorescent materials of 'phosphorus' are also used. Also the introduction of thallium-activated sodium iodide has made an advance in the application of scintillation techniques for gamma counting and energy determination.

Construction

Several types of photo-multiplying system have been constructed. A common type uses non-focusing dynodes, made into a Venetian blind construction, as shown in Fig. 3.7.

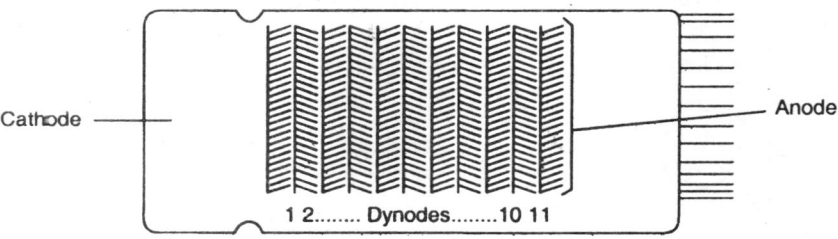

Fig. 7. Photomultiplier tubes.

Normally the cathode is caesium-antimony which is followed by a series of dynodes. Dynodes are made up generally of beryllium-copper alloy, from which the electrons are readily extracted. An accelerating voltage of approximately 150 volts is applied between the cathode and first dynode, and between successive dynodes.

Operation of Scintillation Counters

The following components are required for satisfactory operation:
  (1) Head amplifier
  (2) Main amplifier
  (3) High voltage power unit
  (4) Discriminator, and
  (5) Scaling unit or counting rate meter.

In the head amplifier, high voltage is fed through a high resistor to the anode wire of the counter. High-voltage power unit supplies a stabilized voltage. A pulse height discrimination is used after the amplifier and before the scaling unit to remove unwanted noise pulses. The scaling unit is attached for registering the pulses. It should be remembered that in scintillation counter the high voltage applied to photomultiplier is associated with the amplifying system and not with detectors.

Solid State Detectors

These detectors have been tried to replace conventional ones due to (1) high resolution, (2) compactness, and (3) easy interpretation of output signal. But certain factors like cost and low temperature to be maintained restrict their employment in place of scintillation counter.

Other counters used are pulse ionisation chamber and proportional counter.

Storage of Radioactive Isotopes

In order to have protection from hazards of radiation, utmost care is to be taken in storing the radioactive materials. They must be stored in an area not frequently visited by people. Shielding may be needed. Thick glass or perspex containers usually provide sufficient shielding. To protect from gamma radiations, lead shielding can be used. The storage area must regularly be checked for the radioactivity.

Handling Precautions

The working areas should not be contaminated with radioactive materials. If radioactive liquid is to be handled, it should be carried in trays having absorbent tissue paper so that any spillage will be absorbed by the paper. Rubber gloves must be used when working with radioactive liquids. Pipettes operated by mouth should never be used. Before making use of glass apparatus, it must be ensured that they are inactive. The waste radioactive material must be stored till the activity becomes low before its disposal.

Applications of Radioisotopes

Radioisotopes find their use in medicine, either as the radiation sources or as the radioactive tracer. They are mainly employed as radiation sources and can play an important role in therapy now-a-days. The selection of isotope depends upon the type, energy and properties of the radiation required. When it is used as the radioactive tracer, the chemical identity and form of the nuclide are the most important factors because the tracer has to be isotopic with the element under examination. Radioactive tracers are used in medicine mainly for diagnostic purposes.

I. Radioisotopes in Therapeutics

Radioisotopes are employed as radiation sources which may be used internally or externally. When the radioisotopes are used externally or used as implants in sealed capsules in a tissue, the dose is terminated by removal of the sources. If given internally as unsealed source, the dose cannot be terminated at will by removal of the source. The total dose in therapeutic application is calculated on the basis of effective half-life of the isotope, concentration of the isotope and the type and the energy of radiation emitted.

Gold (^{198}Au) has been used in the treatment of abdominal and pleural effusions associated with malignant tumours. It is used in the form of a colloidal gold suspension. ^{198}Au has also been tried in the treatment of carcinoma of uterus and urinary bladder. Sodium phosphate (^{32}P) is used in the therapy of polycythemia vera to decrease the rate of formation of erythrocytes. It has also been tried in the treatment of chronic granulocytic leukemia. Cobalt labelled cyanocobalamins (vitamin B_{12}) has been used in the diagnosis of pernicious anaemia. The labelled isotopes of cobalt are ^{57}Co, ^{58}Co and ^{60}Co. Sodium iodide (^{131}I) preparation is used in the treatment of thyroid disorders.

II. Radioisotopes in Diagnosis

Labelled cyanocobalamin is used for the measurement of glomerular filtration rate. Ferric citrate (^{59}Fe) injection is used for the diagnosis of haematological disorders. Colloidal gold (^{198}Au) injection is used for diagnostically studying the blood circulation in the liver. Sodium iodide (^{131}I) injection is used to diagnose the functioning of thyroid glands. Iodinated (^{131}I) human serum albumin injection is used to investigate cardiovascular functions. Sodium iodophippurate ^{131}I injection has diagnostic use in the study of renal functions. Sodium rose bengal ^{131}I injection is used as a diagnostic agent to test liver functions. The uptake of labelled compound in the liver is determined by the scintillation counter set up over the liver.

Other Applications

Determination of sterols in natural products:

One always faces a problem in the quantitative determination of stigmasterol in the mixture of sterols present in soybean oil as they are all closely related. The isotope dilution technique appears to be the only solution because this technique does not necessitate quantitative separation. In the direct isotope dilution method, the determination of the component (x) involves the measurement of the ratio of specific activities of (x) before and after dilution. The direct isotope dilution method of analysis consists essentially of the following steps:

(1) adding a known weight of isotopically labelled ions or molecule of a compound to a mixture containing an unknown quantity of unlabelled ions or molecules of the same compound;

(2) allowing complete mixing to occur;

(3) subsequently isolating a portion of purified material being analyzed;

(4) accurately determining the iostopic content. Isotope dilution technique is also used for analysing antibiotics in fermentation broth and in various extracts throughout the recovery processes.

Radioisotopes in Soap, Detergent and Cosmetic Research

The primary use of radioisotopes, with detergents and soaps as a class of compounds, has been for "detergent evaluation" or the determination of detergent's ability to remove oily soils from metal surfaces.

Radioisotopes are also used to study the drug metabolism.

A detailed account of radiopharmaceuticals and their preparations is given in Chapter 13.

PART II

Inorganic Pharmaceutical and Medicinal Compounds and Preparations

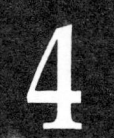

Pharmaceutical Aids and Necessities

Pharmaceutical aids and necessities are substances of chemical nature or of natural origin, that are of little or no therapeutic value, but are important for the preparation, preservation and storage of pharmaceutical products. Included among these are *acids and bases*, often used in the conversion of drugs to chemical forms convenient to the product formulation; *buffers*, that are used to maintain the pH of various formulations within prescribed limits and to deter deterioration; *antioxidants*, to prevent oxidative decomposition of pharmaceutically active compounds; *water*, a primary solvent and vehicle for several liquid preparations; *preservatives; adsorbents; diluents; excipients; suspending agents; colorants*, etc.

ACIDS AND BASES

Relevant to this chapter a consideration of the theories of acids and bases should find a mention here.

Theories of Acids and Bases

Acids and bases may be defined on the basis of various concepts namely the *Arrhenius Concept; Bronsted-Lowry Concept; Lewis Acid-Base Concept; and Hard and Soft Acid-Base Concept.*

Arrhenius Concept

All present concepts of acids and bases have been developed on the basis of this concept.

Arrhenius defined an acid as any substance that yields hydrogen ions (or protons, H) in aqueous solution and a base as a substance yielding or capable of yielding hydroxyl ions (OH) in aqueous solution. According to this definition an acid and base can undergo a neutralization reaction by the combination of these two ions to form water and a salt. The above reaction may be expressed by the following general equation between an acid (HA) and a base (BOH).

$$HA + BOH \leftrightarrow B^+A^- + H_2O$$

Limitation of Arrhenius concept:

- Nonhydroxide compounds which function as bases or produce hydroxide ion in aqueous solution is not covered by the definition.

- It does not consider the behaviour of acids and bases in nonaqueous solvents.

Bronsted and Bjerrum in Denmark and Lowry in England developed the above concept also known as the *proton concept.* According to this theory, an acid is a substance capable of donating a proton (H), while a base is a substance capable of accepting proton. This can be expressed by the equation:

$$A \leftrightarrow H + B$$
$$\text{acid} \qquad \text{base}$$

Thus a Bronsted acid ionizes to form a proton and the conjugate base of the acid and a Bronsted acid accepts a proton to form a conjugate acid of the base. Examples of such pairs are:

Acid			Conjugate base		Base			Conjugate acid
HCl	$\leftrightarrow$ H^+	+	Cl^-		Cl^-	+ H^+	$\leftrightarrow$	HCl
CH_3COOH	$\leftrightarrow$ H^+	+	CH_3COO^-		CH_3COO^-	+ H^+	$\leftrightarrow$	CH_3COOH
H_2O	$\leftrightarrow$ H^+	+	OH^-		OH^-	+ H^+	$\leftrightarrow$	H_2O
H_3O^+	$\leftrightarrow$ H^+	+	H_2O		H_2O	+ H^+	$\leftrightarrow$	H_3O^+
NH_4^+	$\leftrightarrow$ H^+	+	NH_3		NH_3	+ H^+	$\leftrightarrow$	NH_4^+

An acid will not release a proton unless a base capable of accepting it is present. Hence acid-base behaviour involves two sets of conjugate acid-base pairs as represented below. Strong acids have weak conjugate bases and strong bases have weak conjugate acids.

$$A_1 + B_2 \leftrightarrow B_1 + A_2$$
$$\text{acid}_1 \quad \text{base}_2 \qquad \text{base}_1 \quad \text{acid}_2$$

Some typical reactions include:

acid$_1$		base$_2$		base$_1$		acid$_2$
HCl	+	H_2O	$\leftrightarrow$	Cl^-	+	H_3O^+
NH_4^+	+	H_2O	$\leftrightarrow$	NH_3	+	H_3O^+
CH_3COOH	+	OH^-	$\leftrightarrow$	CH_3COO^-	+	H_2O
H_2SO_4	+	OH^-	$\leftrightarrow$	H_2O	+	HSO_4^-

H_2O sometimes behaves as an acid and at other times as a base and is called an *amphiprotic substance.*

Limitation of Bronsted-Lowry Concept:

- Does not indicate the basic reason for proton transfer.
- Does not explain how substances as carbon dioxide, stannic chloride, ferric chloride, sulphur trioxide, boron trichloride, or simple metal cations as Ag^+, Fe^{+2} and Zn^{+2}, which although not capable of donating a proton, can behave as acids.

Lewis Acid-Base Concept

The Lewis concept also called the *electron-pair concept* defines an acid as any substance that can share a pair of electrons made available by another substance called a base, thereby forming a co-ordinate covalent bond. The base is a substance that donates an electron pair to an acid. The following equations illustrate Lewis acid-base reactions.

$$\text{H}^+ \quad + \quad \text{:N:} \quad \text{H} \quad \longrightarrow \quad \left[\text{H :N: H} \right]^+$$

$$\text{Cl :B: H} \quad + \quad \text{:N: H} \quad \longrightarrow \quad \text{Cl :B: N H}$$

$$\text{Ag}^+ + 2 : \text{NH}_3 \rightarrow [\text{H}_3\text{N} : \text{Ag} : \text{NH}_3]^+$$

Hard and Soft Acid-Base Concept

According to this concept, acids and bases are defined as electron acceptor and donor species, respectively. However the HSAB principle further categorizes acids and bases according to the properties of charge, size (e.g. ionic radius), polarizability, etc.

Acid Strength

The strength of an acid can be reflected by the ionization constant K_a. Strong acids have large ionization constants ($K_a > 1$), while weaker acids have successively smaller values. Consider an acid HA dissolved in water. The reaction at equilibrium is expressed as below:

$$\text{HA} + \text{H}_2\text{O} \leftrightarrow \text{H}_3\text{O}^+ + \text{A}^-$$

K_a is expressed as:

$$K_a = \frac{[\text{H}_3\text{O}^+][\text{A}^-]}{[\text{HA}]}$$

K_a may also be expressed as pK_a (the negative logarithm to the base 10 of K) to bring it on the same scale as pH (see below).

Sorenson introduced a practical approach of expressing acidity as the pH, which is defined as the negative logarithm to the base 10 of the hydrogen (or hydronium) ion concentration and is represented by the expression below:

$$pH = -\log [\text{H}] = -\log [\text{H}_3\text{O}^+] = \log 1/[\text{H}_3\text{O}^+]$$

As the concentration of the hydrogen ion increases the acidity increases and the pH decreases.

Importance of Acids and Bases as Pharmaceutical Aids

- Several pharmaceutical drugs are either salts of weak acids or of weak bases. Several weakly acidic drugs like penicillins and basic drugs like atropine are very poorly soluble in water resulting in very poor dissolution rates. Salts have improved solubility and dissociation characteristics in comparison to the original drug. Strong acids and bases are often used in the conversion of such drugs into their salt forms to enhance the aqueous solubility, thereby enabling enhancement of the bioavailability of the drug.

- Acids and bases may be used to obtain the desired pH of pharmaceutical formulations, to ensure maximum stability of the product during storage or to minimize irritation.
- Weak acids like boric acid constitute a portion of what would be needed for a buffer solution.
- Boroglycerin glycerite, which has found some use as a suppository base is produced as a result of the reaction of boric acid with equimolar quantities of glycerin at 140°–150°C.

A number of inorganic acids and bases used as pharmaceutical aids are described below:

INORGANIC ACIDS

BORIC ACID
(Synonym: Boric acid)

Chem. formula: H_3BO_3 Mol. weight: 61.83

Standard: It contains not less than 99.5% and not more than 100.5% of H_3BO_3 calculated with reference to the dried substance.

Preparation: It is prepared from colemanite $Ca_2B_6O_{11}.5H_2O$. Finely powdered colemanite is dissolved in boiling water and sulphur dioxide is passed through the solution when boric acid and calcium bisulphate is formed. The latter being soluble remains in solution while boric acid crystallizes out. The crystals of boric acid separate out on cooling.

$$Ca_2B_6O_{11} + 4SO_2 + 11H_2O \longrightarrow 2Ca(HSO_3)_2 + 6H_3BO_3$$

In the laboratory, boric acid can be prepared by adding a mixture of conc. H_2SO_4 and water (1 : 5) to a boiling solution of borax (60 g in 160 ml of water):

$$Na_2B_4O_7 + H_2SO_4 + 5H_2O \longrightarrow Na_2SO_4 + 4H_3BO_3$$

The solution is filtered and set aside for crystallization. The crystals of boric acid are washed until free from sulphate ions and dried at room temperature.

Description: Boric acid occurs as colourless scales of a somewhat pearl-like lustre as white crystals or white powder. It is odourless with slightly acidic and bitter taste and unctuous touch. Upon being heated, it loses water and is transformed into metaboric acid (HBO_2).

Solubility: 1 g is soluble in 18 ml of water or alcohol; 4 ml of glycerin; 4 ml of boiling water and 6 ml of boiling alcohol.

Tests for identity: (1) A mixture of ethyl alcohol with boric acid burns with a green-edged flame due to the formation of ethyl borate.

$$H_3BO_3 + 3C_2H_5OH \longrightarrow B(OC_2H_5)_3 + 3H_2O$$

(2) Solution in water is acidic in nature.

Tests for Purity: It is tested for arsenic; heavy metals; sulphate and alcohol-insoluble substances (determined by dissolving 1 g in 10 ml of boiling alcohol; when the solution should not be more than faintly turbid).

Assay: This is based upon the titration of boric acid (pK_a 9.24) with sodium hydroxide in the presence of glycerin.

$$H_3BO_3 + NaOH \longrightarrow NaBO_2 + 2H_2O$$

The object of the addition of glycerin is to form a metaborate ion-glycerol complex, which behaves as a monobasic acid and is strong enough to give a satisfactory end point.

Metaborate ion-glycerol complex

I.P. 2007 gives the method of assay by using phenolphthalein solution in the solution of boric acid (2 g) in 50 ml of water and 100 ml of glycerin and titrating the solution with 1 M sodium hydroxide.

Each ml of 1 M sodium hydroxide $\equiv$ 0.06183 g of H_3BO_3.

Uses: It is used as a local anti-infective agent.

Boric acid is a weak germicide and hence it is used as a local anti-infective. Its solutions are not irritating and aqueous solutions are employed as eye wash and mouth wash. Boric acid may be employed as a dusting powder, if diluted with some other inert material.

Boric acid can be very dangerous if ingested and hence its container should bear the warning **"not for internal use"**.

HYDROCHLORIC ACID

Chem. formula: HCl   Mol. weight: 36.46

Hydrochloric acid was commonly called spirit of salt as it was first prepared by distilling sea salt with sulphuric acid. It is an aqueous solution of hydrogen chloride in water and contains not less than 35% w/w and not more than 38% w/w of HCl.

Preparation: (1) Hydrochloric acid is manufactured by the interaction of sodium chloride and sulphuric acid. Calculated quantities of common salt and conc. sulphuric acid are heated in the cast iron pan of a salt cake furnace. Sodium bisulphite in the reaction is mixed with more of common salt and heated strongly in the muffle to get more of HCl.

$$NaCl + H_2SO_4 \longrightarrow NaHSO_4 + HCl$$

$$NaHSO_4 + NaCl \longrightarrow Na_2SO_4 + HCl$$

Hydrochloric acid gas is passed up a tower on which cold water is sprayed, when dilute acid is collected at the bottom. This is again sprayed down the tower to absorb more HCl gas and gets concentrated. The acid so manufactured is purified.

(2) Large quantities of hydrogen and chlorine are obtained as by-products during the manufacture of caustic soda by electrolysis of sodium chloride solution. The gases are combined to give hydrogen chloride.

$$H_2 + Cl_2 \longrightarrow 2HCl$$

Description: It is a colourless fuming liquid with pungent odour. The pungent odour and fumes disappear when it is diluted with double the quantity of water. It is very strongly acidic to litmus even in highly diluted form. Qualitatively it can be recognised by the formation of a white precipitate of silver chloride with silver nitrate. It attacks many metals with the evolution of hydrogen. It is miscible with water or alcohol. Its specific gravity is 1.18.

Tests for Purity: It is tested for weight per ml; As; Pb; bromide and iodide; sulphate; sulphates; free chloride; and residue on ignition.

The test for bromide and iodide is performed by diluting the acid with double amount of its water, adding chloroform (1 ml) and solution of chlorinated lime and noting the colour of chloroform layer, which should not become brown or violet.

Assay: An accurate amount, about 4 g, of HCl is taken in a stoppered flask containing 40 ml of water and the solution is titrated with 1 N sodium hydroxide, using solution of methyl orange as indicator.

$$NaOH + HCl \longrightarrow NaCl + H_2O$$

Each ml of 1 N NaOH is equivalent to 0.03646 g of HCl.

Note: The acid is weighed and not measured because the result is required as percentage of weight by weight. The acid is weighed in stoppered flask containing water, as loss of HCl on being diluted is little.

Uses: It is used as acidifier and hence it is a pharmaceutical necessity for preparing diluted hydrochloric acid.

DILUTE HYDROCHLORIC ACID

Dilute hydrochloric acid contains 10% w/w of HCl (limit 9.5 to 10%). It is prepared by mixing the following ingredients:

Hydrochloric acid .... 274.0 g
Purified water .... 726.0 g

Description: It is a colourless liquid which is strongly acidic and has about 1.05 specific gravity.
Tests for Purity and assay are performed in the same way as for concentrated acid.
Uses: It is used as an acidifier.
Dose: 0.6 to 8 ml.

PHOSPHORIC ACID

Chem. formula: H_3PO_4 Mol. weight: 98.0

Synonym: Concentrated Phosphoric acid; Orthophosphoric acid.
Phosphoric acid contains not less than 88.0% and not more than 90.0% w/w of H_3PO_4.

Preparation:

(1) Phosphoric acid on large scale is prepared from bones or mineral phosphate by digesting the powder with sulphuric acid. The required amount of calcium sulphate is separated by filtration. The filtrate contains phosphoric acid:

$$Ca_3(PO_4)_2 + 3H_2SO_4 \longrightarrow 3CaSO_4 + 2H_3PO_4$$

The acid so obtained is crude and unless purified it cannot be used for medicinal and allied purposes.

(2) A method which gives pure phosphoric acid consists in continuously warming red phosphorus (7 parts) with water (50 parts) and conc. nitric acid (40 parts) in a flask and finally boiling the mixture till the phosphorus is completely oxidised.

$$4P + 10HNO_3 + H_2O \longrightarrow 4H_3PO_4 + 5NO + 5NO_2$$

The above liquid is transferred to a dish and concentrated.

(3) It can also be prepared by converting phosphorus to phosphorus pentoxide in current of hot air and treating the phosphorus pentoxide with water to form phosphoric acid:

$$P_2O_5 + 3H_2O \longrightarrow 2H_3PO_4$$

Description: Phosphoric acid is a colourless and odourless syrupy liquid. It is miscible with water and alcohol. Its specific gravity is about 1.71. It loses water on heating and is finally converted to

---

Phosphorus occurs in nature in the form of phosphates, calcium phosphate mineral being the chief source. Phosphorus occurs in two common allotropic forms, namely (a) yellow or colourless, (b) red or amorphous. Yellow phosphorus, also called white phosphorus, has disagreeable ozone-like odour, emits white luminous fumes which have odour resembling that of garlic. It is insoluble in water but is soluble in chloroform, benzene and carbon disulphide. It is poisonous. Red or amorphous phosphorus as the name suggests is brown to red powder, non-poisonous, non-luminous and is insoluble in any common solvent. Phosphorus compounds are many, like chlorides and trichlorides; oxides and oxyacids; but in I.P. only phosphoric acid and dil. phosphoric acid are included.

Biologically, phosphorus plays an important role as it is one of the essential elements for the life of plants and animals. There is 450–700 gm of phosphorus in the body of an adult. A complex basic $Ca_3(PO_4)_2$ constitutes the main inorganic component of human bones and teeth.

Dihydrogen phosphate and hydrogen phosphate ions circulate in body fluids and are associated with metabolism of various organic materials such as carbohydrate. Glycogen is disintegrated into glucose by a process phosphorolysis. Phosphorylation is the initial step in the synthesis of glycogen from glucose. PO_4 is the principal anion in the intracellular fluid. It plays a part in the regulation of acid base equilibrium in body fluids and the urine. Phosphorylation is also involved in the selective absorption of sugars and fats. Fats are mostly transported in the form of phospholipids and have the highest reactivity. Adinosine phosphate and phosphocreatine in muscles set large amount of energy on disintegration in the course of muscular contraction.

Phosphoric acid is an essential constituent of nucleic acid, nucleotides, phospholipids and hexose phosphate. It is also found in phosphoproteins such as caseine; some of the important enzymes are formed by vitamins combined with H_3PO_4 acid, e.g. phosphoriboflavin is one of the respiratory enzymes. Enzymes which accelerate hydrolysis of monophosphoric ester release phosphoric acid and are called phosphatases. They are found nearly in all the cells and tissues fluids.

Deficient absorption of Ca and P results in rickets in children and osteomalacia in adults.

P is absorbed by plants mainly as H_2PO_4 ions. PO_4 carriers phosphorylation and the energy of phosphate bond are of primary importance in fat and carbohydrate metabolism, respiration, photosynthesis and many other metabollic processes in plants.

The synthesis of proteins does not occur at the usual rate in P deficiency in plants. This leads to accumulation of sugar in the vegetative part of the plant.

The application of PO_4 fertiliser may alter the nitrogen balance of the plant.

The use of inorganic compound in medication now-a-days is quiet common. However, tribasic calcium, magnesium and aluminium phosphates are extensively used as antacids. Dibasic sodium phosphate is an ingredient in a large number of saline cathartic preparations.

metaphosphoric acid, which on cooling forms transparent mass with a composition of $H_3PO_4.\frac{1}{4}H_2O$. The concentrated acid attacks porcelain.

Tests for identity:

(1) Phosphoric acid (and phosphates) gives, in presence of nitric acid, with excess of ammonium molybdate on heating, a yellow precipitate of ammonium phosphomolybdate $(NH_4)_3.(MoO_3).I_{12}PO_4xH_2O$.

(2) Neutral solution of phosphate gives a yellow precipitate with silver nitrate due to the formation of silver phosphate (Ag_3PO_4).

Tests for purity: It is tested for wt. per ml; aluminium and calcium; arsenic; heavy metals; iron chloride; nitrate; alkali phosphate; phosphorus and hypophosphorus acid and sulphate.

Phosphoric acid obtained directly from the natural phosphates (method 1 above) usually contains calcium, iron and sulphate.

Aluminium and calcium can be tested by adding to 1 ml of phosphoric acid, 10 ml of water and diluting the solution till it is alkaline. No precipitate is produced. Nitrate is tested by adding to 5 ml of diluted phosphoric acid, 0.1 ml of solution of indigo carmine and 5 ml of sulphuric acid. The blue colour produced is not discharged within one minute.

Alkali phosphates are tested by transferring 1 ml of phosphoric acid to a graduated cylinder and adding 6 ml of solvent ether and 2 ml of alcohol. No turbidity is produced.

Phosphorus and hypophosphorus acids are tested by diluting 0.5 ml of phosphoric acid with 10 ml of water and warming with 2 ml of solution of silver nitrate. The solution is not brown on warming.

Assay: An accurately weighed amount (about 1.5 g) is mixed with a solution of sodium chloride (10 g in 30 ml H_2O) and titrated with 1 N sodium hydroxide, using solution of phenolphthalein as indicator.

$$H_3PO_4 + 2NaOH \longrightarrow Na_2HPO_4 + 2H_2O$$

Each ml of 1 N sodium hydroxide is equivalent to 0.04900 g of H_3PO_4.

Note: Sodium chloride is used to obtain a more accurate end point.

Uses: It is used as a pharmaceutical aid, to make the dilute acid, which has been employed in lead poisoning. Industrially it is used in dental cements and in beverages as an acidulant.

Preparation: Dilute phosphoric acid.

DILUTE PHOSPHORIC ACID

Dilute phosphoric acid contains 10.0% w/w of H_3PO_4 (limit 9.5 to 10.5).

Preparation: It is prepared by taking 112 g phosphoric acid and mixing it in 888 g of purified water. It is clear, odourless liquid with 1.057 specific gravity. It is miscible with water and alcohol.

Tests for purity: All the tests are same as mentioned under phosphoric acid and tests can be performed by taking nine times the stated amount under phosphoric acid.

Assay: Assay procedure is the same as mentioned under phosphoric acid, except that the amount to be taken should be about 10 g accurately weighed.

Uses: Same as mentioned under phosphoric acid above.

Dose: 0.3–4 ml.

SULPHURIC ACID

Chem. formula: H_2SO_4 Mol. weight: 98.08

Sulphuric acid containing not less than 95.0 per cent w/w of H_2SO_4.

Preparation: Sulphuric acid is perhaps the most important of the inorganic acids, which was called in the earlier days as oil of vitriol. In the free state, it is said to be found in some mineral springs being formed by the action of water on sulphides, for example, iron pyrites as per the reaction given below:

$$2FeS_2 + 2H_2O + 7O_2 \longrightarrow 2H_2SO_4 + 2FeSO_4$$

It is an important chemical in pharmacy and other industries. It is an important pharmaceutical acid.

It is neither required nor possible to discuss the preparation (manufacture) of sulphuric acid here, especially in view of the fact that students for whom this text is written have already been taught the methods of manufacture of sulphuric acid in their previous classes, either in schools, colleges or in the first year of the pharmacy course.

However, it will be worthwhile to mention here that sulphuric acid is manufactured industrially by the following three methods:

1. Lead chamber process
2. Contact process
3. Anhydride process.

The above processes are used only industrially, though it is possible to demonstrate the manufacture of sulphuric acid through contact process on small scale in the laboratory. The industrially produced sulphuric acid is impure and is not suitable for pharmaceutical use. Pure acid required for pharmaceutical purposes is concentrated from its 78% strength to 96.5%. For pharmaceutical purposes, acid produced through contact process is preferred.

Description: Pure sulphuric acid is a colourless, oily liquid, which is highly corrosive. It evolves much heat when added to water (288 K cal per mole of acid) and when dilute acid is to be made, sulphuric acid should be poured into water slowly with constant stirring. The volume of diluted acid is always less than the sum total volume of water and acid mixed. Sulphuric acid solidifies into a crystalline mass at 10.5°C. Its specific gravity at 25°C is about 1.84 g.

Tests for identity: After neutralisation, it yields reaction characteristic of sulphates (App. I).

Tests for purity: It is tested for specific gravity (wt. per ml) oxidisable impurities; nitrate; chloride; arsenic; iron; heavy metals and ash.

The oxidisable impurities: They are tested by treating a cooled diluted solution of 5 ml of acid with 20 ml of water with 0.1 ml of 0.1 N potassium permanganate. The colour of permanganate is not decolourised within five minutes.

The test for nitrate: It is performed by adding 5 ml of acid to a mixture of 5 ml of water and 0.5 ml of solution of indigo carmine and noting the colour, which should not be discharged within one minute.

For chloride test: 5 ml of acid diluted with water and neutralised with dilute solution of ammonia is used.

The test for heavy metals is as follows: Add 1.1 ml of the acid to about 10 mg of sodium carbonate dissolved in a few ml of water and carefully heat over a free flame until nearly dry. Add 1 ml of nitric acid, evaporate to dryness on a water bath. Take up the residue in 20 ml of water and neutralise to solution of phenolphthalein with 0.1 N sodium hydroxide. Add 1 ml of dilute acetic acid and dilute to 40 ml. Prepare a control to contain 0.04 mg of Pb and 1 ml of dilute acetic acid in a volume of 40 ml. Add to each solution 10 ml of solution of hydrogen sulphide. The colour of the solution of the sample is not darker than that of the control solution (20 parts per million).

Assay: An accurately weighed amount, 2 g, is mixed with about 40 ml of water and the solution is titrated with 1 N sodium hydroxide, using solution of methyl red as indicator.

$$H_2SO_4 + 2NaOH \longrightarrow Na_2SO_4 + 2H_2O$$

1000 ml of 1 N NaOH is equivalent to $\frac{1}{2}H_2SO_4$.

Or Each ml of 1 N sodium hydroxide is equivalent to 0.04904 g of H_2SO_4.

Preparations: Dilute Sulphuric Acid.

Aromatic Sulphuric Acid.

DILUTE SULPHURIC ACID (Dil. Sulph. Acid)

Dilute sulphuric acid contains not less than 9.5 per cent and not more than 10.5 per cent w/w H_2SO_4,

Ingredients:

Sulphuric acid	104 g
Purified water	896 g

Preparation: Add the sulphuric acid very gradually to the purified water and cool.

Tests for purity for nitrate: To 15 ml add 0.2 ml of solution of indigo carmine and 15 ml of nitrogen free sulphuric acid, the colour is not discharged within one minute.

Chloride, iron, arsenic, heavy metals, ash: Complies with the requirements stated under sulphuric acid.

Assay: Assay is carried out in the same way as given under sulphuric acid, using about 10 g accurately weighed.

Uses: It is used as a pharmaceutical aid.

Dose: 0.3 to 4 ml.

AROMATIC SULPHURIC ACID (Arom. Sulph. Acid)

Synonym: Elixir* of Vitriol.

Aromatic sulphuric acid contains free and combined sulphuric acid equivalent to not less than 12.2 per cent and not more than 13.5 per cent w/v of H_2SO_4.

Ingredients:

Strong ginger tincture	50 ml
Cinnamon oil	1.5 ml
Sulphuric acid	70 ml
Alcohol (90 per cent) to produce	1000 ml

---

* Elixirs are clear, flavoured oral liquids containing one or more active ingredients dissolved in a vehicle that usually contains a high proportion of sucrose or a suitable polyhydric alcohol or alcohols and may also contain ethanol (95%) or diluted ethanol.

Preparation: Mix the sulphuric acid gradually with 600 ml of the alcohol (90 per cent) and cool; dissolve the cinnamon oil and add the strong ginger tincture and sufficient of the alcohol (90 per cent) to produce the required volume.

Assay: 10 ml of the Aromatic Sulphuric Acid is taken and to this 50 ml of 1 N NaOH is added and the solution is titrated with 1 N H_2SO_4 using solution of methyl orange as indicator.

Each ml of 1 N NaOH is equivalent to 0.04904 g of H_2SO_4.

Uses: It is used as a pharmaceutical aid.

Dose: 0.3 to 1.2 ml.

AMMONIA SOLUTION STRONG (Ammon. sol. strong)

Strong ammonia solution contains not less than 27.0% w/w and not more than 30.0% w/w of NH_3.

Description: It is a colourless, transparent liquid with characteristic strong pungent odour, miscible with water and alcohol; specific gravity about 0.90, strongly alkaline to litmus even when diluted.

Tests for purity: It is tested for As, heavy metals; tarry matter; and non-volatile residue.

Assay: An accurately weighed amount (3 g) of the sample is taken in a flask containing 1 N sulphuric acid (50 ml) and the excess of acid is titrated with 1 N sodium hydroxide, using solution of methyl red as indicator.

Reaction:

$$2NH_2OH + H_2SO_4 \longrightarrow (NH_4)_2SO_4 + 2H_2O$$

$$H_2SO_4 + 2NaOH \longrightarrow Na_2SO_4 + 2H_2O$$

1 ml of H_2SO_4 is equivalent to 0.01703 g of NH_3.

Uses: Strong ammonia solution is used for pharmaceutical purposes, mainly for making ammonia water. It is an ingredient in aromatic spirit of ammonia and strong ammonium acetate solution.

AMMONIA SOLUTION DILUTE

It is prepared by diluting the strong ammonia solution with purified water to contain 10.0% w/w of NH_3.

The solution is tested for purity tests and assayed in the same way as in ammonia solution strong.

CALCIUM HYDROXIDE
(Synonym: Slaked lime)

Chem. formula: $Ca(OH)_2$ Mol. weight. 74.09

Preparation: Calcium hydroxide is made by adding water to calcium oxide (quick lime). The calcium oxide is itself prepared by burning limestone in specially designed kilns.

$$CaCO_3 \xrightarrow{\ 1975\ K\ } CaO + CO_2 \uparrow$$

The reaction being reversible, CO_2 should be removed to favour the forward reaction.

Calcium hydroxide is mixed with excess of water and allowed to settle. The ppt. is air-dried. When an acidic solution of Calcium Hydroxide is warmed with $KMnO_4$, it gives the odour of acetaldehyde.

I.P. requires it to contain not less than 99% of $Ca(OH)_2$. It is not official now in I.P. 2007.

Description: It is a soft, white powder with alkaline and slightly bitter taste. It is slightly soluble in water, soluble in glycerin and insoluble in alcohol.

Tests for identity: A solution in CH_3COOH gives the reactions of Calcium (App. I).

Tests for purity: It is tested for alkalinity; arsenic; heavy metals; Al; Fe; phosphate; acid insoluble matter; chloride; and sulphate.

Alkalinity: A solution is alkaline to phenolphthalein solution.

Arsenic: Not more than 4 ppm.

Heavy metals: Not more than 40 ppm. The solution for this test is prepared by dissolving sample (1 g) in dil. HCl (10 ml) and evaporating to dryness. The residue is dissolved in water (20 ml) and filtered. The filtrate is diluted with water (to 40 ml), and to half of the resulting solution (20 ml) is added dil. HCl (0.1 ml) and water (to make 25 ml).

Aluminium, iron, phosphate and acid-insoluble matter: Dissolve the sample (2 g) in HCl and water (75 ml), boil to remove CO_2 and make alkaline with dil. NH_3 solution using methyl red as an indicator. Boil for one minute, filter, and wash the ppt. with a hot 2% w/v solution of NH_4Cl. The ppt. is dissolved as completely as possible by passing hot dil. HCl (20 ml) through the filter, and wash the filter with sufficient hot water to adjust the volume of the solution (to 50 ml). Boil the solution and make alkaline with dil. NH_3 solution, using methyl red as indicator. Boil for 1 min. filter through the same filter, wash the ppt. with a hot 2% w/v solution of ammonium nitrate, dry and ignite at a temp. not lower than 1000; the residue weighs not more than 20 mg.

Chloride: A specified amount of sample (1 g) dissolved in water with the addition of HNO_3 (4 ml) complies with the limit test for chlorides.

Sulphate: A specified amount of sample (0.15 g) dissolved in water with the addition of dil. HCl (3.5 ml) complies with the limit test for sulphates.

Assay: It is based upon volumetric titration. The titrant used is N HCl and indicator is phenolphthalein.

Shake gently an accurately weighed amount of sample (3 g) with alcohol (10 ml) previously neutralized to phenolphthalein sol. in a 1000 ml flask. Add to this solution a 10% w/v solution of sucrose (490 ml) and shake vigorously for 5 minutes and then frequently for 4 hours. Filter off half of the volume of solution (250 ml) and titrate with N HCl, using phenolphthalein solution as indicator. Alcohol and sucrose solution must be neutralized to phenolphthalein.

$$Ca(OH)_2 + 2HCl \longrightarrow CaCl_2 + 2H_2O$$

Each ml of N HCl $\equiv$ 0.03705 g of $Ca(OH)_2$

Use: It is used as an astringent. It is also used as a protective in various types of lotion for topical application.

Storage: Calcium hydroxide is stored in well-closed containers.

POTASSIUM HYDROXIDE
(Synonym: Caustic potash)

Chem. formula: KOH   Mol. weight: 56.1

It contains not less than 85% of total alkali, calculated as KOH including not more than 40% of K_2CO_3. It has been official in I.P., B.P., U.S.P.

Preparation: It is prepared by electrolysis of a solution of potassium chloride using graphite anode and mercury cathode in a divided cell which will not allow the liberated chloride to react with the newly formed potassium hydroxide. The reaction takes place as under:

At cathode:

$$K^+ \longrightarrow K$$
$$2K + 2H_2O \longrightarrow 2\,KOH + H_2$$

At anode:

$$Cl + Cl = Cl_2$$

The caustic liquid is evaporated and the resulting fused potassium hydroxide is used to prepare either sticks, pellets or fused masses.

Description: It is a dried, white pellets, sticks or fused mass, which is hard or brittle and shows a crystalline fracture. It is very deliquescent, strongly alkaline and corrosive. Soluble in water, alcohol and glycerine.

Tests for purity: It is tested for Cl; SO_4; As; heavy metals; Na and aluminium; iron and matter insoluble in hydrochloric acid.

Assay: An accurately weighed quantity (2 g) of potassium hydroxide is dissolved in water (25 ml) to which $BaCl_2$ solution (5 ml) is added. The solution is then titrated with 1 N HCl using phenolphthalein as indicator.

$$KOH + HCl \longrightarrow KCl + H_2O$$

To the solution is then added bromophenol blue and the titration is continued with 1 N HCl.

The amount of acid consumed in the second titration represents the amount of potassium carbonate present in potassium hydroxide.

$$K_2CO_3 + BaCl_2 \longrightarrow BaCO_3 + 2KCl$$
$$BaCO_3 + 2HCl \longrightarrow BaCl_2 + H_2O + CO_2$$

1000 ml of 1 N HCl is equivalent to $\frac{1}{2}K_2CO_3$.

1000 ml of 1 N HCl is equivalent to 1 KOH.

Or

Each ml of 1 N HCl is equivalent to 0.069 g of K_2CO_3.

Each ml of 1 N HCl is equivalent to 0.05611 g of total alkali calculated as KOB.

The amount of acid used in the combined titration is equivalent to total alkali present.

Storage: It is preserved in a well-closed container. Great care is taken in handling hydroxide as it is highly destructive to tissue. Hence it is not handled with bare hands.

Uses: It is used as a pharmaceutical aid. It is used as caustic chiefly in veterinary practice. It is used in many pharmacopoeial and other preparations like potassium hydroxide solution; cresol solution. soao solution etc.

POTASSIUM HYDROXIDE SOLUTION
(Synonym: Solution of potash)

It is an aqueous solution of KOH containing 5% w/v of total alkali, calculated as KOH (limit 4.75–5.25).

Description: Potassium hydroxide solution is a colourless, strongly alkaline liquid. Its specific gravity is 1.042 g at 20°C.

Assay: It is titrated with 1 N H_2SO_4 using methyl orange as indicator.

$$2KOH + H_2SO_4 \longrightarrow K_2SO_4 + 2H_2O$$

Each ml of 1 N H_2SO_4 is equivalent to 0.05611 g of total alkali calculated as KOH.

Storage: Potassium hydroxide solution is preserved in a well-closed bottle of lead-free glass because alkali reacts with certain kinds of colourless glass containing lead in them. The bottles should be closed with rubber stoppers as the glass stoppers stick.

Uses: It is used as a pharmaceutical aid.

SODIUM HYDROXIDE
(Synonym: Caustic soda)

Chem. formula: NaOH   Mol. weight: 40.0

Sodium hydroxide contains not less than 95% of total alkali calculated as NaOH and not more than 2.5% of Na_2CO_3.

Preparation:

(1) **Soda Lime Process:** It is prepared by heating Na_2CO_3 with milk of lime in large iron tanks.

$$Na_2CO + Ca(OH)_2 \rightleftharpoons CaCO_3 + 2NaOH$$

The reaction is reversible. In the concentrations used in the manufacture more than 90% of the sodium carbonate is converted into hydroxide.

The liquor is filtered and evaporated. The molten product is formed by suitable processes into sticks, pellets or masses. The pellet forms are considered convenient for general use.

(2) **Electrolytic Process:** This process is called Castner-Kellner process. In this sodium hydroxide is prepared on large scale by electrolysis of saturated solution of sodium chloride or brine. Different types of cells are in common use. Most of the cells used employ carbon anode and metallic cathode and are devised in such a way that NaOH is produced in an isolated, brine free, cathode compartment. The electrolytic process is not only simple and economical but it also yields hydrogen and chlorine as valuable by-products.

$$2NaCl \rightleftharpoons 2Na^+ + 2Cl^-$$
$$2H_2O \rightleftharpoons 2OH^- + 2H^+$$

at cathode $\uparrow$ $\uparrow$ at anode

2NaOH $\Big\Updownarrow$ $\Big\Updownarrow$ 2HCl

Or

$$2Na + 2e \longrightarrow 2Na \qquad H^- + 1e \longrightarrow H \longrightarrow H_2$$
$$2OH - 2e \longrightarrow 2OH \qquad Cl^- + 1e \longrightarrow Cl \longrightarrow Cl_2$$

2NaOH   2HCl

These gases are either collected separately or converted into hydrogen chloride. The whole process is summarised as above.

Description: It occurs as white sticks, pellets, fused masses or scales, which are dry, hard or brittle, showing cystalline fracture. Sodium hydroxide is very deliquescent, strongly alkaline and highly corrosive. Its specific gravity is 2.13 and melting point 318°. It is soluble in water (1 g in 1 ml), freely in alcohol and glycerin and generates heat when dissolved. It absorbs moisture and carbon dioxide when exposed to air. The reaction takes place as follows and finally sodium carbonate is formed (other alkali hydroxides also give the same reaction).

$$H_2O + CO_2 \rightleftharpoons H_2CO_3$$

$$2NaOH + H_2CO_3 \rightleftharpoons Na_2CO_3 + 2H_2O$$

Tests for identity: It gives reaction characteristic of sodium.

Tests for purity: Insoluble substances and organic matter; Al, Fe; and matter insoluble in hydrochloric acid; As; heavy metals; Cl; SO_4; and potassium.

The test for insoluble substances and organic matter consists in examining a 5% w/v solution which should be clear and colourless.

The test for Al, Fe and matter insoluble in HCl is based on a gravimetric method. The hydroxides of Al and Fe and insoluble matter are filtered together, warmed with ammonium nitrate, ignited and weighed.

The test is performed by boiling 5 g with 50 ml of dil HCl acid; cooling the solution, making alkaline with dilute solution of NH_3 and again boiling the solution. The mixture is filtered and washed with 2.5% w/v solution of ammonium nitrate. The residue after ignition to constant weight should not be more than 5 mg.

Test for heavy metals: It is performed by taking 1 g of the substance and boiling it in 5 ml of water and 1 ml ofdilute HCl, adding 1 drop of solution of phenolphthalein and sufficient dilute NH_3 solution dropwise to obtain a faint pink colour. The solution is tested for limit of heavy metals (30 parts per million) after adding to it 2 ml of dilute acetic acid and making the volume to 25 ml with water.

Potassium is tested by acidifying 5 ml of a 5% w/v solution with acetic acid and adding 3 drops of sodium cobaltinitrite, when no precipitate should be formed.

Assay: An accurately weighed amount (about 2 g) dissolved in 25 ml of water containing 5 ml of barium chloride solution is titrated with 1 N HCl, using phenolphthalein as indicator. To the solution in the same flask is added bromophenol blue and titration continued with 1 N HCl.

$$BaCl_2 + NaCO_3 \longrightarrow BaCO_3 + 2NaCl$$

$$NaOH + HCl \xrightarrow{\text{Phenolphthalein}} NaCl + H_2O$$

$$BaCO_3 + 2HCl \xrightarrow{\text{Bromophenol blue}} BaCl_2 + CO_2 + H_2O$$

Each ml of 1 N HCl is equivalent to 0.053 g of Na_2CO_3.
Each ml of 1 N HCl is equivalent to 0.040 g of NaOH.

Note: I.P. requires sodium hydroxide to contain not less than 95.0% of total alkali calculated as NaOH and not more than 2.5% of Na_2CO_3. The assay is performed to determine the alkali hydroxide and carbonate together. The assay solution is treated with a quantity of barium chloride which is sufficient to precipitate the soluble alkali carbonate as barium carbonate (see reaction above). Sodium hydroxide is then determined in the solution by titration with Nil hydrochloric acid, using phenolphthalein as indicator. However, the titration is carried out slowly and carefully with stirring.

The alkali carbonate in the solution is determined, using a relatively acid-insensitive indicator, like bromophenol blue (pH range 2.8–4.6) by continuing the titration until a permanent green colour is obtained. In this case also the titration is to be carried out slowly and carefully to avoid overshooting the endpoint (see reaction above). The amount of 1 N HCl used in the second titration using bromophenol blue, is a measure of the carbonate and the amount of 1 N HCl used in both the titrations is a measure of total alkali. In commerce, carbonate free sodium hydroxide (or potassium hydroxide) is not available. Even the best quality sodium hydroxide for analytical use contains about 1% of carbonate. I.P. 2007 has modified the assay method (p. 1723).

Storage: Sodium hydroxide, like potassium hydroxide, should be stored in tightly closed container with stoppers made of rubber, so that moisture and carbon dioxide are not allowed to come in contact with the alkali.

Uses: Sodium hydroxide is too alkaline to be used as a therapeutic agent. It is, however, used to remove warts in a concentration of 2.5% in glycerin. It is also sometimes used in veterinary practice as a caustic and in a 2 to 5% solution as a disinfectant for animal houses.

It is of great value as a pharmaceutical aid and necessity. It is preferred over potassium hydroxide, especially in a pharmaceutical process, as it is less deliquescent and cheaper. Besides, its requirement as compared to potassium hydroxide is less because 40 parts of it are equivalent to 56 parts of potassium hydroxide. It is used in soap, textiles, papers, chemicals and petroleum industries.

SODIUM CARBONATE

Chem. formula: $Na_2CO_3.10 H_2O$ Mol. weight: 286.2

Sodium carbonate contains not less than 99% and not more than equivalent of 105% of $Na_2CO_3.10 H_2O$. I.P. 2007 includes Na_2CO_3 (mol. wt. 106) and $Na_2CO_3.H_2O$ (mol. wt. 124.0).

Preparation: It is prepared by Solvey process, which is also used for making sodium bicarbonate. The bicarbonate is easily converted into carbonate, by heating and the carbon dioxide is returned to carbonating tower. (See also sodium bicarbonate).

$$2NaHCO_3 \longrightarrow Na_2CO_3 + H_2O + CO_2$$

Sodium carbonate can also be prepared by the electrolysis of sodium chloride. Sodium reacts with water to produce sodium hydroxide, which on being treated with carbon dioxide (passed through the sodium hydroxide solution) gives sodium carbonate.

$$NaCl \longrightarrow Na^+ + Cl^-$$
$$2Na + 2H_2O \longrightarrow 2NaOH + H_2\uparrow$$
$$2NaOH + CO_2 \longrightarrow Na_2CO_3 + H_2O$$

Description: It is a white colourless crystalline powder which is odourless with Decahydrate is stable below 32°C; hepta is stable between 32°–35°C. Monohydrate is stable above 35°C.

Tests for identity: It is tested for reactions characteristic of sodium and carbonates (App. I).

Tests for purity: It is tested for As; Fe; Cl; SO_4; heavy metals; and aluminium; calcium; and insoluble matter.

Assay: It is assayed by titrating accurately weighed amount with 0.5 N sulphuric acid using methyl orange as indicator (see also I.P. 2007, p. 1708).

$$Na_2CO_3 + H_2SO_4 \longrightarrow Na_2SO_4 + H_2O + CO_2\uparrow$$

1000 ml 0.5 N H_2SO_4 is equivalent to ¼Na_2CO_3.

Each ml of 0.5 N sulphuric acid is equivalent to 0.07154 g of $Na_2CO).10\ H_2O$.

Storage: It is preserved in a well-closed container.

Uses: It is used as an antacid and as a pharmaceutical aid. Sometimes it is used topically as lotion for dermatitis. It is also used as a mouth wash and as a vaginal douche. As a chemical it is used for preparing sodium salts of many acids.

SODA LIME

Soda lime is a mixture of sodium hydroxide and potassium hydroxide fused with calcium hydroxide. The fused mass is then granulated. During granulation an indicator like methyl violet or potassium permanganate, inert towards anaesthetic gases, is added to know its absorbing capacity. The I.P. and B.P. do not prescribe an indicator, but permit the use of an indicator, which changes its colour, when the pH falls to a level at which the soda lime may be considered as exhausted.

Description: It is white or greyish-white granules, which may be coloured if an indicator is added. It is partially soluble in water, but completely soluble in dilute acetic acid. It absorbs carbon dioxide and water on being exposed to air. It is not included in new I.P.

Tests for purity: It is tested for definite size and hardness of granules; loss on drying; moisture absorption; and carbon dioxide absorption.

The test for moisture absorption is carried out in a state of constant vapour pressure. It is usually carried out in a desiccator containing dilute H_2SO_4 (14% w/v) and finding out the increase in weight in the sample in 24 hours. The increase in weight should not be more than 7.5%.

Tests for CO_2 absorption: It is carried out by passing the stream of dry air and CO_2 through two interconnected tubes, first one containing weighed quantity of soda lime and the second containing dried $CaCl_2$. The moisture removed from soda lime is absorbed by anhydrous $CaCl_2$.

The test tube containing H_2SO_4 is attached at the end to prevent the absorption of moisture from atmosphere. The gain in weight of two tubes gives the weight of CO_2 absorbed.

I.P. prescribes the exhaustive power for soda lime for CO_2 to be not less than 20% of its weight. The I.P. method is as follows:

Plug with cotton wool one end of a straight glass tube about 12 cm long and 1 cm internal diameter. Introduce into it about 2 g of soda lime, accurately weighed and close the free end with a plug of cotton wool. Connect by means of a short wide rubber tube to a similar tube packed with anhydrous calcium chloride and close both ends of the apparatus with rubber caps and weigh the complete apparatus. Pass a slow stream, about 3 bubbles per second, of carbon dioxide mixed with an approximately equal volume of air for about 90 minutes, first through a wash bottle containing sulphuric acid, then through the soda lime and calcium chloride in the prepared tube in order, and finally through another wash bottle containing sulphuric acid. Disconnect the supply of carbon dioxide, aspirate a little air through the apparatus, allow to attain laboratory temperature, disconnect from the wash bottles, fit on the rubber caps and weigh. The increase in weight is not less than 20 per cent of the amount taken for test.

Storage: It is preserved in a well-closed container.

Uses: It is used as a carbon dioxide absorbent.

BUFFERS

Buffer systems are pairs of chemically related compounds capable of resisting large changes in the pH of a solution caused by the addition of small amounts of acids or base. It may be composed of a weak acid and its salt or a weak base and its salt.

It is necessary to control the pH in solutions within certain specified limits to improve the chemical stability and solubility of the drug and in patient comfort. Even though the pH of a solution has been carefully adjusted using acid and base to the prescribed level, with storage, the pH may change. This change in pH may occur as a result of leaching of alkali from certain glass containers, and gases in air, such as CO_2 and NH_3, which can dissolve in the solution accompanied by acidic or basic reactions. This can result in poor stability of the dissolved drug. This effect can be controlled through the use of a buffer system. Buffers are sometimes used for creating the right atmosphere for drug dissolution as in the case of buffered aspirin tablets. It is necessary to select the right buffer system to prevent the inhibitory effect of various buffer cations on drug transfer rate across the intestinal epithelium. Hence, buffer system for a salt of a drug should contain the same cation as the drug salt and introduce no additional cations.

It may also be recognized that solutions of drugs that are weak electrolytes exhibit buffer action. Salicylic acid solution in a soft glass bottle is influenced by the alkalinity of the glass to form a buffer system of salicylic acid and sodium salicylate.

Buffer systems may be used in pharmacy for roughly two purposes namely:

1. Standard buffer systems, designed to provide a solution having a specific pH for analytical purposes.
2. Pharmaceutical buffers designed to maintain pH limits in drug preparations.

The selection of a buffer system for pharmaceutical purposes is controlled by the following criteria:

A. **Chemical criteria:**
   1. The buffer system should not:
      - React with other chemicals in the preparation.
      - Participate in oxidation-reduction reactions.
      - Alter the solubility of other components.
      - Form complexes with active ingredients.
      - Participate in acid-base reactions other than that required for its buffer action.
   2. The buffer system must exhibit reasonable chemical stability.
   3. Volatile species e.g. NH_3, CO_2 should be avoided as their loss may cause change in pH.
   4. Buffer range and capacity is to be considered.

B. **Pharmacological criteria:**
   1. The buffer should neither contribute nor detract from the pharmacological properties of the active ingredient.

2. Toxicity of the buffer system. Ex. Borate buffers are toxic systematically but may be used topically or in ophthalmic preparations.

3. The salt form of the drug is to be considered so as to introduce a buffer system with the same cation/anion.

The theory behind mixtures of compounds as buffers is that the buffer pair will complement each other. When small amounts of H^+ are introduced, they will react with the basic member of the buffer pair to produce the weak acid (only slightly ionized). Similarly when a small amount of OH^- (base) is added, it will react with the acidic member of the buffer pair to produce water and the conjugate base.

An example of a buffer system is the phosphate buffer system composed of potassium dihydrogen phosphate, $H_2PO_4^-$, as the acid member and dipotassium hydrogen phosphate, HPO_4^{-2}, as the basic member of the buffer pair. The following equations represent what happens when small quantities of HCl are added to a phosphate buffer system.

$$HCl + H_2O \longrightarrow H_3O^+ + Cl^-$$

$$HPO_4^{-2} + H_3O^+ \longrightarrow H_2PO_4^- + H_2O$$

Since dihydrogen phosphate ion is a weak acid, the equilibrium in this reaction will lie strongly to the right.

Similarly, in the following equation also the equilibrium will lie strongly to the right, when a small quantity of a base (NaOH) is added to the same system.

$$NaOH \longrightarrow Na^+ + OH^-$$

$$H_2PO_4^- + OH^- \longrightarrow HPO_4^{-2} + H_2O$$

Buffer solution can be formulated to produce specific pH's within particular ranges by varying the concentrations of the components of the system. Some of these methods of preparation, for the standardizing of pH meters and other analytical procedures, can be obtained from the official books like the I.P., the U.S.P. and the N.F., etc.

Examples of some buffer systems and their pH ranges are given in the table below:

Buffer systems	pH range
KCl/HCl (Clark and Lubs)	1.0–2.2
K biphthalate/HCl (Clark and Lubs)	2.4–4.0
K biphthalate/NaOH (Clark and Lubs)	4.2–6.2
Citric acid/phosphate (McIlvaine)	2.2–8.0
Na acetate/acetic acid (Walpole)	3.8–5.6
Phosphate (Sorensen)	5.8–8.0
Na borate/HCl (Sorensen)	7.8–9.2
Na tetraborate/boric acid (Gifford's)	6.0–7.8
Na borate/NaOH (Sorensen)	9.4–10.6
Na tetraborate/boric acid (Feldman's)	7.0–8.2
Na tetraborate/boric acid (Pantin)	7.6–11.0
$NaCO_3$/$NaHCO_3$ (Delory and King)	9.2–10.8

The hydrochloric acid buffer cannot be considered a buffer, since HCl is a strong acid. Buffer systems containing potassium are biologically undesirable and are used mostly for analytical procedures. Sorensen phosphate buffer is a phosphate buffer system that has been modified to include the addition of NaCl to make it isotonic with physiological fluid.

ANTIOXIDANTS

Antioxidants are used to prevent oxidative decomposition of pharmaceutically active compounds, for example, the development of rancidity in oils and fats or the inactivation of some medicine in the environment of their dosage forms. They have the capability of acting as reducing agents through an oxidation-reduction or redox reaction. They may either be oxidized in place of the active constituent or reduce an oxidized active constituent to its normal state. Antioxidants possess a higher oxidative potential than the drug they are to protect. Antioxidants may be water soluble or oil soluble (e.g. ascorbyl palmitate, butylated hydroxy toluene). Most water soluble antioxidants are inorganic compounds that act by preferentially undergoing in place of the drug.

Official antioxidants include hypophosphorus acid, sulphur dioxide, sodium bisulphite, sodium metabisulphite, sodium thiosulphate, sodium nitrite and nitrogen.

HYPOPHOSPHOROUS ACID

Chem. formula: H_3PO_2 Mol. weight: 66.0

It contains not less than 30% and more than 32% w/w of phosphorous acid, H_3PO_2.

Preparations: (1) It is obtained by treating a hypophosphite, e.g. calcium hypophosphite with an acid, like sulphuric acid or oxalic acid, resulting in the insoluble calcium salt and hypophosphorous acid. Acid is used in excess.

$$Ca(H_2PO_4)_2 + H_2C_2O_4 \longrightarrow CaC_2O_4 + 2H_3PO_2$$

Calcium   Oxalic acid   Calcium   Hypophosphorous
hypophosphite   oxalate   acid

$$Ca(H_2PO_4)_2 + H_2SO_4 \longrightarrow CaSO_4 + 2H_3PO_2$$

Purer hypophosphorous acid can be obtained by using barium hypophosphite in place of calcium hypophosphite.

Hypophosphorous acid can also be prepared from potassium hypophosphite by treating with tartaric acid:

$$KH_2PO_2 + C_4H_6O_6 \longrightarrow H_3PO_2 + KHC_4H_4O_6$$

Potassium   Tartaric   Hypophos-   Potassium
hypophosphite   acid   phorous   bitartrate
                          acid

Description: Hypophosphorous acid is a clear or slightly yellowish liquid having slight odour and strongly acid taste. The acid is miscible with water and alcohol. Its specific gravity at 25° is 1.32.

Tests for identity: The acid (0.3 ml) gives with $HgCl_2$ solution (10 ml) a white precipitate which changes to grey on heating and finally deposits a globule of mercury.

On being warmed (0.3 ml) with a solution of copper sulphate (5 ml) a reddish brown ppt. is produced.

Tests for purity: It is tested for As; heavy metals; barium; calcium; oxalic acid; phosphoric acid; Fe; Cl; SO_4.

Phosphoric acid and oxalic acid can be tested by diluting 0.3 ml with water (10 ml), adding solution of calcium chloride (1 ml) and dilute ammonia solution (2 ml) and noting the turbidity, which should not be more than a slight.

Assay: It is assayed by diluting an accurately weighed quantity (5 g) with water (50 ml) and titrating with 0.5 N NaOH using methyl orange as indicator.

One ml of 0.5 N NaOH is equivalent to 0.033 g of H_3PO_2.

Uses: It is used as a pharmaceutical aid and as an antioxidant in pharmaceutical preparation. Earlier hypophosphites were quite favourably used as source for phosphorus. But it is now believed that they pass out of the body unchanged. They were and are still regarded as brain tonics.

SODIUM METABISULPHITE

Chem. formula: $Na_2S_2O_5$ Mol. weight: 190.1

Sodium metabisulphite contains not less than 90.0% of $Na_2S_2O_5$.

Preparation: It is prepared by passing sulphur dioxide through a hot solution of sodium hydroxide. when sodium bisulphite, $NaHSO_3$ is formed. This $NaHSO_3$ is not considered stable and decomposes to give $Na_2S_2O_5$. The solution is then cooled to crystallization. The $NaHSO_3$ is also unstable in solid state and decomposes to give sodium metabisulphite.

$$NaOH + SO_2 \longrightarrow NaHSO_3$$
$$2NaHSO_3 \longrightarrow \underset{\substack{\text{Sodium} \\ \text{metabisulphite}}}{Na_2S_2O_5} + H_2O$$

Description: It is a white or slightly yellow white crystalline solid or fused mass, deliquescent. When dissolved in water it will give back $NaHSO_3$.

$$Na_2S_2O_5 + H_2O \longrightarrow 2NaHSO_3$$

It is slightly acidic in reaction and has sulphurous odour and an acid and saline taste.

Tests for identity:

(i) A solution decolourises the solution of iodine and this resulting solution gives reactions characteristic of sulphates.

(ii) It gives reactions characteristic of sodium.

Tests for purity: It is tested for acidity; arsenic; lead; and thiosulphate.

Thiosulphate is tested by dissolving about 1 g of the substance in 10 ml of dilute HCl. The solution should not give more than a faint opalescence on heating. The reaction is as follows:

$$Na_2S_2O_3 + 2HCl \longrightarrow 2NaCl + S + SO_2\uparrow + H_2O$$

The opalescence is due to sulphur.

Assay: It is assayed by titrating an accurately weighed amount of the substance with a known excess of N/10 I_2 (the $Na_2S_2O_5$ being a reducing agent. the reaction is an oxidation reaction and so sulphite is converted to sulphate) in which small amount of HCl is added. Excess of I_2 is then determined by titration with N/10 $Na_2S_2O_3$ using starch (added towards the end) as indicator.

$$Na_2S_2O_5 + H_2O \longrightarrow 2NaHSO_3$$

or

$$2NaHSO_3 + 2I_2 + 2H_2O \longrightarrow 2NaHSO_3 + 4HI$$

$$Na_2S_2O_5 + 2I_2 + 3H_2O \longrightarrow 2NaHSO_4 + 4HI$$

$$\underset{\substack{\text{Sod.} \\ \text{thiosulphate}}}{2Na_2S_2O_3} + I_2 \longrightarrow \underset{\substack{\text{Sod.} \\ \text{tetrathionate}}}{Na_2S_4O_6} + 2NaI$$

The assay as given in I.P. is described below:

Weigh accurately about 0.2 g and dissolve in 50 ml of 0.1 N iodine, add 1 ml of hydrochloric acid and titrate the excess of iodine with 0.1 N sodium thiosulphate using solution of starch as indicator, added towards the end of the titration.

1000 ml of N/10 I_2 is equivalent to 1/40 $Na_2S_2O_5$.

Each ml of 0.1 N I_2 is equivalent to 0.004753 g of $Na_2S_2O_5$.

Uses: It is a powerful reducing agent and is used as an antioxidant.

It is used as a stabilizer in adrenaline and apomorphine injections. It is also used as preservative. It is used for preservation of food materials for its antimicrobial action.

Storage: Sodium metabisulphite is preserved in tight container.

SODIUM THIOSULPHATE

Chem. formula: $Na_2S_2O_3 \cdot 5H_2O$ Mol. weight: 248.2

Sodium thiosulphate contains not less than 99.0% and not more than the equivalent of 101% of $Na_2S_2O_3 \cdot 5H_2O$. It is also known as sodium hyposulphate or antichlor or hypo.

Preparation: It can be prepared by boiling sodium sulphite with sulphur. Sodium sulphite is obtained by a reaction between sodium carbonate, water and sulphur dioxide.

First sodium bisulphite (i) is obtained, which is then treated with a further quantity of Na_2CO_3 to obtain sodium sulphite, Na_2SO_3, (ii). Sodium sulphite, on heating with powdered sulphur, gives sodium thiosulphate, (ii). The solution is evaporated to crystallization and the crystals obtained through centrifugation (freed from mother liquor through washings) and powdered to the required size:

$$Na_2CO_3 + H_2O + 2SO_2 \longrightarrow 2NaHSO_3 + CO_2\uparrow$$

$$2NaHSO_3 + Na_2CO_3 \longrightarrow 2Na_2SO_3 + H_2O + CO_2\uparrow$$

$$Na_2SO_3 + S \longrightarrow Na_2S_2O_3$$

Description: It occurs as large, colourless crystals or as a coarse crystalline powder or as transparent, monoclinic prismatic crystals. It is odourless and has an alkaline taste. It is efflorescent in dry air while deliquescent in moist. It melts at 50°C, while decomposes on being heated at 100°C.

It is decomposed by dilute acids, liberating sulphur dioxide with precipitation of sulphur as under:

$$Na_2S_2O_3 + 2HCl \longrightarrow 2NaCl + S + SO_2 + H_2O$$

It is soluble in water (0.5 parts) and insoluble in alcohol. The aqueous solution decomposes slowly in cold, but rapidly, if heated.

$$4Na_2S_2O_3 \longrightarrow 3Na_2SO_4 + Na_2S_5$$
Polysulfide

$$Na_2S_5 \longrightarrow Na_2S + 4S$$

Alkaline solutions are stable and thus if a solution is to be stored, a sufficient amount (0.1 to 0.2 g per litre) of sodium carbonate or borax is added to make the solution stable.

Sodium thiosulphate is known as '*hypo*' in the photographic field and is an important chemical, being required as a fixing material for negatives and prints. It is used because of its solvent action on silver halides.

$$AgBr + Na_2S_2O_3 \longrightarrow NaAgS_2O_3 + NaBr$$

Sodium thiosulphate is used as an antichlor in bleaching, as it reacts with chlorine or hypochlorite as under:

$$Na_2S_2O_3 + 4HOCl + H_2O \longrightarrow Na_2SO_4 + H_2SO_4 + 4HCl$$

Sodium thiosulphate acts as a reducing agent and reduces ferric chloride and iodine as follows:

$$2FeCl_3 + 2Na_2SO_3 \longrightarrow 2FeCl_2 + 2NaCl + Na_2S_4O_6$$
$$Na_2S_2O_3 + I_2 \longrightarrow Na_2S_4O_6 + 2NaI$$
Sod. tetrathionate

Tests for identity: It gives reactions characteristic of sodium and thiosulphates (App. I).

Tests for purity: Reaction; As; Ca; and heavy metals.

Reaction: A 10% solution is tested, which should be neutral or faintly alkaline to litmus.

Calcium is tested by taking 5 ml of 5% solution of the salt and adding to it 5 ml of solution of ammonium oxalate and setting aside for five minutes. No turbidity should be produced.

Heavy metals test is performed by dissolving 1 g of the substance in 10 ml of water and slowly adding to the solution 5 ml of dilute hydrochloric acid and evaporating the mixture to dryness on a water bath. The residue is boiled gently with 15 ml of water for two minutes and the solution filtered. The filtrate is boiled and to it sufficient solution of bromine is added to produce clear solution, adding a slight excess of solution of bromine. The solution is boiled to expel bromine completely, cooled to room temperature and to the cooled solution are added a drop of solution of phenolphthalein and solution of hydroxide until a slight pink colour is produced. 2 ml of dilute acetic acid is added and the solution diluted with water to 25 ml and the limit test for heavy metals performed. Limit of heavy metals is 25 parts per million.

Assay: An accurately weighed (about 1 g) of sodium thiosulphate is dissolved in water (20 ml) and titrated with standard iodine solution (0.1 N I_2 sol.)

$$2Na_2S_2O_3 + I_2 \longrightarrow Na_2S_2O_6 + 2NaI$$

1000 ml of N/10 I_2 is equivalent to 1/10 $Na_2S_2O_3$.

Or each ml of N/10 I_2 is equivalent to 0.02482 g of $Na_2S_2O_3$.

Storage: Sodium thiosulphate is preserved in a well closed container.

Uses: The most important use of sodium thiosulphate is as an antidote in the treatment of cyanide poisoning. In fact it is given intravenously in conjunction with sodium nitrite. It is immediately followed by the injection of sodium nitrite. Cyanides are highly poisonous and the poisoning is instantaneous and fatal. The sodium thiosulphate inactivates cyanide by forming thiocyanate. It is also an effective antidote in poisonings resulting from iodine preparations. Sodium thiosulphate is an effective antifungal drug and is useful in skin infections including dermatophytosis. It is used as an antichlor in bleaching and a fixer in photographic work under the name of '*Hypo*' as mentioned above.

Dose: 0.3 to 1 g by intravenous or intramuscular injection.

Preparation: Sodium thiosulphate injection.

SODIUM THIOSULPHATE INJECTION

Sodium thiosulphate injection is a sterile solution of sodium thiosulphate in freshly boiled water for injection and contains sodium thiosulphate, $Na_2S_2O_3.5H_2O$, not less than 95% and not more than 105% of the stated amount of sodium thiosulphate. The air in the ampoules is replaced by nitrogen or other suitable gas and the injection is sterilised by heating in autoclave.

Tests for identity: Complies with the tests described under sodium thiosulphate.

Tests for purity: Reaction; As; calcium; heavy metals.

Reaction: The pH is between 8.0 to 9.5.

Other requirements: The sodium thiosulphate injection should comply with the requirements stated under injections.

Assay: The assay is carried out in the same way as described under sodium thiosulphate above, using an accurately measured volume equivalent to about 0.75 g of sodium thiosulphate and neutralising the solution, if necessary, before performing the assay.

Uses: Same as described under sodium thiosulphate.

Dose: 0.3 to 1 g of sodium thiosulphate by intramuscular or by intravenous injection.

WATER

Water is such a simple and common material that to many who do not know its importance in pharmaceutical industry and hospitals, its inclusion here or for that matter in other books including pharmacopoeias, may look quite comical or ridiculous. But water is an unusual liquid, whose physical and chemical properties play important role in life and living processes. Water is unique in its ability to form strong hydrogen bonds with other water molecules. Water is of great biological significance. It is a predominant constituent of human body and animals (constituting upto 70%) and since it has a high dielectric constant it is the best vehicle for liquid dosage forms. It is thus the best solvent and stabilizer for macromolecules, e.g. proteins. Chemically, water may be regarded as unreactive. It hardly dissociates and is a poor reducing agent.

$$2H_2O \rightleftharpoons H_3O^+ + OH^-$$

Water is capable of oxidising any element which can displace one or both of its protons as hydrogen gas, e.g. rusting of iron:

$$2Fe + 3H_2O \longrightarrow Fe_2O_3 + 3H_2$$

Pure water is a clear liquid, which is devoid of any odour and taste. Water looks greenish blue or bluish in depth, e.g. pond water, canal water and sea water. Many times people attribute taste and flavour to drinking waters, which are due to additives from nature or man. Mineral water, which is natural water has dissolved electrolytes, indicative of ions like Na^+, K^+, Ca^{+2}, Ba^{+2}, Fe^{+3}, Cl^-, HCO_3^-, CO_2^{-2}, SO_4^{-2} etc. Water may be saline, carbonated, alkaline, chalybeate and give characteristic reactions for different electrolytes. A more detailed general account of water is beyond the scope of this book.

I.P. includes water as:

(1) Purified water

(2) Water for injection

(3) Water for injection in bulk

(4) Sterile water for injection.

Purified water and water for injection are given under separate monograph not only in I.P. but also in other international pharmacopoeias.

PURIFIED WATER

Chem. formula: H_2O Mol. wt.: 18.02

Purified water is prepared from suitable potable water by distillation or treatment with ion-exchange materials. During production and subsequent storage, it is recommended that adequate measures are taken to ensure that the microbial quality is controlled and monitored. Appropriate alert and action limits are set so as to detect adverse trends.

Description: It is a clear, colourless, odourless and tasteless liquid. It has 4.5 to 7.0 pH.

Tests for purity: It is tested for reaction; copper; iron and lead; Cl, SO_4; albuminoid ammonia; ammonia; oxidisable matter; and non-volatile matter.

Test for albuminoid ammonia: It is performed by placing 500 ml of purified water in a distillation flask, adding 0.2 g of $MgCO_2$ and distillating 200 ml and rejecting the distillate. To the flask is then added 25 ml of an alkaline solution of potassium permanganate and collecting 100 ml of the distillate. To the distillate (100 ml) is added 4 ml of alkaline solution of potassium mercuric iodide and the colour noted. The colour produced is not deeper than that produced by adding 4 ml of alkaline solution of potassium mercuric iodide to a mixture of 100 ml of ammonia-free water and 4 ml of dilute ammonium chloride solution.

Test for ammonia: It is performed by adding to 50 of purified water 2 ml of alkaline solution of potassium mercuric iodide and viewing the solution in a Nessler cylinder placed on a white tile. The colour in Nessler cylinder is not more intense than that given by 50 ml of ammonia-free water with the addition of 2 ml of dilute ammonium chloride solution (when tested under similar condition).

Tests for oxidisable matter: It is performed by boiling 100 ml of purified water with 3 ml of sulphuric acid and 1 ml of 0.01 N potassium permanganate for 10 minutes. The colour of potassium permanganate is not completely discharged.

Tests for non-volatile matter: It is done by evaporating to dryness on water bath and then to constant weight at 105°C. The residue should not be more than 0.001% w/v.

Test for copper, iron and lead: It is performed by adding to 100 ml of purified water one drop of solution of sodium sulphate. The liquid remains clear and colourless.

Test for chloride: It is performed by adding to 100 ml of purified water 1 ml of solution of silver nitrate and allowing to stand for five minutes. The liquid should remain clear and colourless.

Test for sulphate: It is performed by adding to 10 ml of purified water 1 ml solution of barium chloride and allowing to stand for five minutes. The liquid should remain clear and colourless.

Test for aluminium: It is performed as per I.P. 2.3.8. Not more than 10 ppb should be found (I.P. 1870).

Bacterial endotoxins: It is performed as per I.P. 2.2.3. Not more than 0.25 endotoxin unit per ml should be detected (I.P. 1870).

Uses: Purified water is used for preparation of most of the test reagents and as a solvent for many preparations. It is the water of choice for various types of extemporanious preparation in compounding.

When distilled water is prescribed or demanded, purified water shall be dispensed or supplied. Injections are made with water for injection. Purified water is unsuitable for parenteral administration.

WATER FOR INJECTION

WATER FOR INJECTION IN BULK

Water for injection is prepared by distilling potable water from a natural glass or metal still fitted with an efficient device for preventing the entrainment of droplets. The first portion of the distillate is rejected and the remaining distillate is received in a suitable container.

The distilled water collected above is sterilised immediately in an autoclave or by filteration without the addition of any bacteriostatic.

When water for injection free from carbon dioxide is required the distillate is boiled for 10 minutes with as little exposure to air as possible. It is then cooled and distributed in the final container and sterilised by heating in an autoclave.

Description: It occurs as a clear, colourless and odourless liquid. It has no added substance. It meets all the requirements, i.e. tests for purity, which are called for in the monograph of purified water with the exception of bacteriological purity.

Test for sterility is performed as given in I.P. 2.2.11, p. 52.

The test for pyrogens is performed as given in I.P. 2.2.8, p. 34 using not less than 10 ml per kg of rabbit's weight.

Note: The above tests for sterility and pyrogens are covered under pharmaceutics syllabi.

Uses: Water for injection is used as a solvent for the preparation of parenteral solutions. The finished preparations are required to be sterilised. Water for injection is to be stored in tight containers and in I.P. there is no specific temperature mentioned at which it should be stored.

Sterile water for injections (I.P. p. 1871): It is water for injection in bulk that has been distributed in suitable containers of glass or any other material, sealed and sterilised by heat to ensure that it complies with tests for bacterial endotoxins.

PRESERVATIVES

A preservative is, in the common pharmaceutical sense, a substance that prevents or inhibits microbial growth and may be added to a pharmaceutical preparation for this purpose to avoid consequent spoilage of the preparations by microorganisms.

An ideal preservative is one that must be effective against a broad spectrum of microorganisms and is physically, chemically and microbiologically stable for the lifetime of the product. It must be nontoxic, nonsensitizing, adequately soluble, compatible with other formulation components, and acceptable with respect to taste and odour.

Some pharmaceutically useful preservatives are phenol (0.2–0.5%), chlorocresol (0.05–0.1%), benzoic acid and its salts (0.1–0.3%), boric acid and its salts (0.5–1.0%), sorbic acid and its salts (0.05–0.2%), benzyl alcohol, thiomersal, benzalkonium chloride and cetylpyridinium chloride.

SODIUM BENZOATE
(Abbr.: Sod. Benz)

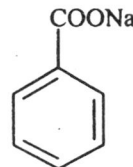

Chem. formula: C_6H_5COONa Mol. weight: 144.1

Sodium benzoate contains not less than 99.0 per cent of sodium benzoate, $C_7H_5O_2Na$ calculated with reference to the substance dried to constant weight at 105°.

Method of preparation: It is prepared by adding sodium carbonate to a hot conc. solution of benzoic acid. The liquid should be just alkaline to litmus. The solution is then evaporated to crystallisation.

$$2C_6H_5COOH + Na_2CO_3 \longrightarrow 2C_6H_5COONa + H_2O + CO_2\uparrow$$
Benzoic acid   Sodium benzoate

Description: It occurs as a white, amorphous or crystalline powder. It is either colourless or has a faint odour of benzoin. It has an unpleasant, sweetish and saline taste. It is freely soluble in water (2 parts), but sparingly in alcohol (75 parts).

Tests for identity:

(1) On being heated it fuses, emitting vapour with characteristic odour chars and yields a residue of sodium carbonate and carbon.

(2) A 10% solution of sodium benzoate, when treated with:

(a) Ferric chloride solution gives a buff-coloured precipitate of ferric benzoate.

$$3C_6H_5COONa + FeCl_3 \longrightarrow Fe(C_6H_5COO)_3 + 3NaCl$$

(b) Dilute hydrochloric acid gives a white-coloured crystalline precipitate of benzoic acid.

$$C_6H_5COONa + HCl \longrightarrow C_6H_5COOH + NaCl$$

(3) It yields reactions characteristic of sodium ions (App. I).

Tests for purity: It is tested for acidity and alkalinity; As; heavy metals; Cl; SO_4; chlorinate compounds; and loss on drying.

Test for chlorinated compounds: It is necessitated because of the fact that usually benzoic acid is prepared from toluene, which is first chlorinated to benzyl chloride followed by the oxidation of benzyl chloride by nitric acid to benzoic acid as follows:

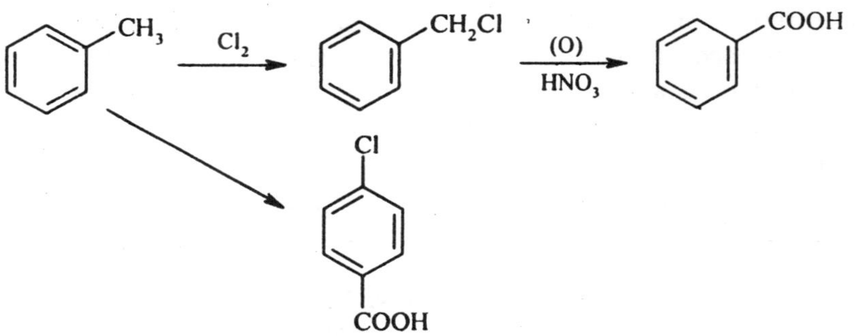

Chlorobenzoic acid (impurity)

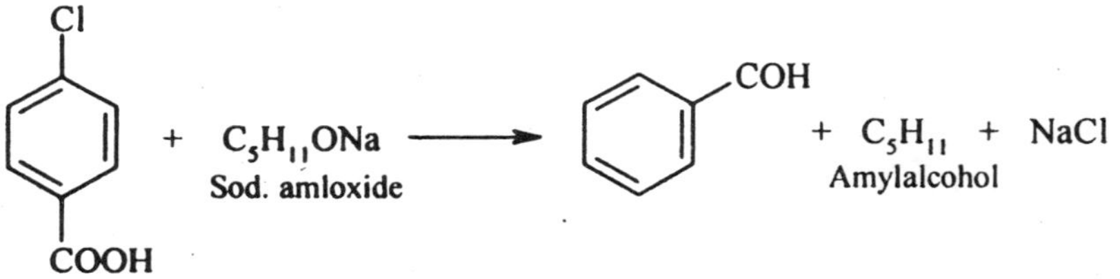

The test for chlorinated compounds is described under benzoic acid (I.P. p. 1707).

Assay: Sodium benzoate is assayed by titration and gives a slight alkaline reaction in solution. It is carried out in a separating funnel. A sufficient quantity of sodium benzoate is taken in a separating funnel to which ether is added. It is titrated against 0.5 N H_2SO_4 with strong shaking, using bromophenol blue as indicator. During titration the benzoic acid liberated is taken up by ether layer. When most of benzoic acid has been liberated the colour of this indicator will change to green.

The partition coefficient of sodium benzoate is low and most of it will be taken up by ether layer.

$$2C_6H_5COONa + H_2SO_4 \longrightarrow 2C_6H_5COOH + Na_2SO_4$$

The aqueous phase is separated and treated with 20 ml of ether. The ether phase is washed with sufficient quantity of water to remove any traces of C_6H_5COONa dissolved in it. The washing is then added to the separated aqueous phase. The ether phase is rejected. The colour will change now to blue violet. The titration is continued with H_2SO_4 till the colour becomes green.

I.P. 85 method is as follows:

Weigh accurately about 3 g and dissolve in 50 ml of water, and neutralise the solution, if necessary with 0.1 N sulphuric acid using solution of phenolphthalein as indicator; and 50 ml of solvent ether and a few drops of solution of bromophenol blue, and titrate with 0.5 N sulphuric acid, with constant shaking, until the colour of the indicator begins to change; separate the lower layer, wash the ethereal layer with 10 ml of water, and to the separated aqueous layer and the washings add a further 20 ml of solvent ether; complete the titration with the 0.5 N sulphuric acid shaking constantly.

Each ml of 0.5 N sulphuric acid is equivalent to 0.07205 g of $C_7H_5O_2Na$.

I.P. 2007 gives a new method for assay which is given below.

An accurately weighed about 0.25 g of sodium benzoate is dissolved in 20 ml of anhydrous glacial acetic acid, warming the solution to 50°C and cool the same. The solution is titrated with 0.1 M perchloric acid, using 0.05 ml of 1-naphthobenzein solution as an indicator. A blank titration is also carried out.

1 ml of 0.1 M perchloric acid is equivalent to 0.01441 g of $C_7H_5NaO_2$.

Uses: Sodium benzoate is a fungistatic and diagnostic agent. It is used as an expectorant and antiseptic, especially in urinary tract infections. It is sometimes used for liver function test and is excreted as hippuric acid in urine.

It is very popular with household ladies as a food preservative and is as such sold legally as a preservative for all kinds of food products. It should, however, be used in an acid media not above 4 pH. It is a bacteriostatic and (slets) bactericidal.

Dose: 0.3 to 2 g.

ADSORBENTS

An adsorbent is a material used to adsorb. Adsorption is a surface phenomenon where added molecules are partitioned in favour of (or towards) the interface (solid-gas, solid-liquid or liquid-liquid). Adsorbents are chemically inert powders that have the ability to adsorb gases, toxins and bacteria. The high adsorptive capacity is dependent on the fine state of subdivision.

Certain relatively inert and insoluble substances are used in a finely subdivided form as dusting powders to cover and protect epithelial surfaces, ulcers and wounds. Such powders adsorb moisture and act as cutaneous dessicants. It is also held that the adsorptive capacity is important to the gastrointestinal protective action of chemically inert powders taken internally. Many nonsystemic antacids may serve as internal protectives and adsorbents.

Examples of adsorbents used as pharmaceutical practice are bentonite, kaolin, magnesium trisilicate, pectin, bismuth subcarbonate, bismuth subnitrate, purified talc, titanium dioxide and zinc oxide. Activated charcoal is used as a detoxicant and emergency antidote by virtue of its adsorptive capacity. It is also used for the relief of intestinal gas and diarrhoea with associated GI distress.

ACTIVATED WOOD CHARCOAL
(Synonym: Medicinal charcoal, Carbo ligni, Wood charcoal)

The activated charcoal is nearly pure carbon which is undergone activation process in order to remove substances previously adsorbed on the charcoal and also breaking down the granules of carbon into smaller ones to get greater total surface area. After activation process, the adsorptive-powers of charcoal will increase tremendously. It was official in I.P. 1966 but omitted from I.P. 1985. Since it plays an important role in medicinal chemistry, it is needed to be mentioned here.

Preparation: It is prepared by burning wood in absence of air, the residue obtained consisting of nearly pure carbon. In order to increase its adsorptive power, one should treat it with various substances such as steam, air, CO_2, oxygen, zinc chloride, H_2SO_4, phosphoric acid or a combination of some of these substances at a temp. between 500° to 900°.

Description: It occurs as a fine, black, odourless, tasteless powder, free from gritty matter.

Solubility: Insoluble in water or the other known solvents.

Tests for identity:

(1) On being heated in absence of air, it does not change its appearance and properties.

(2) On being burnt in presence of air it produces carbon monoxide and carbon dioxide.

Tests for purity: It is tested for acidity or alkalinity; chloride; sulphate; sulphide; cyanogen compounds; water soluble matter; uncarbonised constituents; heavy metals; loss on drying; absorptive capacity; and sulphated ash.

Acidity and alkalinity is determined by boiling 3 g of the substance with 60 ml of water for five minutes, allowing the mixture to cool and filtering the solution after diluting it to the original volume with water. The filtrate should be colourless and neutral to both red and blue litmus papers.

Chloride and sulphate purity tests are performed as usual with 2 ml and 3 ml of filtrate respectively, obtained in the above test.

Sulphide is tested by boiling 0.5 g of activated charcoal with a mixture of 20 ml of water and 5 ml of hydrochloric acid and exposing the lead paper to the vapours of the boiling mixture. The lead paper is not blackened on being exposed to the vapours.

Cyanogen compounds are tested by adding 5 g of activated charcoal to a solution of 2 g of tartaric acid in 50 ml of water contained in a flask. The flask is fitted to a condenser with the outlet tube dipping below the surface of 10 ml of 1 N sodium hydroxide. About 25 ml of the liquid is distilled in the receiver and to the liquid in receiver is added 2 ml of solution of ferrous sulphate and the solution acidified to litmus paper with hydrochloric acid. No blue colour or precipitate is produced.

Test for water soluble matter is carried out by boiling about 2 g accurately weighed activated charcoal with 40 ml of recently boiled and cooled water for one minute and filtering the solution. 20 ml of the filtrate is evaporated to dryness and then the residue is dried to constant weight at 105°. The residue should not weigh more than 0.05 per cent of the weight taken.

Test for uncarbonised constituents depends upon noting the colour of the filtrate obtained after boiling 0.25 g of the activated charcoal with 10 ml of 1 N sodium hydroxide and filtering the solution. The solution should be colourless.

Loss on drying: It loses not more than 15.0 per cent of its weight, when dried at 105° to constant weight.

Sulphated ash: It should not be more than 10.0%.

Heavy metals: The I.P. method for heavy metals is reproduced hereunder: Boil 1 g with a mixture of 8 ml of hydrochloric acid, 12 ml of water and 5 ml of solution of bromine for five minutes, filter and wash the charcoal with 50 ml of boiling water. Evaporate the filtrate and washing to dryness and extract the residue with mixture of 1 ml of 1 N hydrochloric acid, 20 ml of water and 5 ml of solution of sulphuric acid. Boil the solution until all the sulphur dioxide is expelled, then dilute it to 50 ml with water. To 10 ml of the solution add 5 ml of solution of hydrogen sulphide; the solution does not show a darker coloration in ten seconds than that produced by the addition of 10 ml of solution of hydrogen sulphide to 7 ml of water to which 2 ml of 0.1 N hydrochloric acid and 1.0 ml of standard solution of lead have been added.

Absorptive capacity: This is determined by following the I.P. method which is reproduced hereunder:

(a) Weigh accurately about 0.3 g and add to 50 ml of a 0.4 per cent w/v solution of phenazone contained in stoppered flask. Keep for twenty minutes shaking at frequent intervals, filter through a dry filter paper and reject the first 15 ml of the filtrate. To next 25 ml of the filtrate in a stoppered flask add 2 g of sodium acetate and 30 ml of 0.1 N iodine, shake occasionally for half an hour, add 10 ml of chloroform, shake until the precipitate is dissolved and titrate the excess of iodine with 0.1 N sodium thiosulphate using solution of starch as indicator.

Repeat the experiment with the same quantities of the same reagent in same manner omitting activated wood charcoal. Twice the difference between the two titrations represents the amount of iodine required by the phenazone absorbed by the charcoal. Each ml of 0.1 N iodine is equivalent to 0.00945 g of phenazone. Determined by the above method activated wood charcoal absorbs from solution not less than 30 per cent of its weight of phenazone calculated with reference to the substance dried at 105°.

(b) Weigh accurately about 1 g in a shallow glass fitted with a ground-in stopper. Place the dish, with stopper removed in a closed vessel containing chloroform in an open dish, allow to stand for twenty four hours at 16° to 20°, withdraw the dish and the stopper and weigh. Determined by the above method, 1 g of Activated Wood Charcoal absorbs not less than 0.4 g of chloroform calculated with reference to the substance dried at 105°.

Uses: It is included under the category of adsorbents, which are used to remove toxic substances before they get absorbed in the body. Activated charcoal adsorbs alkaloids, amines, gases (ammonia, carbon monoxide, carbon dioxide, nitrous oxide etc.) and some salts of heavy metals. It is one of the constituents of "universal antidote", which consists of two parts of activated charcoal, one part of magnesium oxide and one part of tannic acid. The universal antidote is normally kept in first-aid kits. However, it has now been found out that activated charcoal alone is a better adsorbent than in the universal antidote. Although the activated charcoal has broad spectrum of activity, yet it cannot be considered a universal adsorbent. Hence it is necessary that its limitations be kept in mind before administering it as a first-aid material in poisoning cases. In vivo it gets effectively bound with compounds like aspirin, barbitone, chloroquine, chlorpromazine, kerosene, mercuric chloride, strychnine, sodium salicylate etc.

Its poisoning ratio is 5 : 1 to 10 : 1, usually dispersed in water. Sometimes tablets of charcoal are given, which are much less effective than powdered charcoal. It should be given soon after the ingestion of the poison. Charcoal is available in the market in different dosage forms like granules, tablets, powder. Sometimes it is given with Kaolin. It is also given in diarrhoea and dysentery. Externally it is used as a deodorant in foul smelling wounds and ulcers.

In the industry it is used as a decolorizer.

Dose: 5 to 50 g usual, adult, oral 50 g, children, oral, 25 g.

Storage: Activated wood charcoal is preserved in a dry, well closed container.

HEAVY KAOLIN (CHINA CLAY)

Chem. formula: $Al_2O_3.2SiO_2.2H_2O$ (!)

Heavy Kaolin is also known as china clay and consists mainly of a hydrated aluminium silicate of the approximate composition mentioned above. Heavy Kaolin is powdered and freed from gritty particles and other impurities by elutriation. It is said to contain traces of compounds of magnesium, calcium and iron. It loses not more than 1.5 per cent of its weight when dried to constant weight at 105°.

Preparation: Heavy Kaolin is prepared by powdering the natural substance, which is freed from most of its impurities by elutriation and dried.

Description: It is soft, whitish odourless and tasteless powder, free from gritty particles and is insoluble in water and mineral acids.

Tests for identity: It gives tests similar to bentonite, i.e. for aluminium.

Tests for purity: It is tested for As; Cl; Fe; CG_3; loss on drying; loss on ignition; soluble matter and heavy metals.

For iron the test is performed by triturating 2 g of Kaolin in a mortar with 10 ml of water adding 0.5 g of sodium salicylate to the mixture, which should not acquire more than a slight reddish colour.

Soluble matter is tested by boiling heavy Kaolin with 5 ml of 0.2 N hydrochloric acid for five minutes, filtering the solution and evaporating the filtrate. The residue after gentle ignition weighs not more than 10 mg.

Absorption power: I.P. 2007 includes this test (p. 1265).

Swelling factor: 2 g is triturated with 2 ml of water. The mixture should not flow.

Uses: It is used as a pharmaceutical aid, e.g. in the preparation of Kaolin Poultice. When Kaolin is prescribed, light Kaolin is to be dispensed.

Preparation: Kaolin Poultice.

LIGHT KAOLIN

Light Kaolin is nothing but finely divided form of Kaolin, which is lighter and is used for internal administration. Its approximate chemical formula is the same as that mentioned under the Heavy Kaolin.

Preparation: It is prepared from the natural substance by electrical sedimentation. It must be free from gritty and other impurities.

Description: It is light, odourless, tasteless, white powder, insoluble in water and mineral acids.

Tests for identity: It gives tests similar to that mentioned under bentonite, i.e. for Aluminium (App. 1).

Tests for purity: Same as for Heavy Kaolin. It is also required to comply with a test for coarse particles; particles larger than 10 microns in diameter; particles larger than 3 microns in diameter and sedimentation volume. These tests given in I.P.

Coarse particles: Transfer 5 g to a stoppered cylinder about 35 mm in diameter and 16 cm in length, add 60 ml of a 1 per cent w/v solution of sodium pyrophosphate and shake thoroughly. Allow the suspension to stand for five minutes, draw off 50 ml of the suspension by means of a pipette from a point about 5 cm below the surface of the liquid without disturbing the sediment. To the remaining liquid add 50 ml of water, shake thoroughly, allow to stand for five minutes and draw off 50 ml of the suspension in the same way as before. Repeat the operation until a total of 400 ml of suspension have been drawn off. Evaporate the remaining liquid on a water-bath, transfer the residue to a tared evaporating dish; the residue after drying to constant weight at 105° weighs not more than 25 mg.

Particles larger than 10 microns in diameter: Transfer 20 g to a 1000 ml stoppered cylinder, add sufficient water at 20° to produce 1000 ml and shake thoroughly for two minutes. Allow the suspension to stand at 200 for twenty minutes. By means of a pipette, draw off 25 ml from a point 10 cm below the surface of the liquid, the weight per ml at 20° of the sample of suspension removed is not less than 1.0086 g.

Particles larger than 3 microns in diameter: Return the sample taken in the test for particles larger than 10 microns in diameter to the suspension remaining in the cylinder, shake vigorously for two minutes. Allow to stand for three and a half hours at 20°. Draw off 25 ml of the suspension from a point

10 cm below the surface of the liquid; the weight per ml at 20° of the sample of suspension removed is not less than 1.0063 g.

Sedimentation volume: Mix 2 g with 0.1 g light magnesium oxide, transfer to a 50 ml stoppered graduated cylinder with water and make the volume to 50 ml. Shake thoroughly for five minutes and allow to stand for one hour. The volume occupied by the sediment should not be below 10 ml.

Uses: It is given orally to adsorb toxins and other substances from gastrointestinal tract. It increases the bulk of faeces. It is administered in the symptomatic treatment of colitis, cholera, dysentery and diarrhoea and in the treatment of food and alkaloidal poisoning. It finds widespread use in pharmaceutical industry as it is used as a dusting powder, as an ingredient of toilet powders, as an excipient for pills etc.

If Kaolin is prescribed or demanded, only light Kaolin should be dispensed or supplied.

Dose: 15–60 g orally.

KAOLIN POULTICE

Kaolin poultice contains 50.5% w/w of Kaolin (limit 48 to 53) per cent. It contains the following ingredients:

Heavy Kaolin, finely sifted, dried at 100° .... 527 g
Boric acid, finely sifted .... 45 g
Methyl salicylate .... 2 ml
Mentha oil .... 0.5 ml
Thymol .... 0.5 g
Glycerin ....425 g

It is prepared by mixing the heavy Kaolin and the Boric acid with glycerin; heating the mixture at 120° for one hour with occasional stirring; allowing the mixture to cool and adding the thymol, previously dissolved in the methyl salicylate followed by the mentha oil. The mixture is mixed thoroughly.

Assay[1]: An accurately weighed amount of Kaolin poultice is mixed with hot water, till thoroughly disintegrated; filtered through a tared Gooch crucible and the residue of Kaolin is washed with hot water until free from all water soluble matter. The residue of Kaolin is then dried in an oven to constant weight at 105°.

---

[1] Since Kaolin poultice also contains boric acid and glycerin in appreciable amounts, I.P. prescribed limits and tests for these ingredients as well. These assays are therefore, given below.
Boric acid: Not less than 4.2 per cent and not more than 4.7 per cent, when determined by the following method: Weigh accurately about 20 g and warm with 20 ml of water in a 250 ml glass beaker. Stir with a glass until thoroughly disintegrated and filter through a Buchner funnel. Wash the residue several times with water. To the combined filtrate add an equal volume of glycerin previously neutralised to solution of phenolphthalein and mix. Titrate the solution with 0.5 N potassium hydroxide using solution of phenolphthalein as indicator. Each ml of 0.5 N potassium hydroxide is equivalent to 0.03092 g of boric acid.
Glycerin: Not less than 39.5 per cent and not more than 45 per cent when determined by the following method: Weigh accurately about 20 g and heat with 50 ml of water in a 250 ml glass beaker. Stir with a glass until thoroughly disintegrated and filter through a Buchner funnel and wash until complete extraction of glycerin is effected. Evaporate the combined filtrate and washings to less than 30 ml, cool transfer into a 50 ml volumetric flask, and make up the volume to 50 ml at 15° and determine its specific gravity at that temperature. Make necessary corrections in the specific gravity by subtracting 0.0035 for each one per cent of boric acid found in the test for boric acid. From the corrected specific gravity, the percentages of glycerin is calculated (as per table given in App. II).

Storage: Kaolin poultice is preserved in a well closed container.

Uses: It is used as an anti-inflammatory and counter-irritant.

EXCIPIENTS

Excipients are certain classes of components other than the active ingredient added to various formulations as pharmaceutical aids.

Excipients may be classified as diluents; suspending agents; emulsifying agents; binders and adhesives, like acacia, glucose and gelatin; disintegrants, like clays, cellulose and starch; lubricants, like talc, stearic acid and its derivatives; glidants and flow promoters, like silica derivatives and talc, colourants, flavours and sweeteners.

DILUENTS

Diluents are inert substances, and vehicles used in pharmaceutical preparation to dilute, and decrease the concentration of the active ingredient or increase the bulk of the formulation. In liquid preparations, the diluent commonly employed is the vehicle or solvent. Tablet and capsule formulations may contain a diluent to improve formulation properties such as improved cohesion, promoting flow or permitting use of direct compression manufacturing.

In solid preparations like powder, capsules and tablets commonly employed diluents are lactose, directly compressible starches, microcrystalline cellulose, dibasic calcium phosphate dihydrate, mannitol, sorbitol, sucrose, calcium sulphate dihydrate and dextrose. Diluents used in ointments, semi-solid formulations and suppositories are their respective bases.

CALCIUM SULPHATE
(Plaster of Paris)

Chem. formula: $CaSO_4, 1/2H_2O$ or $CaSO_4, 2H_2O$ (Gypsum)   Mol. weight: 145.2

Preparation: Calcium sulphate can be prepared by adding dilute H_2SO_4 to a solution of calcium chloride.

$$CaCl_2 + H_2SO_4 + 2H_2O \longrightarrow CaSO_4.2H_2O + 2HCl$$

Calcium sulphate being sparingly soluble in water gets precipitated and is filtered.

Description: It is a white hygroscopic powder, which is odourless and tasteless.

Solubility: It is only sparingly soluble in water, solubility decreases sharply with rise of temperature. It is insoluble in alcohol but dissolves in dilute hydrochloric acid.

Tests for identity: It gives tests for calcium and sulphate ions.

Tests for purity: It is tested for acidity or alkalinity; acid insoluble matter; loss on drying and setting properties.

Storage: Plaster of Paris is preserved in a sound, clean, dry and water-tight container.

Uses: It is a surgical aid and is used in making casts in plaster* of paris bandages. It is also used as a diluent in the manufacture of compressed tablets.

---

* Plasters are materials which are only used for external applications and are such materials prepared from certain materials which have adhesive properties enabling the plaster to stick to the skin and help in fixing the bandage and dressing in position. They thus protect the wounds and provide the mechanical support. Besides they have an occlusive and macerating action and being medicaments come into close contact with the wounds and skin.

CALCIUM CARBONATE

Chem. formula: $CaCO_3$ Mol. weight. : 100.09

The calcium carbonate is the precipitated Calcium Carbonate and contains not less than 98% and not more than equivalent of 100.5% $CaCO_3$, calculated with reference to the dried substance.

Preparation:

(1) It is prepared by passing CO_2 through lime-water.

$$Ca(OH)_2 + CO_2 \longrightarrow CaCO_3\downarrow + H_2O$$

(2) It is also prepared by adding boiling sodium carbonate solution to calcium chloride.

$$CaCl_2 + NaCO_3 \longrightarrow CaCO_3\downarrow + 2NaCl$$

The precipitate is allowed to settle. It is then collected on calico filter (a) printed cotton cloth, washed with freshly double-distilled water and freed from CO_2 and chloride. The washing is continued till the filtrate is free from chloride ions. The precipitate is dried in an oven at a temp. not exceeding 105°C.

Description: It is a fine, white, microcrystalline powder without odour and taste.

Solubility: Practically insoluble in water and alcohol, but slightly soluble in water in presence of CO_2 or any ammonium salt.

$$\text{Insoluble } CaCO_3 + CO_2 + H_2O \longrightarrow Ca(HCO_3)_2 \text{ soluble in water.}$$

It dissolves with effervescence in dil. acetic acid, hydrochloric acid and in dil. nitric acid.

$$CaCO_3 \xrightarrow{\text{acid}} H_2CO_3$$
$$H_2CO_3 \longrightarrow H_2O + CO_2\uparrow$$

Tests for identity:

(1) It gives with dil. HCl and dil. HNO_3 effervescence due to the liberation of CO_2 (see reactions above).

(2) The resulting solution from test No.1 gives the reactions for calcium (App. I).

Tests for purity: It is tested for barium; iron; arsenic; heavy metals; chloride and sulphate.

Tests for insoluble matters: Not more than 0.2% determined by dissolving the sample (5 g) in water (l0 ml) and adding HCl, dropwise with shaking until effervescence ceases. Boil for 2 minutes, allow to cool, dilute with water (to about 200 ml) and filter through a sintered-glass filter. Wash the residue with hot water (4 × 5 ml) and dry the residue at 105° for 1 hour.

Magnesium and alkali metals: Not more than 1.0% determined by dissolving the sample (1 g) in dil. HCl (10 ml), neutralising the solution by adding dil. ammonia solution, heating to boiling and adding hot ammonium oxalate solution (50 ml). The solution is cooled, diluted with water (to 100 ml) and filtered. To a specified volume of the filtrate (50 ml) is added dil. H_2SO_4 (1.5 ml) and evaporated to dryness on a water bath. The residue is heated to redness. allowed to cool and weighed.

Soluble alkali: A specified amount of the sample (5 g) in water (100 ml) is boiled for 5 minutes, filtered immediately and cooled. The amount of 0.1 N H_2SO_4 required for neutralizing the above solution does not exceed the desired volume (2.5 ml) using methyl orange as indicator.

Barium: An acidic solution of the sample is made by dissolving (0.6 g) in dil. CH_3COOH (10 ml).

It is then boiled. cooled and to it is added $CaSO_4$ solution (10 ml). The solution must remain clear for 15 minutes.

Iron: A solution of the sample (0.2 g), prepared in water (5 ml) and iron-free HCl (0.5 ml) after boiling and diluting with water (to 40 ml) complies with the limit test for iron.

Arsenic: Not more than four parts per million.

Heavy metals: Not more than 20 parts per million (I.P. 2.3.13).

The solution is prepared by dissolving the sample (1 g) in water (5 ml), and by slowly adding dil. HCl (8 ml), shaking and evaporating to dryness on a water-bath. The residue is then dissolved in water (20 ml), filtered and to the filtrate is added dil. CH_3COOH (3 ml) and water to make 25 ml.

Chloride: The sample (1 g) is dissolved in water with the help of HNO_3 (3 ml) and it complies with the limit test for chlorides (250 ppm).

Calcium carbonate is insoluble in water but dissolves in the presence of carbon dioxide, which is formed by addition of acid to the calcium carbonate.

$$CaCO_3 + 2HNO_3 \longrightarrow Ca(NO_3)_2 + H_2CO_3$$
$$H_2CO_3 \longrightarrow CO_2\uparrow + H_2O$$
$$CaCO_3 + CO_2 + H_2O \longrightarrow Ca(HCO_3)_2$$
$$\text{Soluble in water}$$

Sulphate: The solution of the sample (0.5 g) in water (5 ml) is prepared by adding dropwise dil. HCl (2 ml). The resultant solution complies with the limit test for sulphates (0.3 per cent).

Loss on drying: Not more than 2% determined by drying the sample (1 g) in an oven at 200°.

Assay: This is based on the basic principle of complexometric titration. Disodium ethylenediamine tetraacetate is used as sequestering agent. Dil. HCl is used in order to dissolve calcium carbonate in water because as such it is insoluble in water.

Acid will generate CO_2 which is formed as follow:

$$2HCl + CaCO_3 \longrightarrow CaCl_2 + H_2CO_3$$
$$H_2CO_3 \longrightarrow H_2O + CO_2$$
$$CaCO_3 + H_2O + CO_2 \longrightarrow Ca(HCO_3)_2$$
$$\text{Insoluble} \qquad\qquad\qquad \text{Soluble}$$

Disodium edetate is also called complexone III.

Disodium edetate [HOOC $CH_2 \cdot$ N($CH_2 \cdot$ COONa)$\cdot$ $CH_2]_2$ can be represented as Na_2H_2Y yielding the complex-forming ion H_2Y in aqueous solution.

The reaction of H_2Y^{2-} with Ca^{2+} may be written as follows:

$$Ca^{2+} + H_2Y^{2-} \rightleftharpoons CaY^{2-} + 2H^+$$

Calcium-disodium edetate complex

The sample (0.1 g) is dissolved in dil. HCl (3 ml) and water (10 ml). The solution is boiled for 10 minutes in order to remove CO_2 formed, cooled and diluted with water (to 50 ml), The solution is titrated with 0.05 M disodium edetate. Near the end-point is added NaOH solution (8 ml) and calcon mixture (0.1 g) and the titration is continued until the colour from pinkish changes to a full blue colour.

Each ml of 0.05 M disodium edetate is equivalent to 0.005004 g of $CaCO_3$.

0.05 M disodium edetate is available in the market and can be standardised against $ZnSO_4.7H_2O$.

Uses: It is used as an antacid, food additive, excipient and dentifrice.

Dose: 1 to 5 g 6 times a day.

CALCIUM PHOSPHATE

Chem. formula : $Ca_3(PO_4)_2$ Mol. weight: Variable

It consists of a mixture of normal basic and acid calcium phosphate in different proportions which should contain calcium equivalent to not less than 85% of calcium phosphate.

Description: It occurs as a white amorphous powder, odourless, tasteless and stable in air. It is insoluble in water and alcohol but soluble in dilute nitric acid and dilute hydrochloric acid.

Tests for identity: It gives reactions characteristics of calcium and phosphates (App. I).

Tests for purity: It is tested for As; heavy metals; iron; carbonate; chloride; sulphate; and hydrochloric acid-insoluble matter.

Assay: An accurately weighed amount (about 2 g) is dissolved in a mixture of water (15 ml) and hydrochloric acid (2 ml) and to this is added dilute solution of ammonium acetate (25 ml), followed by a slight excess of solution of ammonium oxalate. The mixture is heated for one hour on a water bath, filtered and the residue after washing with warm water is suspended in water (15 ml) and acidified to litmus paper with dilute sulphuric acid. The solution is heated to 70° and titrated with 0.1 N potassium permanganate keeping the solution at 70° during the titration.

Factor: 1 ml of 0.1 N potassium permanganate is equivalent to 0.00517 g of $Ca_3(PO_4)_2$.

Uses: It is used as a pharmaceutical aid.

DIBASIC CALCIUM PHOSPHATE
(Calcium Hydrogen Phosphate)

Chem. formula: $CaHPO_4$ Mol. weight. 136.1 (anhydrous)
Chem. formula: $CaHPO_4.2H_2O$ Mol. weight. 172.1 (dihydrate)

It is anhydrous or contains two molecules of water of hydration. It contains 30.9 to 31.7% of calcium (Ca) calculated with reference to the ignited substance.

Description: It is a white powder, odourless and tasteless.

Solubility: It is insoluble in water and alcohol, but is soluble in dil. HCl and dil. HNO_3.

Tests for identity:

(1) It gives the reactions of calcium when a solution of sample (0.1 g) is prepared by using dil. HCl (5 ml) and water (5 ml) (App. I).

(2) It gives the reactions of phosphates when a solution of sample (0.1 g) is prepared by using dil. HNO_3 (App. I).

Tests for purity: It is tested for acid insoluble substances; pH; carbonate; iron; chloride; sulphate; arsenic; heavy metals; loss on drying; loss on ignition; proteinous impurities; monocalcium; and tricalcium phosphates.

(1) **Acid insoluble substances:** Not more than 0.1% determined by heating the sample (5 g) with a mixture of water (40 ml) and HCl (10 ml) until no more dissolves, followed by dilution with water (to 100 ml). Filter the mixture and wash with hot water until the washing is free from chloride. The residue is dried at 105° for one hour.

(2) **pH:** Between 6.0 to 7.0 determined in a 20% w/v suspension in water.

(3) **Carbonate:** When sample (1 g) is dissolved in water (5 ml) and dil. HCl (2 ml), it does not produce effervescence.

(4) **Iron:** Dissolve the sample (0.1 g) in water (5 ml) and HCl (0.5 ml) with the addition of citric acid (1 g). The solution is diluted to 40 ml with water. This resulting solution complies with limit test for iron (400 ppm).

Chloride: 0.3 g of the sample is dissolved in water by the addition of 2 ml of nitric acid. The solution complies with the limit test for chlorides.

Sulphate: 0.1 g of the sample is dissolved in water by the addition of 1 ml of hydrochloric acid. The solution complies with the limit test for sulphates (0.5 per cent).

Arsenic: Not more than 10 ppm, determined by following the limit test for arsenic (p. 6).

Heavy metals: Not more than 40 parts per million, determined by taking 1.0 g of the sample, warming it with 3 ml of dil. HCl, cooling and diluting the solution to 50 ml (p. 14).

Loss on drying: Not more than 1.0% determined by drying a definite amount (1.0 g) "in vacuo at 60°C for three hours (I.P. 85, App. IV).

Loss on ignition: Between 6.6% and 8.5% for anhydrous and between 24.5% and 26.5% for the dihydrate. It is determined by igniting a definite amount of the sample (1.0 g) in a muffle furnace at 800° to 825°.

Proteinous impurities: Heat 0.5 g in a dry test tube. No change in colour should take place. Also no unpleasant odour is emitted.

Monocalcium and tricalcium phosphates: It is determined by following the I.P. method.

Assay: An accurately weighed amount of about 0.2 g of the sample is dissolved with the aid of gentle heat in a mixture of 5 ml of HCl and 3 ml H_2O. To this solution is added 125 ml of water and 0.5 ml of triethanolamine, 0.3 g of hydroxynaphthol blue indicator and from a burette about 23 ml of 0.05 M disodium ethylenediamine tetraacetate. To the solution is added sodium hydroxide solution until the initial red colour changes to clear blue. Dropwise addition is continued until the colour changes to violet and then an additional 0.5 ml is added. The titration is continued till a clear blue end-point which persists for not less than 60 seconds is obtained.

Each ml of 0.05 M disodium ethylenediamine tetraacetate $\equiv$ 0.002004 g of Ca.

I.P. 2007 gives another assay method using disodium edetate, titrating with 0.1 M zinc sulphate in the presence of mordant black II as an indicator (p. 846).

Use: It is used as a calcium supplement and pharmaceutical aid (excipient).

Dose: 1 to 5 g.

TRIBASIC CALCIUM PHOSPHATE
(Calcium hydroxide phosphate, Calcium Phosphate)

It consists of a variable mixture of calcium phosphates having the composition $10CaO3P_2O_5.H_2O$. It contains between 34 to 40% of Calcium, Ca and Phosphate, PO_4, equivalent to not less than 90.0% and not more than 100.5% of calcium phosphate, $Ca_3(PO_4)_2$, calculated with reference to the ignited substance.

Description: It is a white, amorphous powder, odourless and almost tasteless.

Solubility: It is insoluble in water and in alcohol but soluble in dil. HNO_3 and dil. HCl.

Tests for identity: Same as for Dibasic Calcium Phosphate (App. I).

Tests for purity: Same as in Dibasic Sodium Phosphate and water soluble substances; dibasic sodium phosphate and water.

Acid-insoluble substances: Not more than 0.2%, when diluted with water (to 40 ml).

Iron: Complies with the limit test for iron (p. 5).

Chloride: A solution of sample (0.3 g) in water by the addition of HNO_3 (2 ml) complies with the limit test for chlorides (p. 4).

Sulphate: A solution of sample (0.15 g) in water (25 ml) by the addition of HCl (1 ml) complies with the limit test for sulphates (p. 5).

Arsenic: Not more than 5 ppm.

Heavy metals: Not more than 30 ppm determined by dissolving sample (1 g) with HCl (3 ml) in water (50 ml).

Dibasic salt and calcium oxide: An accurately weighed amount of sample (2 g) is dissolved by warming in 1 N HCl (50 ml). The solution is cooled and it is titrated with 1 N NaOH by shaking constantly to a pH 4.0, determined potentiometrically. Not less than specified sample of 1 N HCl (13–14 ml) is consumed for each g, calculated with reference to the ignited substance.

Water: Not more than 2.5% w/v.

Loss on ignition: Not more than 8.0%, determined by igniting 1.0 g in a muffle furnace at 800° for thirty minutes.

Water-soluble substances: Not more than 0.5% determined by using 2 g of sample, digesting in water to 100 ml for 30 minutes on a water bath, cooling and adding sufficient water to restore the original volume, stirring well and filtering. Evaporating then to 1/2 volume and drying at 105° to constant weight.

Carbonate: No effervescence should be produced when HCl (10 ml) is added to 10% w/v solution of sample (5 g in 50 ml of water).

Assay: It is assayed for calcium and phosphate.

 (A) **For Calcium:** Same as in Dibasic Calcium Phosphate.

 (B) **For Phosphate:** PO_4.

Phosphates are detected in analysis by addition of HNO_3, followed by excess ammonium molybdate. On warming a canary yellow ppt. of ammonium phosphomolybdate $(NH_4)_3(MO_3)_{12}PO_4.xH_2O$ is formed.

An accurately weighed amount of sample (0.2 g) is dissolved in a mixture of water and dil. HNO_3 (25 ml : 10 ml). Filter and wash any ppt. with water. To the filtrate add sufficient strong NH_3 solution to produce as slight ppt. and then dissolve the ppt. by the addition of dil. HNO_3 (1 ml). Adjust the temp. to about 50°, add ammonium molybdate solution (75 ml) and heat the solution at about 50° for 30 minutes, stirring occasionally. Wash the ppt. with water (30 ml) by decantation. Wash the ppt. with 1% w/v solution of KNO_3 until it is neutral to litmus paper. Transfer the ppt. and filter paper to the precipitation vessel into water (50 ml) and add 1 N NaOH (40 ml), agitate until the ppt. is dissolved, add phenolphthalein solution and titrate the excess of alkali with 1 N H_2SO_4.

Each ml of 1 N NaOH $\equiv$ 0.006743 g of $Ca_3(PO_4)_2$.

I.P. 2007 gives another assay method (p. 846). About 1 g accurately weighed sample dissolved in 10 ml of HCl by heating on water bath is diluted with 50 ml of water. The solution is cooled and further diluted to 250 ml with water. To the 25 ml of the resulting solution, 30.0 ml of 0.05 M disodium edetate is added followed by 10.0 ml of ammonia buffer, pH 10.9, and 100 ml of water. The excess of disodium edetate is titrated with 0.05 M zinc chloride using mordant black II as an indicator.

1 ml of 0.05 M disodium edetate is equivalent to 0.00517 g of $Ca_3(PO_4)_2$.

Use: It is used as a pharmaceutical aid (excipient).

LUBRICANTS

Lubricants are substances added to the granules during the tabletting procedure to enable the easy ejection of the tablets from the mould.

MAGNESIUM STEARATE

According to I.P. requirements, magnesium stearate is a mixture of varying proportions of magnesium stearate $(C_{17}H_{35}COO)_2Mg$ and magnesium palmitate $(C_{15}H_{31}COO)_2Mg$. It contains equivalent of not less than 6.5% and not more than 8.5% of MgO and not less than 3.8% and not more than 5.0% of Mg, calculated on the dried basis.

Preparation: A weighed quantity of stearic acid is added gradually, with constant stirring, to a hot solution of sodium hydroxide. The resulting solution is cooled and to it is added a solution of magnesium sulphate. The precipitated magnesium stearate is then collected on filter paper, washed and dried.

$$C_{17}H_{35}COOH + NaOH \longrightarrow C_{17}H_{35}COO^-Na^+ + H_2O$$

$$2C_{17}H_{35}COO^-Na^+ + MgSO_4 \longrightarrow (C_{17}H_{35}COO^-)_2Mg^+ + Na_2SO_4$$

Description: It is white, impalpable powder with faint and characteristic odour. It is greasy to touch and free from grittiness.

Solubility: It is insoluble in water, alcohol and solvent ether.

Tests for identity:

(1) 5.0 g of magnesium stearate is heated by shaking with 40 ml of dil. H_2SO_4 and cooled. The fatty acid liberated is filtered off. The filtrate gives the reactions of magnesium (App. I).

(2) The fatty acid obtained in test (1) above melts at a temp. not below 54° (I.P. 85, p. 292).

(3) I.P. 2007 gives a new freezing point test (2.4.11).

Tests for purity: It is tested for pH; zinc stearate; heavy metals; loss on drying; chloride; sulphate; acid value of the fatty acids; free stearic acid.

pH: Between 6.2 and 7.4 determined in a solution obtained by mixing 1 g of drug with 20 ml freshly boiled and cooled water, boiling for 1 minute with continuous shaking and filtering.

Zinc stearate: 5.0 g of the substance is shaken with a mixture of 50 ml of water and 50 ml of dil. H_2SO_4, until the fatty acid separates as an oily layer. After cooling the aqueous layer is filtered off and the residue is washed with two successive volumes of 5 ml of hot water. The washings are combined with the filtrate and the liquid is made up to 100 ml with water. To 5 ml of the resulting solution is added 0.5 ml of ammonium mercurithiocyanate solution and one drop of 0.1% w/v sol. of copper sulphate. The wall of the test tube is scratched with a glass rod and the test tube with sol. is allowed to stand for 15 minutes. No violet ppt. should be formed.

Heavy metals: Not more than 20 ppm (I.P. 2.3.13).

Loss on drying: Not more than 6% determined by drying 0.5 g magnsium stearate in an oven at 105° (App. IV).

Assay: It is based on simple acid-base volumetric titration. An accurately weighed amount of about 1.0 g of magnesium stearate is boiled with 50.0 ml of 0.1 N H_2SO_4 for 10 min. or until the fatty layer is clear, adding water if necessary to maintain the original vol. The contents are cooled, filtered and the filter and flask are washed with water until the washing is not acidic to litmus paper. To the solution is added a few drops of methyl orange sol. and it is titrated for the excess of acid with 0.1 N NaOH.

$$\text{Each ml of } 0.1 \text{ N } H_2SO_4 \equiv 0.002015 \text{ g of MgO.}$$

I.P. gives a new method of assay using 0.1 M disodium edetate in presence of mordant black II mixture as an indicator.

Storage: It is stored in well-closed containers.

Uses: Magnesium stearate is used as a lubricant (pharmaceutical aid).

SUSPENDING AGENTS

A suspension is a biphasic system containing finely divided insoluble solid suspended in a liquid medium. A suspending agent is used in suspensions to overcome agglomeration of dispersed particles and to increase the viscosity of the medium so that sedimentation of the particles takes place more slowly.

Examples of commonly used suspending agents are acacia, bentonite, carboxymethylcellulose sodium and powdered cellulose.

BENTONITE

Chem. formula: $Al_2O_3 4SiO_2.H_2O$ (!)

Bentonite is a colloidal, hydrated aluminium silicate. Bentonite, obtained from different localities, was originally known as Tarylosite and is commonly called as soap clay.

Description: Bentonite occurs as a very fine, white, pale buff or cream-coloured powder, devoid of any gritty particles. It is odourless with slightly earthy taste.

Bentonite is insoluble in water, but it swells in it to about 12 times its volume (hence I.P. includes a test for its swelling power). It neither dissolves nor swells in organic solvents.

Tests for identity:

(1) It gives tests for its identification based on reactions characteristic of aluminium (App. I).

(2) I.P. 2007 gives a new test for identification again based on reactions on aluminium salts and obtaining a gelatinous precipitate.

A two per cent solution is alkaline (pH 9 to 10.5).

Tests for purity: It is tested for alkalinity; arsenic; gel formation; swelling power; gritty particles; loss on drying; coarse particles; sedimentation volume; and microbial contamination.

Gel formation: 6 g of bentonite is mixed thoroughly with 0.3 g of light magnesium oxide and the mixture is added in many divided doses to 200 ml of water contained in 500 ml glass-stoppered cylinder. The water in the cylinder is then agitated thoroughly for one hour and 100 ml of this mixture is transferred to a 100 ml cylinder. The 100 ml cylinder is allowed to remain undisturbed for 24 hours, and the volume of the clear supernatant liquid appearing on the surface in the cylinder is noted. The volume should not be more than 2 ml.

Swelling power: It is determined by dropping from the top 2 g of bentonite in divided portion upon the surface of water (100 ml) contained in 100 ml capacity glass-stoppered cylinder and allowing each portion to get settled before the next is added. Bentonite swells generally at the bottom and it should occupy a volume of not less than 24 ml.

Gritty particles (fineness of powder): 2 g of bentonite sample is sprinkled upon 20 ml of water contained in a mortar and allowed to swell. The swollen mass is evenly dispersed with a pestle and diluted with water to 100 ml. The suspension is poured through a No. 200 sieve and sieve washed thoroughly with water. The test passes if no grit is felt when the figures are rubbed over the wire mesh of the sieve.

Microbial contamination: 1 g should be free from *Escherichia coli* (I.P. 2.2.9).

Loss on drying: On being dried to constant weight at 105°, bentonite should not lose less than 5% and not more than 12% of its weight.

Uses: It is a good pharmaceutical aid and is used as a protective colloid for the stabilization of suspensions. It is used as an emulsifier for oil in water emulsions and as a base for many pharmaceutical preparations, including plasters and ointments. It is used in the well-known preparation calamine lotion (I.P. 85) which is used as a protective.

COLOURANTS

The use of colours and dyes in pharmaceutical formulations has served three main purposes: distinguishing of off-colour drugs, product identification and the production of a more elegant product.

The choice of a suitable colourant will depend on the desired colour, its stability, toxicity, reaction with other ingredients, etc. The legally approved dyes, which may be used in pharmaceutical preparations, are FD&C dyes, D&C dyes and external D&C dyes. The choice of a dye is very important since even a very low concentration of a water-soluble dye can have an inhibitory effect on dissolution rate of several crystalline drugs. The dye molecules adsorbed on to the crystal faces inhibit drug dissolution - for example, brilliant blue retards dissolution of sulfathiazole.

Mineral colours or pigments are used to colour preparations for external application like lotions, and cosmetics. Examples are red ferric oxide, yellow ferric oxide, titanium dioxide and carbon black.

Several plants also contain pigments that can be extracted and used as colourants, e.g., chlorophyll and natural beta-carotene, alizarin and indigo. Colourants are also obtained from animal sources. Synthetic colouring principles are also widely used, like the coal tar dyes.

FERRIC OXIDE, RED

Chem. formula: Fe_2O_3 Mol. weight: 159.7

Its contains not less than 90% Fe_2O_3.

Description: It is a dark or light reddish brown powder. It is not official in new I.P.

Preparation: Ferric oxide is made by heating native ferric oxide or hydroxide at a ternperature which will yield a product of the desired colour. The colour depends on the temperature at the time of heating, the presence and kind of other metals and the particle size of the oxide. A dark-coloured oxide is favoured by prolonged heating at high temperature and the presence of manganese. A light-coloured oxide is favoured by the presence of aluminium and by finer particle size.

Uses: Ferric oxide is used for imparting colour to calamine and cosmetics.

FERRIC OXIDE, YELLOW

It contains not less than 97.5% Fe_2O_3. It is prepared by heating ferrous hydroxide or ferrous carbonate in air at a low temperature.

TITANIUM DIOXIDE

Titanium dioxide (TiO_2) is described under 'topical agents' as a topical protectent in ointments and creams.

Major Intra- and Extracellular Electrolytes

Water is a predominant constituent of the body (60–70%). The body fluids are solutions of inorganic and organic solutes that are distributed in the three major fluid compartments namely:

1. Intracellular fluid (45–50% of body weight)
2. Interstitial fluid (12–15% of body weight)
3. Plasma or vascular fluid (4–5% of body weight)

Semi-permeable membranes separate the body fluids, and each fluid compartment has its unique concentration of electrolytes. The membranes are permeable to water and many organic and inorganic solutes. They are nearly impermeable to macromolecules like proteins and selectively permeable to certain ions such as Na^+, K^+ and Mg^{++}, thereby enabling each compartment to have its own distinct solute pattern.

The distribution of ions in the various body fluid compartments is constant in a healthy individual and is graphically represented below.

Distribution of electrolytes in body fluids

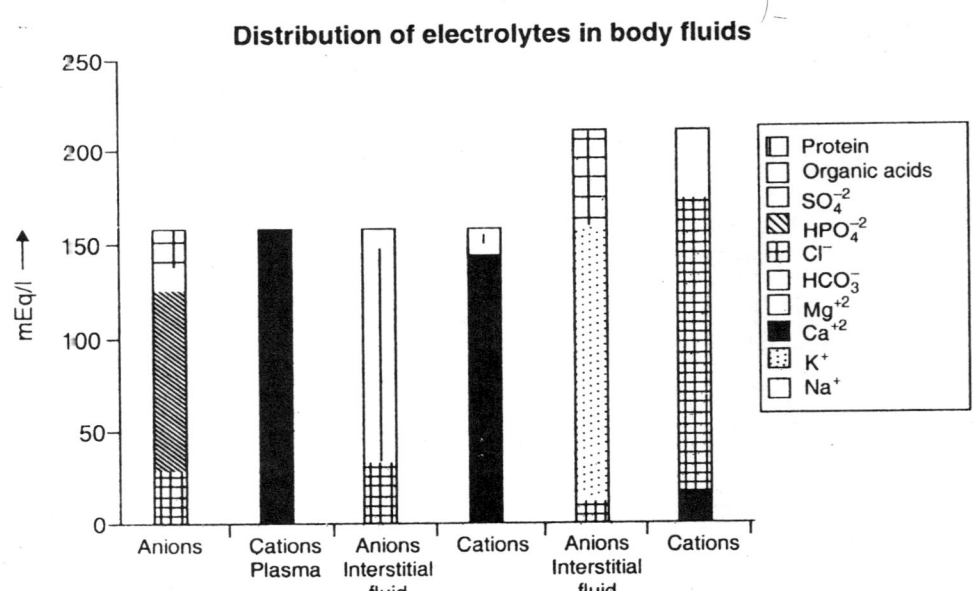

90

COMPARISON BETWEEN THE INTRACELLULAR AND EXTRACELLULAR CONCENTRATIONS OF ELECTROLYTES

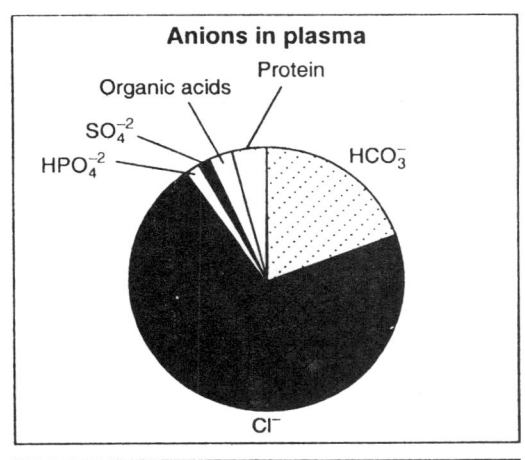

Anions in plasma

Organic acids · Protein · SO_4^{-2} · HPO_4^{-2} · HCO_3^- · Cl^-

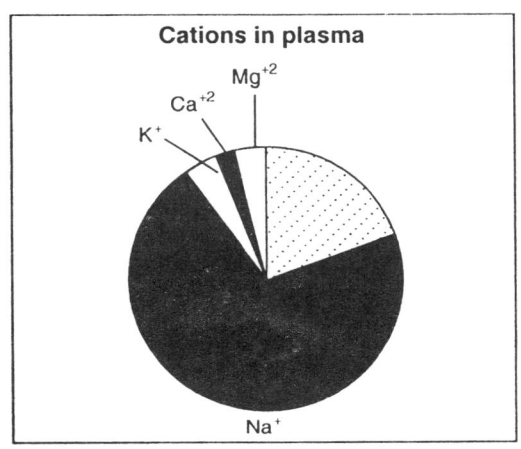

Cations in plasma

Mg^{+2} · Ca^{+2} · K^+ · Na^+

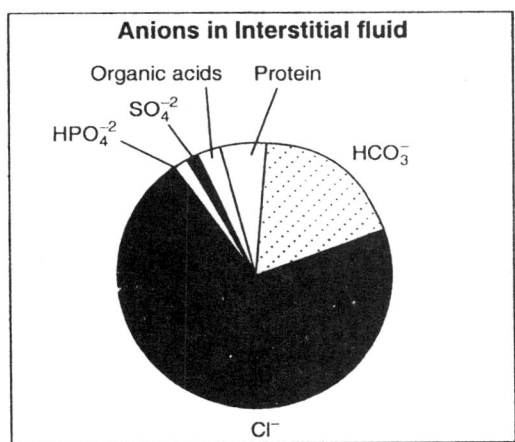

Anions in Interstitial fluid

Organic acids · Protein · SO_4^{-2} · HPO_4^{-2} · HCO_3^- · Cl^-

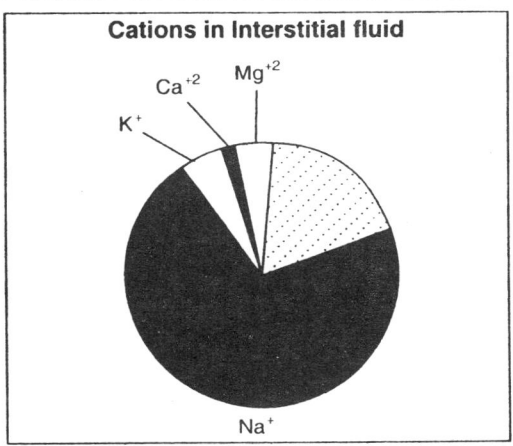

Cations in Interstitial fluid

Ca^{+2} · Mg^{+2} · K^+ · Na^+

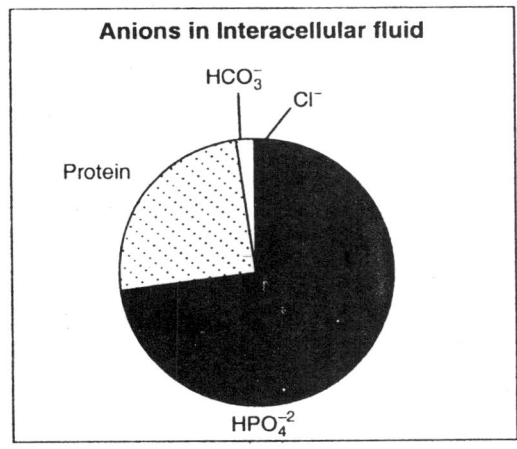

Anions in Interacellular fluid

HCO_3^- · Cl^- · Protein · HPO_4^{-2}

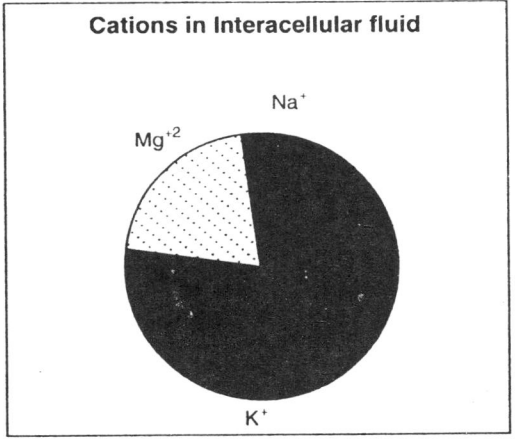

Cations in Interacellular fluid

Na^+ · Mg^{+2} · K^+

While the major ions in the extracellular fluid (plasma and interstitial fluid) are Na^+ and Cl^-, the major ions in the intracellular fluid are K^+, Mg^{+2} and HPO_4^{2-}. The differences in the ionic composition are essential to life and are maintained by ionic pumps within the cell membrane. Osmotic activity is believed to be almost identical in the fluid compartments, in spite of the differences in ionic composition.

PHYSIOLOGICAL IONS

The major physiological ions in the human body are sodium, potassium, calcium, magnesium, chloride, phosphate and bicarbonate.

Sodium

Sodium is the principal cation in the extracellular fluid compartments. The ionic balance of sodium depends on the amount of Na^+ absorbed and excreted. It also depends greatly on the intake and excretion of water, the blood volume status, and to a lesser degree on the renal regulation of sodium. Kidneys regulate the sodium content in the body by the process of excretion and reabsorption. Sodium depletion results more from excessive salt loss rather than inadequate intake. Loss of Na^+ is almost always accompanied by a reduction in body water.

Hyponatremia or low serum sodium level can occur as a result of large losses of salt and water due to extreme urine loss, as in diabetes insipidus; diarrhea and vomiting; excessive sweating; kidney damage; metabolic acidosis, in which sodium is excreted; Addison's disease, with decreased excretion of aldosterone, a diuretic hormone; and the use of thiazide diuretics, which induces Na and K loss. Symptoms of hyponatremia include nausea and vomiting, muscular weakness, headache, lethargy and ataxia. In severe conditions seizures, coma and respiratory depression may occur. Treatment involves identification and correction of the cause and appropriate fluid and salt replenishment.

Hypernatremia (increased serum sodium concentration) may result from severe dehydration, with excessive loss of water relative to sodium; increased sodium intake; from hypertonic dialysis solutions; hyperadrenalism (Cushing's syndrome) with increased aldsoterone production; and certain types of brain injury. It can also occur in temporary conditions as in prernancy. Hypernatremia may result in water retention in tissues to maintain osmotic balance, resulting in edema, and excessive burden on the heart. Treatment is directed at correction of the condition that caused sodium retention or water depletion; low salt diets; diuretics; cardiotonic drugs or a combination of the above.

Potassium

Potassium is rapidly absorbed from the diet and is the principal intracellular cation with a concentration over 20 times greater inside the cells than outside. Functions of potassium in the body include transmission of nerve impulse (during transmission, K leaves the cell and Na enters). Potassium functions to regulate neuromuscular excitability, contraction of the heart, ICF volume, and hydrogen ion concentration. It has a major effect on contraction of skeletal and cardiac muscles.

Hypokalemia (low serum potassium) decreases cell excitability that can result in arrhythmias or paralysis. It causes changes in myocardial function, and blood pressure.

It also affects the hydrogen ion concentration in the blood, since its loss results in movement of Na^+ and H^+ into the cells to maintain the ionic balance, decreasing the H^+ concentration in the ECF. This leads to alkalosis. Alkalosis can also result in hypokalemia, due to the movement of K^+ into the cells to compensate the movement of protons out of the cell to the proton deficient ECF. Other conditions that can lead to hypokalemia are vomiting, diarrhea, burns, and hemorrhage; use of intravenous solutions lacking potassium; diabetic coma and overuse of thiazide diuretics.

Hyperkalemia is less common since the kidneys rapidly excrete excess potassium (refer use of potassium salts as inorganic diuretics). Hyperkalemia may occur as a result of kidney damage, diabetes mellitus or metabolic acidosis. It is thought that an increase in potassium levels may displace calcium ions in the heart with K^+, causing the heart muscle to become flaccid. This may cause cessation of heart beat (potassium arrest).

Note: The above reason may explain why calcium gluconate is effective in hyperpotassemic conditions.

Calcium

Only about 1% of body calcium is present in extracellular fluids as Ca^{+2}, 99% of it being found in bones. The absorption of calcium is controlled by the parathyroid hormone and a metabolite of vitamin D. Ionic calcium is involved in neurohormonal functions, blood clotting and muscle contraction. The deleterious effects of excess potassium on the heart may be due to the displacement of Ca^{+2} from the heart muscle. Ionic calcium is necessary for the release of acetylcholine from preganglionic nerve endings.

Hypocalcemia can be caused by decreased calcium absorption, hypoparathyroidism, vitamin D deficiency, osteoblastic metastasis (spreading bone cancer), Cushing's syndrome (hyperactive adrenal cortex), acute hyperphosphatemia, and acute pancreatitis. Low serum calcium levels may result in hypocalcemic tetany.

Symptoms of hypercalcemia include fatigue, muscle weakness, constipation, anorexia (loss of appetite) and cardiac irregularities. Calcium salts may also get deposited in the kidneys and blood vessels. Hypercalcemia is found in hyperparathyroidism, hypervitaminosis D, and some bone neoplastic diseases.

Magnesium

Magnesium is the second most abundant cation in the intracellular fluid. Approximately 53% of total body magnesium (10–20 g in an adult) is combined with calcium and phosphorus in the bone, 46% in other organs and soft tissues and less than 1% in the blood, 1/3rd of which is bound to protein. Magnesium is required for protein synthesis, smooth functioning of the neuromuscular system, and is an essential component of several enzymes involving phosphate metabolism.

Disorders of magnesium deficiency are widespread and are responsible for certain puzzling clinical features. The causes of magnesium deficiency are:

- *Reduced intake* – due to protein calorie malnutrition or prolonged administration of Mg^{++} free parenteral fluids.
- *Loss from GIT* – due to vomiting, diarrhea or aspiration of gastrointestinal secretions.
- *Increased excretion* – due to ketoacidosis, hyperparathyroidism, hyperaldosteronism, hypercalcemia, chronic alcoholism, renal disease and certain drugs, e.g. loop diuretics, gentamycin, cisplatin, cyclosporin and digitalis.
- Excess lactation, pregnancy and acute pancreatitis.

Magnesium depletion may be confirmed if the plasma magnesium is less than 0.75 mmol/L. Since most of the Mg^{++} is intracellular, serum plasma levels may be misleading. Administration of intravenous solution of magnesium may reveal deficiency as only a small portion (less than 40%) is excreted. Magnesium deficiency (hypomagnesia) exhibits clinical features, which are *neuromuscular*, with tremor, seizure, weakness, cramps, paralysis etc.; *cardiovascular* disturbances – arrhythmias, hypertension; *psychiatric* symptoms – personality changes, depression, confusion, agitation, hallucinations; failure to gain weight properly; and *metabolic* symptoms – hypokalemia. hyponatremia, hypocalcemia and hypophosphatemia. Treatment involves administration of $MgCl_2$ as an infusion with isotonic saline or glucose.

Hypermagnesemia occurs in acute and chronic renal disease and contributes to central nervous features associated with uremia. Hence injections of magnesium salts should not be carried out on patients with impaired renal function. Other causes of hypermagnesemia include decreased excretion of magnesium due to hypothyroidism, hypopituitarism, hypoaldosteronism, increased intake of antacids, cathartics and enemas; dehydration and bone carcinoma. Its treatment is that of the primary disorder and the discontinuation of the source of magnesium.

Chloride

Chloride is the major extracellular anion. Its function in the body involves maintaining proper hydration, osmotic pressure, electrical neutrality in the extracellular fluid compartments and blood volume. As such Cl^- has no pharmacological activity (the chloride ion, when administered as NH_4Cl, may be used as an urinary acidifier).

Cl^- is removed from the body by glomerular filtration and also reabsorbed by the tubules. *Hypochloremia* can be caused by conditions leading to a probable lack of tubular reabsorption of Cl^- like nephritis; metabolic acidosis as found in renal failure and diabetes mellitus; and prolonged vomiting.

Hyperchloremia can occur when there is an excessive loss of bicarbonate ion, in dehydration and decreased renal blood flow in cases of congestive heart failure and severe renal damage.

Phosphate

HPO_4^{2-} is the principal anion in the intracellular fluid compartment. Like chlorides, phosphate is not considered to have any specific pharmacological action. Phosphate esters of biochemical interest are derived from phosphoric acid. The $HPO_4^{2-}/H_2PO_4^-$ is an important biochemical buffer. The phosphoric acid anhydrate linkage is the body's means of storing potential chemical energy as ATP (adenosine triphosphate). The hydrolysis of a pyrophosphate bond releases approximately 8000 calories/mole of energy. Phosphorus is essential for normal bone and tooth development, and proper calcium metabolism. It is also hypothesized that serum inorganic phosphate has a role in regulating erythrocyte glucose metabolism.

Hyperphosphatemia may occur due to inappropriate excretion as a result of renal failure, increase in absorption due to hypervitaminosis D, and hypoparathyroidism. Hyperphosphatemia may lead to formation of phosphatic urinary calculi (a form of kidney stone).

Serum calcium and phosphate levels appear to correlate and there is also correlation in their absorption pattern. Hypophosphatemia is seen in vitamin D deficiency (rickets), hyperparathyroidism and lack of phosphate reabsorption by kidney tubule due to infections, cancer etc.

Bicarbonate

Bicarbonate is the second most prevalent anion in the extracellular fluid compartments and functions as the body's most important buffer system. A lack of bicarbonate causes metabolic acidosis while an excess causes metabolic alkalosis.

ELECTROLYTES USED IN REPLACEMENT THERAPY
Sodium Replacement

Sodium chloride is the salt of extracellular fluids and is used in replacement therapy as isotonic solutions or hypertonic injections. The various preparations of NaCl that may be used in replacement therapy are described in the following pages.

SODIUM SALTS

Sodium: Sodium is one of the five alkali metals which are included in periodic group I. It is perhaps the most important alkali metal which in the form of its compounds is not only widely distributed and is met with in abundance, but even therapeutically or otherwise its salts/compounds have great significance. A large number of compounds of sodium are official in Indian Pharmacopoeia. Sodium and potassium have great similarity as far as the therapeutic action of the an anion part of any of these metals is concerned. Hence some of their salts can be substituted for one another, i.e. potassium bromide can be given in place of sodium bromide or vice versa. However, sodium compounds are preferred as they are considered to be more therapeutically active (because of lower equivalent weight of sodium) and less expensive.

Because sodium ions are present in the organism in abundance, the administration of these from outside has no action. It is because of this reason that most of the remedies are used as sodium salts. It is, therefore, the action of the ions, whom the characteristic properties of the sodium salts can be attributed. Since the sodium salts promote retention of water in tissues, they are used with great caution in the treatment of cardiac ailments and renal diseases, which are accompanied by oedema.

The most abundant, yet the most important, naturally occurring compound of sodium is its chloride, i.e. sodium chloride, which is also considered to be the most important source for isolation of free metal. Sodium chloride occurs in sea water and in solid deposits as rock salt. Another naturally occurring sodium compound of great significance is sodium nitrate (Chile saltpeter).

SODIUM CHLORIDE

Chem. formula: NaCl   Mol. weight: 58.5

It contains not less than 99.0% and not more than 100.5% of NaCl calculated with reference to the substance dried to constant weight at 130°.

Preparation: It is prepared by evaporating a solution of concentrated sea water or purified saline deposits. By this only crude salt is obtained. For purification salt is dissolved in a small quantity of water and hydrogen chloride (HCl) is passed through it till saturation takes place. Sodium chloride is insoluble in HCl and thus whatever HCl gas is passed combines with water. Hence less H_2O is available to dissolve NaCl, which gets precipitated leaving impurities in solution. (The less solubility of NaCl in HCl is explained by the fact that it forms hydrates with the water present and since less water is available for dissolving sodium chloride, crystals are separated out which are dried).

Description: It is a white colourless crystalline powder, odourless and has saline taste. It is freely soluble in water, soluble in glycerin (10 parts) and insoluble in HCl.

Tests for identity: It yields reactions characteristic for sodium and chlorides (App. I).

Tests for purity: It is tested for acidity; alkalinity; As; Ba; Ca; and Mg; Fe; for heavy metals, bromide and iodide and sulphate. Bromide and chloride are detected by extraction (digestion) with warm alcohol. The alcoholic extract is then evaporated to dryness and the residue is taken up in chloroform and chlorine is added drop by drop.

$$Cl_2 + 2I^- \longrightarrow I_2 + 2Cl^-$$

$$Cl_2 + 2Br^- \longrightarrow Br_2 + 2Cl^-$$

The chloroform should not acquire violet, yellow or orange colour.

Assay: It is assayed by Mohr's method. An accurately weighed quantity (0.25 g) of substance is dissolved in sufficient quantity of water (50 ml) and the solution is then titrated with N/10 $AgNO_3$, using solution of potassium chromate as indicator. The reaction is as follows:

$$NaCl + AgNO_3 \longrightarrow AgCl\downarrow + NaNO_3$$

$$2AgNO_3 + K_2CrO_4 \longrightarrow Ag_2CrO_4 + 2KNO_3$$

1000 ml of N/10 $AgNO_3$ is equivalent to 1/10 NaCl.

Or each ml of 0.1 N $AgNO_3$ is equivalent to 0.005845 g of NaCl.

The K_2CrO_4 should be used in neutral medium because in acidic and alkaline medium its sensitivity is affected.

New I.P. uses a modified assay method (p. 1709).

Uses: It is used as an electrolyte replenisher in the treatment of shock.

Storage: Sodium chloride is preserved in a well-closed container, protected from light.

SODIUM CHLORIDE INJECTION

Sodium chloride is the most important of all the salts which is found in the body fluids, especially in the extracellular fluid of the body. Sodium is the main cation of the extracellular fluid which amounts to more than 90%, while chloride as anion amounts to more than 60%. 0.9% solution of sodium chloride is isotonic, i.e. it has the same osmotic pressure as body fluids. Besides, solution of sodium chloride, i.e. isotonic solution is non-irritating to body tissues and can be administered parenterally containing drugs. All the solutions, whether they are mixed with sodium chloride solution or not, especially for intravenous administration, should be sterile and pyrogen-free. Sodium chloride is given as such or as injection in many diseases to make up its depletion in the body. It increases excretion of calcium, if given in hypercacemia, by increasing glomerular filtration. It is the common table salt and is used as a condiment.

Pyrogens: The injection should comply with the test for pyrogens.

Arsenic: It is tested for As and heavy metals.

Other requirements: It should comply with all other I.P. requirements for parenteral preparations.

Assay: The assay is carried out in the same way as described under sodium chloride above, using an accurately measured volume equivalent to about 0.16 g of sodium chloride.

Each ml of 0.1 N silver nitrate is equivalent to 0.005845 g of sodium chloride.

Storage: The hypertonic injection of sodium chloride on keeping may cause separation of small solid particles from glass container. Solution containing such particles must not be used.

Uses: For uses see sodium chloride above.

Labelling: The label should state (1) the strength as the percentage w/v of sodium chloride; (2) solution with visible solid particles must not be used.

COMPOUND SODIUM CHLORIDE INJECTION

Synonym: Ringer's Injection.

Compound sodium chloride injection is a sterile solution of sodium chloride, potassium chloride and calcium chloride hydrated in water for injection, containing in each 100 ml not less than 0.82 g and not more than 0.90 g of sodium chloride, NaCl, not less than 0.025 g and not more than 0.035 g of potassium chloride, KCl, not less than 0.30 and not more than 0.36 g of calcium chloride, $CaCl_2$, $6H_2O$.

Ingredients:

Sodium chloride	8.6 g.
Potassium chloride	0.30 g.
Calcium chloride hydrated	0.33 g.
Water for injection, sufficient to produce	1000 ml

Preparation: The three salts are dissolved in water for injection and the solution is sterilised by heating by an autoclave or by filtration.

Description: The solution is clear and colourless with mild saline taste. It has pH 5.0 to 7.5.

Tests for identity: The compound sodium injection gives the reaction characteristic of sodium and chlorides. It also gives the reaction characteristic of potassium and calcium when the injection is concentrated to 1/2 of its original volume (App. I).

Tests for purity: It is tested for As and heavy metals. For heavy metals, to the 20 ml of injection 2 ml of dilute acetic acid is added and sufficient water to make the volume upto 25 ml and the limit test applied. Limit of heavy metal is 0.3 parts per million.

Pyrogens: Injection should comply with the test for pyrogens.

Other requirements: It complies with the requirements stated under injection.

Assay: The compound sodium chloride injection, since it contains three different salts, is assayed for individual salt. The procedures for the three assays as outlined in I.P. are reproduced here.

For $CaCl_2$.$6H_2O$: Measure 50 ml into a 250 ml beaker. Add 50 ml of water, 15 ml of solution of sodium hydroxide, 40 mg of murexide indicator preparation and 3 ml of solution of naphthol green and titrate with 0.005 M disodium ethylene diamine tetraacetate until the solution is deep in colour.

Each ml of 0.005 M disodium ethylene diamine tetraacetate is equivalent to 0.001095 g of $CaCl_2$, $6H_2O$.

For calcium chloride new I.P. 2007 gives a new method.

For KCl: Measure 5 ml and place into a centrifuge tube containing 1.5 ml of alcohol. Mix well. Add dropwise with continuous shaking 2 ml of solution of sodium cobaltinitrite and allow to stand for one hour at room temperature. Centrifuge the mixture until the precipitate is firmly packed in the bottom of the tube. Decant the supernatant liquid and allow the precipitate to drain for five minutes. Carefully wash the precipitate with 5 ml of alcohol (70 per cent) from a pipette using the fine stream of the wash solution to break up the precipitate. Centrifuge for five minutes and drain again. Dry at 80° for one hour. Add 10 ml of 0.2 N ceric sulphate and 1 ml of sulphuric acid (50 per cent v/v) and heat on a water bath until all the precipitate disappears. Cool to room temperature, add one drop of solution of ortho-phenanthroline ferrous complex and titrate the excess of ceric sulphate with 0.02 N ferrous ammonium sulphate. See new I.P. for an atomic absorption spectrophotometry i.e. method.

Each ml of 0 20 N ceric sulphate is equivalent to 0.000248 g of KCl.

For NaCl: Measure 25 ml and place in a 250 ml glass-stoppered flask. Add 60 ml of water and shake. Add 50 ml of 0.1 N silver nitrate, 3 ml of nitric acid and 5 ml of nitrobenzene, shake well and titrate the excess of silver nitrate with 0.1 N ammonium thiocyanate, using 2 ml of solution of ferric ammonium sulphate as indicator. Each ml of 0.1 N silver nitrate is equivalent to 0.003546 g of Cl. Calculate the sodium chloride content in each 100 ml of injection by the formula 1.648 (3.546 (4V)-0.4823 (Ca)-0.4756 (K) in which V is the volume in ml of 0.1 N silver nitrate required for total Cl in the portion of the injection taken, Ca and K represent respectively, the quantities, in mg in each 100 ml of calcium chloride hydrated and potassium chloride found in the assays for these constituents. See I.P. 2007 method on p. 1713.

Uses: It is an electrolyte replenisher.

Storage: Compound sodium chloride injection when kept in glass container for a long time may cause the separation of small solid particles. Such solutions must not be used.

(See also Sodium Chloride above, p. 169.)

COMPOUND SODIUM CHLORIDE SOLUTION

Synonym: Ringer's solution.

Compound sodium chloride contains in each 100 ml not less than 0.82 g and not more than 0.90 g of sodium chloride, NaCl, not less than 0.25 g and not more than 0.35 g of potassium chloride, KCl and not less than 0.30 g and not more than 0.36 g of calcium chloride hydrated, $CaCl_2, 6H_2O$.

Ingredients:

Sodium chloride	8.6 g
Potassium chloride	0.3 g
Calcium chloride hydrated	0.33 g
Purified water recently boiled, sufficient to produce	1000 ml

Preparation: The Ringer's solution is prepared by dissolving the three salts in sufficient quantity of recently boiled, purified water and making the volume 1000 ml with more water. The solution is filtered, repeating the filtration until free from suspending particles.

Description: The solution is clear and colourless with mild saline taste.

Tests for identity, reaction, tests for purity and other tests are same as those mentioned under the constituent salts and Ringer's injection.

Assay: The assay is carried out in the similar way as described under compound sodium chloride injection.

Uses: Like Ringer's injection, Ringer's solution is also used as fluid and electrolyte replenisher.

SODIUM CHLORIDE TABLETS
(Sod. Chlor. Tab.)

The tablets are prepared with sodium chloride and some lubricant and binding agents. The weight of sodium chloride in each tablet of average weight, as determined by the assay, is not less than 95% and not more than 105.0% of the stated amount of sodium chloride.

Tests for identity: The powdered tablets give the reactions characteristic of sodium and chlorides (App. I).

Tests for disintegration: The tablets are not required to comply with this test because they are mainly used in the form of a solution.

Clarity of solution: The solution should be clear if a quantity of the powdered tablets equivalent to 0.65 g of sodium chloride is dissolved in 100 ml of water.

Assay: As usual 20 tablets are weighed and reduced to a fine powder. The assay is carried out by using an accurately weighed quantity of the powdered tablets equivalent to about 0.25 g of sodium chloride in the same way as described under sodium chloride. The weight of sodium chloride, NaCl, in each tablet of average weight is calculated.

The usual strength of the tablet is 0.3 g and the tablets are dissolved in water before administration.

Uses: Same as mentioned under Sodium Chloride.

POTASSIUM REPLACEMENT

Potassium chloride is the drug of choice for oral replacement of potassium preferably as solution. Potassium gluconate is also used. Some of the preparations for potassium replacement are described here.

POTASSIUM SALTS

Potassium ions like sodium ions are essential components of the organisms and they exchange themselves in the living cells. This so happens, because the living cells are in a position to push out sodium ions out of the cells wall by utilising energy, while potassium ions are taken into the cells from the solution surrounding the living cell. In the blood plasma of all the animals one finds a constant ratio of sodium, potassium and calcium ions, which is as follows:

$$Na^+ : K^+ : Ca^{2+} = 25 : 1 : 1 \text{ in chemical equivalence}$$
$$\text{or in other words } 300 : 20 : 10 \text{ in mg/100 g}$$

A human being takes on an average about 2.6 g of potassium specially through vegetable nourishment. The absorption is quite quick. At first, potassium is stored in the liver but after a few hours it is distributed in the body. Its maximum amount is excreted from the kidneys. About 15 g of KCl, if given by mouth, can result in extremely toxic indications. One has to be very careful with an injection of calcium salt which is almost forbidden because there may result a large number of undesirable circulatory reactions. Bradycardia may result if the concentration of potassium in blood reaches 30 mg/100 g of blood plasma; with a concentration of 40 mg/100 g heart blocking results while with 80 mg/100 g of blood plasma would not be tolerated. The normal blood level is 20 mg/100 g.

Potassium is the alkali metal cation found in the intercellular fluids and one of its commercial sources includes potash derived from ashes of beet sugar residues. The chief mineral for potassium compounds is carnallite, which is a double salt of potassium and magnesium chlorides having molecular formula $KCl, MgCl_2 6H_2O$. The compound is fractionally crystallised from water, potassium chloride separating first.

There are a large number of potassium salts of which the official ones are given below in the tabulated form with their molecular formula and molecular weights. Individual salts are detailed separately as per usual scheme.

POTASSIUM CHLORIDE

Chem. formula: KCl   Mol. weight: 74.6

Potassium chloride contains not less than 99.5% and not more than 100.5% of KCl calculated with reference to the substance dried at 105° for two hours.

Preparation: It can be prepared in laboratory by the action of hydrochloric acid on K_2CO_3 or $KHCO_3$.

$$K_2CO_3 + 2HCl \longrightarrow 2KCl + CO_2\uparrow + H_2O$$

$$KHCO_3 + HCl \longrightarrow KCl + CO_2\uparrow + H_2O$$

It is industrially manufactured from the mineral carnallite ($KCl.MgCl_2 6H_2O$). This salt deposit is ground up and treated with steam while the less soluble potassium chloride crystillises out on cooling the solution.

Description: It occurs as colourless, odourless crystals or prismatic or crystalline powder, with saline taste. It is soluble in water; insoluble in alcohol and solvent ether. Its solution is neutral to litmus.

Tests for identity: Gives tests for potassium and chlorides (App. I).

Tests for purity: It is tested for acidity or alkalinity; As; Ba; Fe; Ca and Mg; heavy metals; Na; bromides and iodides; SO_4; and loss on drying and appearance of solution.

Assay: Argentometric titration method called Mohr's method is used.

An accurately weighed quantity (0.25 g) of substance dissolved in water (50 ml) is titrated with 0.1 N silver nitrate using potassium chromate as indicator.

$$KCl + AgNO_3 \longrightarrow AgCl + KNO_3$$

1000 ml N/10 $AgNO_3$ is equivalent to 1/10 KCl.

Or Each ml of N/10 $AgNO_3$ is equivalent to 0.007455 g of KCl.

Uses: It is used as an electrolyte replenisher. It is used when hypokalemia of hypochloremic alkalosis exists as is the case after prolonged diarrhoea or vomiting. It is sometimes used as diuretic. Potassium chloride is an ingredient of sodium chloride compound injection, Ringer's solution etc. It has to be administered very cautiously, especially in cardiac and renal diseases.

Preparations: (i) **Potassium chloride and dextrose injection.** (ii) **Potassium chloride, sodium chloride and dextrose injection.** The I.P. includes full monographs on both the above preparations (p. 1571 and 1572). They are sterile solutions, require labelling instructions and may be dispensable as individual dose injections (containers).

CALCIUM REPLACEMENT
CALCIUM

Chem. formula: Ca   At. wt.: 40.08

Calcium is very abundantly available in nature. Even in the body its percentage compared to other elements is enormous. About 98% of calcium in the body is found in the bones and of the remaining about one per cent of calcium is present in the extracellular fluids. Calcium is highly essential for biochemical processes and its compounds are indispensable for life and hence are extensively used for their therapeutic values.

The effect of calcium in the body is due to the ionic calcium, whose percentage in the commonly used calcium compounds is given below:

Calcium carbonate 40%
Calcium gluconate 9%
Calcium lactate 13%

The daily requirement of calcium for an adult is about 1 g Ca^{2+}. The absorption of calcium from the alimentary canal is erratic and incomplete as phosphate, carbonate and fatty acid salts, which are not easily soluble, are formed. It is believed that absorption of calcium is promoted by vitamin D. Calcium plays an important role in blood coagulation. Hypercalcaemic and hypocalcaemic conditions result in serious diseases. A detailed account of biochemical functions of calcium, which is important and interesting and may run into pages, is not envisaged here. Readers are advised to consult other relevant books.

CALCIUM CHLORIDE
CALCIUM CHLORIDE DIHYDRATE

Chem. formula: $CaCl_2 \cdot 2H_2O$ Mol. wt.: 147

It contains not less than 97% and not more than the equivalent of 103% of $CaCl_2 \cdot 2H_2O$.

Preparation: It can be prepared in the laboratory by the action of hydrochloric acid on calcium, its oxide (lime) or carbonate.

$$2HCl \longrightarrow 2H^+ + 2Cl^-$$
$$Ca^{++} + 2Cl^- \longrightarrow CaCl_2$$

On evaporating the resulting solution to a syrup and then cooling, colourless hexagonal crystals of the hexahydrate, $CaCl_2 \cdot 5H_2O$ are obtained. On heating, it first loses four molecules of water at 200°C to give the dihydrate $CaCl_2 \cdot 2H_2O$ and finally becomes anhydrous on fusion. The dihydrate and the anhydrous salt dissolve in water with evolution of heat while the hexahydrate dissolves with lowering of temperature.

Description: It is a white, crystalline powder, odourless, deliquescent. It is freely soluble in H_2O and alcohol.

Tests for identity: A 10% w/v solution of the sample gives the reaction of calcium and of chloride (App. I).

Tests for purity: It is tested for clarity and colour of solution; acidity or alkalinity; arsenic; heavy metals; aluminium and phosphate; magnesium and alkali salts and iron.

Clarity and colour of solution: A 10% w/v solution is clear and colourless.

Acidity or alkalinity: It is determined by titrating a 10% w/v fresh solution with 0.01 N HCl or 0.01 N NaOH using phenolphthalein solution as an indicator. Not more than 0.2 ml is required for each 10 ml of solution of the sample.

Arsenic: Not more than three parts per million.

Heavy metals: Not more than 10 parts per million. A solution of the sample is prepared by taking 2 g in 25 ml of water.

Aluminium and phosphate: A specified volume of solution (10 ml of a 5% solution) is taken to which two drops of dil. HCl and one drop of phenolphthalein solution are added. Solution of NH_4OH - NH_4Cl is added dropwise to the above test solution until the colour of solution is faintly pink. A few drops in excess are added and the liquid is heated to boiling. No turbidity or precipitate is produced.

Magnesium and alkali salts: Not more than 1.0 per cent. It is determined by taking a specified amount of the sample (1 g), dissolving it in water (50 ml) and adding NH_4Cl (0.5 g). The test is performed as per the procedure given under calcium carbonate starting from "the sol. is boiled to which 50 ml of hot ammonium oxalate is added....".

Iron: A specified amount of the sample (0.3 g) is dissolved in HCl (0.5 ml) and water (25 ml) and the resulting solution shall comply with the limit test for iron.

Assay: An accurately weighed amount of the sample (0.15 g) is dissolved in water (50 ml) and the assay is carried out by following the procedure given in Calcium Carbonate beginning at the words "is titrated with ....". Each ml of 0.05 M disodium edetate $\equiv$ 0.007351 g of $CaCl_2.2H_2O$.

Storage: It is stored in tightly-closed containers.

Uses: As a calcium replenisher, it provides calcium ions in the treatment of hypocalcaemic tetany. As antispasmodic to smooth muscle for treatment of colic arising from lead poisoning. It is used as a specific antidote in case of magnesium poisoning. It is also used in the treatment of hyperkalemia, since it antagonizes the cardiac effects of potassium. As an antiallergic to prevent severe sickness after injection of antitoxins and antisera.

Dose: 1 to 2 g by mouth, 5 to 10 ml of a 10% solution by slow intravenous injection.

Dosage forms: Injection (50 to 100 mg/ml).

CALCIUM CHLORIDE HYDRATED

Chem. formula: $CaCl_2.6H_2O$ Mol. wt.: 219.1

I.P. 85 requires it to contain not less than 98% and note more than the equivalent of 102% of $CaCl_2.H_2O$.

Preparation: Calcium chloride hydrated is prepared by the addition of pure calcium carbonate in slight excess to a hot diluted hydrochloric acid. When the reaction is over, the solution is filtered and evaporated to crystallization.

$$CaCO_3 + 2HCl \longrightarrow CaCl_2 + H_2O + CO_2\uparrow$$

Crystallization is a little difficult and hence the concentrated syrupy liquid is cooled to about $10°$ or even to much lower temperature (refrigeration is sometimes necessary). The crystals are separated by suction and since it is highly hygroscopic, it is transferred immediately to stoppered bottles.

Description: Calcium chloride occurs as white deliquescent odourless crystals or granules with a slight bitter taste. It is soluble in water and alcohol. It reacts with ammonia and combines with eight molecules of ammonia. It has cooling effect.

42.5 g of $CaCl_2$ per 100 g of water freezes at 55°C and hence it is used as refrigerant.

Tests for identity:

(a) On being heated in a dry test tube it melts and expels water.

(b) It gives reactions for Ca and Cl ions (App. I).

Tests for purity: It is tested for alkalinity or acidity; Al; Fe; PO_4; matter insoluble in hydrochloric acid; As; heavy metals; SO_4 and alcohol insoluble matter.

Assay: It is assayed in the same way as calcium carbonate.

1.0 ml of M/20 disodium ethylenediamine tetraacetate is equivalent to 0.01095 g of $CaCl_2.6H_2O$.

Uses: Calcium chloride is considered of value as an acid-forming diuretic and for this purpose it is used like ammonium chloride. It is also antispasmodic to smooth muscle and is indicated in the treatment of colic and in lead poisoning. It is supposed to be an immediate source of calcium ion in the treatment or hypocalcemic tetany. As an electrolyte replenisher, calcium chloride is used for Ringer's solution. Calcium chloride is not preferred over other calcium salts, because it is contraindicated in many ailments and renal insufficiency.

Dose: 1–5 g per day in divided oral doses and 0.6 to 2 g by intravenous injection.

CALCIUM GLUCONATE

Chem. formula: $C_{12}H_{22}CaO_{14}.H_2O$ 　　　　　　　　　　　　　　　　　　Mol. wt.: 448.40

It contains not less than 98% and not more than equivalent of 102% of $C_{12}H_{22}CaO_{14}.H_2O$.

Synthesis: It is prepared by boiling a solution of gluconic acid with a slight excess of calcium carbonate, filtering and crystallizing the product from the filterate.

$$2CH_2(OH)[CH(OH)]_4COOH + CaCO_3 \longrightarrow \left[HOCH_2 - \overset{\overset{\displaystyle H}{|}}{C} - \overset{\overset{\displaystyle H}{|}}{\underset{\underset{\displaystyle OH}{|}}{C}} - \overset{\overset{\displaystyle OH}{|}}{\underset{\underset{\displaystyle OH}{|}}{C}} - \overset{\overset{\displaystyle H}{|}}{\underset{\underset{\displaystyle H}{|}}{C}} - \overset{\overset{\displaystyle H}{|}}{\underset{\underset{\displaystyle OH}{|}}{C}} - COO \right]_2 Ca$$

Description: It is stable in air. Its solution is neutral to litmus paper. It is decomposed by mineral acids into gluconic acid and the calcium salts of the mineral acid used.

It is soluble in water and its solubility increases by boiling the water. It is insoluble in organic solvents.

Tests for identity:

(1) When a drop of $FeCl_3$ test solution is added to 1 ml of a 3% w/v solution of cal. gluconate, it gives a yellow colour.

(2) To a specified amount of sample (0.75 g) in water (7.5 ml) add glacial acetic acid (1 ml) and freshly distilled phenyl hydrazine (1.0 ml). Heat the mixture on a water bath for 30 minutes and allow to cool. Scratch the inner surface of the tube with a glass rod until crystals of

gluconic acid phenyl hydrazide begin to form. Set aside for 10 minutes, filter, dissolve the ppt. in hot water (10 ml), add a small amount of decolourising charcoal and filter in a test tube. Allow the filtrate to cool and scratch the inner surface of the tube. White crystals are obtained, which melt at about 200° with decomposition.

(3) A 10% w/v solution of sample gives the reactions of calcium (App. I).

(4) I.P. 2007 give a new test for identification. It is a thin layer chromatography test. A solution of 2% w/v solution of calcium gluconate RS in water is used as a reference solution for spotting on TLC-plate.

Tests for purity: It is tested for As; clarity and colour of solution; acidity or alkalinity; heavy metals; chloride; sulphate; sucrose and reducing sugar.

Arsenic: Not more than 2 ppm.

Clarity and colour of solution: Dissolve a specified amount of the sample (2 g) in water at a temp. below 60° and dilute with water (to 100 ml). The solution is clear at 60° and is colourless.

Acidity or alkalinity: Dissolve a specified amount of sample (0.5 g) in water (20 ml), add 0.01 N HCl (0.1 ml) and phenolphthalein (0.1 ml). No colour is produced. On addition of 0.01 N NaOH (0.3 ml) a pink colour is produced.

Heavy metals: Not more than 20 ppm. Determined by dissolving a specified amount of sample (1 g) in dil. HCl (4 ml) and sufficient water (to 25 ml).

Chloride: A specified amount of sample (0.5 g) complies with the limit test for chlorides.

Sulphate: A specified amount of sample (2 g) complies with limit test for sulphates.

Sucrose and reducing sugar: Sucrose is not a reducing sugar. It does not reduce Fehling's solution, neither does it yield an osazone. Fehling's solution is potassium cupritartrate solution. When Fehling's solution is warmed with an aldehyde, it is reduced with loss of the blue colour and formation of brown-red cuprous oxide, Cu_2O.

A sufficient amount of the sample (10 ml of 5% w/v) is dissolved in hot water to which is added dil. HCl (2 ml) and is boiled for about 2 minutes. The mixture is cooled and to it is added Na_2CO_3 (15 ml) solution. It is allowed to stand for 5 minutes and filtered. Potassium cupritartrate solution (2 ml) is added to the filtrate (5 ml) and the filtrate is boiled for 2 minutes. No red ppt. is formed, indicating that sucrose and reducing sugar are absent.

In the above test, **sucrose** is boiled with dil. mineral acid and then made alkaline with Na_2CO_3 which leads **sucrose** to be inverted in which form it is capable of reducing Fehling's solution.

$$Sucrose \xrightarrow{\text{Inversion}} D\text{-glucose} + D\text{-fructose}$$
$$(+) \qquad\qquad (-)$$
$$(-) \text{ Invert sugar}$$

Assay: It is based upon the basic principle of complexometric titration.

Dissolve a specified amount of the sample (0.5 g) in warm water (50 ml), cool, add 0.05 M magnesium sulphate (5 ml) and strong NH_3–NH_4Cl solution (10 ml) and titrate with 0.05 M disodium ethylenediamine tetraacetate, using mordant black II mixture as an indicator. Substract the volume of 0.05 M magnesium sulphate from the volume of 0.05 M disodium edetate.

ml of disodium edetate used – ml of magnesium sulphate used = Remainder.

Each ml of remainder = 0.022420 g of $C_{12}H_{22}CaO_{14}.H_2O$.

Use: It is used as a calcium replenisher.

Dose: By I.M. or I.V. injection, 1 to 2 g.

Orally: 1 to 5 g.

CALCIUM GLUCONATE INJECTION

Calcium gluconate injection is a sterile solution of calcium gluconate in water for injection. Upto 5% of calcium gluconate is allowed to be replaced by other suitable calcium salt in order to make a stabilized preparation. The amount of calcium is between 8.5 to 9.4% of the stated content of calcium gluconate.

Tests for identity: Same as calcium gluconate, including TLC test.

pH: Between 6.0 and 8.2.

Pyrogens: When it is tested in a dose of 0.2 g/kg body wt. of rabbit, it passes the test for pyrogens.

Other requirements: Same as stated under injections in Pharmacopoeia of India 85.

Assay: Prepare a solution equivalent to 0.5 g of cal. gluconate in 50 ml of water and carry out the assay as stated under calcium gluconate beginning at the words "add 5.0 ml of 0.05 M $MgSO_4$....".

Each ml of the remainder is equivalent to 0.002004 g of Ca.

Storage: Calcium gluconate injection must be completely free from solid particles, because it is a super-saturated solution and any solid particle can act as a nuclei for crystallization.

Labelling: The following information must be written on the container:

(1) The strength as the percentage w/v of calcium gluconate equivalent to the total amount of calcium present;

(2) The solution containing visible solid particles must be rejected; and

(3) The percentage of stabilising agent.

Use: It is used as a calcium replenisher. It is the calcium salt of choice for I.V. use.

Dose: I.M. or I.V. injection, 1 to 2 g.

Usual strength: 1 g in 10 ml.

CALCIUM GLUCONATE TABLETS

The amount of calcium gluconate in calcium gluconate tablets is between 95% and 105% of the stated amount of $C_{12}H_{22}O_{14}Ca.H_2O$.

Tests for identity: Prepare a 10% w/v warm filtered solution of the tablets. It must comply with tests described under calcium gluconate, including TLC test.

Other requirements: It complies with the requirements stated under tablets in Pharmacopoeia of India, 1985 (p. 500).

Assay: Weigh 20 tablets and powder them. Weigh accurately an amount of the powder equivalent to 0.5 g of calcium gluconate and ignite it gently at first, until free from carbon, cool, add water (10 ml) and sufficient dil. HCl to effect complete solution of the residue. Add dil. NH_3 solution to neutralise the acid and complete the assay stated under calcium gluconate, beginning with "add 0.05 M magnesium sulphate....".

Each ml of the remainder is equivalent to 0.022420 g of $C_{12}H_{22}O_{14}Ca.H_2O$.

Use: It is used as a calcium replenisher.

Dose: 1 to 4 g.

Usual strengths: 0.325 g, 0.5 g, 0.65 g and 1 g.

Storage: The cal. gluconate tablets are stored in well-closed containers.

CALCIUM LACTATE

$$Ca^{++} \begin{bmatrix} H & OH \\ & X \\ H_3C & COO^- \end{bmatrix}_2$$

Chem. formula: $C_6H_{10}CaO_6 \cdot xH_2O$ Mol. wt.: 218.22 (anhydrous)

Calcium lactate is hydrated calcium (RS)–2–hydroxy-propionate or mixtures of the calcium salts of (R)–, (S)– and (RS)–2–hydroxypropionic acid.

Preparation: It is prepared by adding a slight excess of calcium carbonate to hot dil. lactic acid and boiling the resulted mixture for half an hour.

$$2CH_3CH(OH)COOH + CaCO_3 \longrightarrow [CH_3CH(OH)COO]_2Ca + CO_2 + H_2O$$

The hot solution is filtered and the filtrate is evaporated to crystallization.

Description: Calcium lactate is the hydrated calcium salt of 2-hydroxy propionic acid. It contains not less than 98.0% and not more than 102.0% of $C_6H_{10}CaO_6$, calculated with reference to the anhydrous substance.

Calcium lactate occurs as colourless crystals or white granular powder. It is odourless. It is soluble in water and more readily in hot water.

Tests for identity:

(1) A solution of 1:20 in water gives the reactions of calcium (App. I).

(2) A solution acidified with H_2SO_4 and warmed with $K_2Cr_2O_7$ develops the odour of acetaldehyde.

Tests for purity: Calcium lactate is tested for acidity or alkalinity; arsenic; iron; heavy metals; chloride; sulphate; reducing sugars and water.

Acidity or alkalinity: To a solution of sample (10 ml of 5% w/v) and 0.01 N HCl (0.1 ml) add phenolphthalein solution (2 drops), no colour is developed. On addition of 0.01 N NaOH (0.6 ml), however, a pink colour is produced.

Arsenic: Not more than 2 ppm.

Iron: A specfied amount of sample (0.5 g) complies with the limit test for iron.

Heavy metals: Not more than 20 ppm. The solution is prepared by dissolving specified amount of sample (1 g) in dil. HCl (2.5 ml) and water to produce required volume (25 ml).

Chloride: Dissolve a specified amount of the sample (0.5 g) in water by adding HNO_3 (2 ml). The solution complies with the limit test for chloride.

Sulphate: Dissolve a specified amount of the sample (1 g) in water by the addition of HCl (2 ml). The solution complies with the limit test for sulphates.

Reducing sugars: Prepare a 10% w/v sol. of sample in water, add potassium cupritartrate solution and boil. Not more than a slight brick-red ppt. is produced.

Water: Not more than 30% determined on specified amount (1 g) of sample by drying in an oven at 120° for 4 hours.

Assay: An accurately weighed sample (0.3 g) is dissolved in water (50 ml) and the assay is completed as described under calcium gluconate, beginning at the words "add 0.05 M magnesium sulphate (5 ml)....".

Each ml of the remainder $\equiv 0.01091$ g of $C_6H_{10}CaO_6$.

Use: It is used as a calcium replenisher.

Dose: 1 to 5 g.

Storage: It is stored in well-closed containers.

CALCIUM LACTATE TABLETS

Chem. formula: $C_6H_{10}CaO_6.5H_2O$

Calcium lactate tablets contain 95 to 105% of the stated amount of calcium lactate.

Tests for identity:

(1) An aqueous filtered extract of the powdered tablets when warmed with H_2SO_4 and $KMnO_4$ gives odour of acetaldehyde.

(2) The powdered tablets when moistened with HCl is introduced on a platinum wire into the flame of Bunsen burner gives a brick-red colour to the flame.

Disintegration: Maximum time for the tablets to disintegrate is 30 minutes.

Other requirements: Comply with the requirements stated under tablets.

Assay: Assay procedure is same as mentioned under calcium lactate. Take 20 tablets and powder them. Weigh accurately a specified amount of powder (equivalent to 0.3 g) of calcium lactate and dissolve as completely as possible in water (50 ml) and complete the assay described under calcium gluconate beginning at the words "add 5.0 ml of 0.05 M $MgSO_4$....".

Each ml of the remainder is $\equiv 0.01542$ g of $C_6H_{10}CaO_6.5H_2O$.

Use: It is used as a calcium replenisher.

Dose: 1 to 5 g, usual strength of a tablet 0.3 g.

Store: It is stored in air-tight containers.

Labelling: The label on the container should state the quantity of cal. lactate in terms of calcium lactate pentahydrate.

CALCIUM LEVULINATE

Chem. formula: $(CH_3CO.CH_2CH_2COO^-)_2 Ca^{2+}, 2H_2O$ Mol. wt.: 306.3

Calcium levulinate is the dihydrate of calcium 4-oxopentanoate.

It contains 97.5% to 100.5% of $C_{10}H_{14}CaO_6$ in dry state.

Preparation: It is prepared by action of levulinic acid on calcium carbonate.

$$2CH_3COCH_2CH_2COOH + CaCO_3 \longrightarrow (CH_3COCH_2CH_2COO^-)_2 Ca^{2+} + H_2CO_3$$

Description: It is a white, crystalline or amorphous powder with faint and burnt sugar-like odour, bitter and salty taste.

Solubility: It is freely soluble in water and slightly soluble in alcohol but insoluble in ether and chloroform.

Tests for identity:

(A) Prepare a 10% solution of sample in water (0.5 g in 5 ml), add NaOH (5 ml) and filter. To the filtrate add iodine solution (5 ml). A ppt. of iodoform is produced.

(B) Dinitrophenylhydrazine derivative melts at 198°–206°.

(C) A 10% solution in H_2O gives the reactions of calcium (App. I).

Tests for purity: It is tested for melting range; pH; As; heavy metals; reducing sugars and loss on drying.

M. P.: 199°–125°C.

pH: A 10% w/v solution has pH between 7.0–8.5.

Arsenic: Not more than 3 ppm.

Heavy metals: Not more than 20 ppm determined by using 1 g of the substance.

Reducing sugars: It does not give red ppt. with potassium cupritartrate solution. Dissolve the sample (0.5 g) in water (10 ml), add dil. HCl (2 ml), boil for 10 minutes and cool. Add Na_2CO_3 (5 ml) to neutralize free HCl, allow to stand for 5 minutes, dilute with water (20 ml) and filter. The clear filtrate (5 ml) does not give red ppt. with pot. cupritartrate (2 ml) when they are boiled together for one minute.

Loss on drying: 10.5%–12%, determined by using a specified amount of the sample (0.5 g) by drying in vacuo at 60° for 5 hrs.

Assay: An accurately weighed amount of the sample (0.6 g) is dissolved in water (50 ml) and the assay is carried out as described under Calcium Gluconate, beginning at words "add 0.05M Magnesium sulphate (5 ml) ..... "

Each ml of the remainder $\equiv 0.01351$ g of $C_{10}H_{14}CaO_6$.

Storage: It is stored in a well-closed container.

Use: It is used as a calcium replenisher. It is superior to calcium gluconate because of less irritating effect and is hence more suitable for I.M. or S.C. administration.

Dose: Oral, I.V., I.M., S.C. Adults 1 g once a day.

Dosage form: Injection (100 mg).

CALCIUM LEVULINATE INJECTION

Calcium levulinate injection is a sterile solution of Calcium Levulinate in water for injection. It contains 95% to 105% of the stated amount of Calcium Levulinate, $C_{10}H_{14}CaO_6$, $2H_2O$.

Identification: Same as in Calcium Levulinate.

pH: Same as in Calcium Levulinate.

Pyrogens: Complies with the test for pyrogens.

Other requirements: Complies with the requirements stated under injections.

Assay: Same as Calcium Gluconate.

Each ml of remainder $\equiv 0.01532$ g of $C_{10}H_{14}CaO_6$, $2H_2O$.

Storage: Stored in single dose containers.

Use: It is used as a Calcium replenisher.

Dose: I.M. or I.V., 1 g once a day.

Usual strength: 100 mg/ml.

DIBASIC CALCIUM PHOSPHATE

Chem. form: $CaHPO_4$ Mol. wt. 136.1 (anhydrous)

Chem. form: $CaHPO_4.2H_2O$ Mol. wt. 172.1 (dihydrate)

Dibasic Calcium Phosphate is anhydrous or contains two molecules of water of hydration.

Description: White, crystalline powder; odourless.

Solubility: Practically insoluble in water and in ethanol (95%). It dissolves in dilute hydrochloric acid and in nitric acid.

Standards: Dibasic Calcium Phosphate contains not less than 98.0 per cent and not more than 105.0 per cent of $CaHPO_4$ (for anhydrous material) or of $CaHPO_42H_2O$ (for the dihydrate).

Tests for purity: It is tested for acid-insoluble substances; arsenic; heavy metals; barium; iron; carbonate; chloride; sulphate; nitrate; reducing substances; proteinous impurities; and monocalcium and tricalcium phosphates. The limits of the above substances should be within the limits prescribed in the I.P. (p. 845).

Assay: Weigh accurately about 0.3 g and dissolve in a mixture of 5 ml of water and 1 ml of 7 M hydrochloric acid, add 25.0 ml of 0.1 M disodium edetate and dilute to 200 ml with water. Neutralise with strong ammonia solution, add 10 ml of ammonium chloride buffer pH 10.0 and 50 mg of mordant black II mixture and titrate the excess of disodium edetate with 0.1 M zinc sulphate. Each ml of 0.1 M disodium edetate is equivalent to 0.01361 g of $CaHPO_4$ or 0.01721 g of $CaHPO_4,2H_2O$. It is assayed as per I.P. method (p. 846).

Use: It is used as a calcium supplement and as a pharmaceutical aid (excipient).

MAGNESIUM

Magnesium ions like potassium, K^+, occur in the organism especially intracellularly and compete with Ca^{++}. The proportion in weight in the blood plasma of Ca^{2+} to Mg^{2+} is known to be 10:3 and in the erythrocytes about 2:4. There does not occur any deficiency in magnesium, as the diet contains Mg^{2+} in richer amount. In meat and corn the content of magnesium is higher than that of calcium; in vegetables and fruits the proportion is fluctuating. The adults need 0.2 to 0.5 g Mg daily. In the organism the Mg ions are absorbed slowly. Magnesium salts are mostly given orally.

MAGNESIUM REPLACEMENT

Magnesium sulphate can be used orally or as magnesium sulphate injection in the treatment of eclampsia (convulsions and coma) as a central nervous system depressant. Over treatment can cause respiratory paralysis and cardiac depression.

MAGNESIUM SULPHATE
(Synonym: Epsom salt)

Chem. formula: $MgSO_4, 7H_2O$ Mol. weight: 246.47

Magnesium sulphate contains not less than 99.5% and not more than the equivalent of 100.5% of $MgSO_4$ calculated with reference to the substance dried to constant weight at 300°C.

Preparation:

(1) Magnesium sulphate can be prepared on the laboratory scale by neutralising hot, dilute sulphuric acid with magnesium or its oxide or carbonate and evaporating the filtered solution to crystallisation.

$$MgCO_3 + H_2SO_4 \longrightarrow MgSO_4 + H_4O + CO_2\uparrow$$

(2) It is manufactured by the action of sulphuric acid on the native carbonate (magnesite) or on previously powdered and calcined dolomite. When dolomite is used magnesium sulphate passes into solution and sparingly soluble calcium sulphate is deposited.

$$MgCO_3 \cdot CaCO_3 + 2H_2SO_4 \longrightarrow MgSO_4 + CaSO_4\downarrow + 2H_2O + 2CO_2\uparrow$$

The liquid is filtered and the filtrate is evaporated to crystallization.

The crystals have the composition $MgSO_4.7H_2O$.

It is also produced in large quantities from magnesium salt occurring in brine, used for the extraction of bromine. The liquors after removal of bromine are treated with milk of lime, thus precipitating magnesium salt as magnesium hydroxide. Sulphur dioxide and air is passed through the suspension of magnesium hydroxide.

$$Mg(OH)_2 + SO_2 + O \longrightarrow MgSO_4 + H_2O$$

Description: It occurs as colourless crystals which are usually needlelike. It is odourless and has cool, saline and bitter taste. It effloresces in warm dry air. It is soluble in one part of water, sparingly soluble in alcohol and dissolved slowly in one part of glycerin.

Tests for purity: It is tested for arsenic; iron; heavy metals; loss on drying and chloride.

Assay: An accurately weighed amount of about 0.3 g of the sample is taken in water (50 ml) and strong ammonia-ammonium chloride solution (10 ml) and titrated with 0.05 M disodium EDTA using mordant black II mixture (0.1 g) as indicator. The end point is achieved when the pink colour is discharged to the blue.

Each ml of 0.05 M disodium EDTA ≡ 0.00602 g $MgSO_4$.

Storage: It is stored in well-closed containers.

Uses: It is used as cathartic, osmotic laxative and in the treatment of elecrolyte deficiency.

Dose: 2 to 16 g.

PHYSIOLOGICAL ACID-BASE BALANCE

Most metabolic reactions in the body occur within a very narrow pH range. During metabolism, acids like carbonic acid (from CO_2) and lactic acid are constantly being produced. Hence the body utilizes several efficient buffer systems that can maintain the acid-base balance.

The major buffer systems in the body are:

- Bicarbonate/carbonic acid system (HCO/H_2CO_3) in plasma and kidneys.
- Monohydrogen phosphate/dihydrogen phosphate system $HPO_4^{2-}/H_2PO_4^-$) in cells and kidneys.
- Haemoglobin (Hb) buffer system in red blood cells - for every millimole of oxygen that dissociates from Hb 0.7 millimole H^+ is removed.
- Plasma proteins (especially the imidazole group of histidine). Circulating proteins have a net negative charge and are capable of binding H^+.

Acid-Base Disorders

Acid-base disorders can occur due to a variety of reasons. The normal pH of arterial blood is 7.35–7.45. When the pH of blood is less or more than the normal values, it is termed *acidemia* and *alkalemia* respectively. A disorder due initially to respiratory dysfunction is termed primary respiratory acidosis or alkalosis. If the disorder is due to a change in bicarbonate level (a renal or metabolic function), it is termed as a *nonrespiratory (metabolic) disorder.*

Because the body's cellular and metabolic activities are pH dependent, the body tries to return the pH towards normal whenever an imbalance occurs. This action is termed *compensation.*

Acidosis

When the body's acid level increases (and/or alkalie level decreases) below normal, and the pH drops slightly below 7.35, the condition is called acidosis. If the cause is respiratory, then the condition is called respiratory acidosis.

Metabolic acidosis can occur as a result of diabetes, renal failure or excessive loss of bicarbonate from diarrhea or drainage from a biliary, pancreatic, or intestinal fistula. Non-respiratory acidosis may also be caused by the direct administration of an acid-producing substance, such as ammonium chloride or calcium chloride. Respiratory acidosis can occur due to cardiac disease, lung damage or drowning.

The compensatory mechanism of the body in acidosis includes hyperventilation, causing increased excretion of carbonic acid as CO_2, increased acid excretion by $Na^+ - H^+$ exchange, increased NH_3 formation, and HCO^{3-} reabsorption.

Alkalosis

Alkalosis is the condition where the body's acid level decreases below normal, and the pH rises slightly above 7.45.

Metabolic alkalosis can occur as a result of vomiting, administration of excess alkali or potassium ions. Respiratory alkalosis can occur due to fever, hysteria, anoxia and salicylate poisoning.

The body compensates for alkalosis by retention of CO_2 causing increased H_2CO_3 concentration. decreased $Na^+- H^+$ exchange, decreased NH_3 formation. The kidneys compensate by excreting HCO_3^- and retaining H^+.

ELECTROLYTES USED IN ACID-BASE THERAPY

Various salts may be used in acid-base therapy. Metabolic acidosis may be treated with the sodium salts of bicarbonate, lactate, acetate and citrate. These salts decrease the bicarbonate deficit in the body either by providing the bicarbonate ion or by providing anions which will be degraded in the body to CO_2 (by the TCA cycle or citric acid cycle or Krebs cycle). The carbon dioxide, by the action of carbonic anhydrase, will form bicarbonate and thereby reduce the bicarbonate deficit.

Salts used in the treatment of metabolic acidosis are:

Sodium acetate, potassium acetate, sodium bicarbonate, potassium bicarbonate, sodium biphosphate, potassium citrate, and sodium lactate. They are administered either as tablets, infusions, injections or as a combination therapy with other electrolytes.

Metabolic alkalosis has been treated with NH_4Cl. It acts in the kidney to retard Na^+-H^+ exchange. It is rarely recommended as it may cause potassium and sodium depletion.

POTASSIUM ACETATE

Chem. formula: CH_3COOK Mol. weight: 98.14

Potassium acetate contains not less than 99% of CH_3COOK calculated with reference to the substance dried to constant weight at 105°.

Preparation: It is prepared by the reaction between acetic acid and potassium carbonate or bicarbonate till effervescence ceases. The filtered solution is evaporated to dryness. The residue is fused and allowed to solidify.

$$CH_3COOH + KHCO_3 \longrightarrow CHO_3COOK + CO_2 + H_2O$$

Description: It is a white powder with acetous odour. Its taste is saline or slightly alkaline. It is very deliquescent. It melts at 290°C and on strong heating it leaves residue of K_2CO_3 along with carbon residue.

$$2CH_3COOK + 4O_2 \longrightarrow K_2CO_3 + 3CO_2 + 3H_2O$$

This salt gets dissolved in H_2O (0.5 parts); the solution is alkaline. It dissolves in 3 parts of alcohol.

$$CH_3COOK + K-OH \longrightarrow CH_3COOH + KOH$$

Tests for identity: It gives reactions for potassium and ions (App. I).

Tests for purity: It is tested for Cl; SO_4; heavy metals; Ca; Al; Na; alkalinity and loss on drying.

Assay: An accurately weighed quantity (about 2 g) of the substance is heated until it is fully carbonised. To the cooled and carbonised residue is then added a mixture of water (50 ml) and excess of 0.5 N sulphuric acid (50 ml). It is then boiled, filtered and washed with water. The excess of acid in the filtrate and washings is titrated against 0.5 N sodium hydroxide using methyl orange as indicator.

1000 ml of N/2 H_2SO_4 is equivalent to $\frac{1}{2}CH_3COOK$.

Or each ml of N/2 H_2SO_4 is equivalent to 0.04907 g of CH_3COOK.

Storage: Potassium acetate is preserved in a well-closed container.

Uses: It is used as diuretic and diphoretic. It is a systemic and urinary alkaliser. It is also used for effects of potassium ion. Indiscriminate use sometimes produces toxic manifestations of hyperkalemia.

Dose: 1–3 g in divided doses in solution form.

SODIUM BICARBONATE
(Synonym: Baking soda)

Chem. formula: $NaHCO_3$ Mol. weight: 84.0

It contains not less than 99% of $NaHCO_3$.

Preparation: It is commonly prepared by Solvay process which is also known as ammonia soda process. In this process brine is saturated with ammonia to remove traces of impurities, like Mg and Fe, solution filtered and heated to a temperature of 30°C.

The warm solution is then allowed to descend the carbonating tower and meets an ascending current of carbon dioxide. The following reactions occur:

$$2NH_3 + Mg^{++} + 2H_2O \longrightarrow Mg(OH)_2 + 2NH_4^+$$
$$H_2O + CO_2 \longrightarrow H_2CO_3$$
$$NH_3 + H_2CO_3 \longrightarrow 2HN_4^+ + HCO_3^-$$
$$Na^+ + HCO_3^- \longrightarrow NaHCO_3$$

or

$$H_2O + CO_2 + NH_3 \longrightarrow NH_4HCO_3$$
$$NH_4HCO_3 + NaCl \longrightarrow NaHCO_3 + NH_4Cl$$

Since it is sparingly soluble in water at a temperature of about 15°C or below, the face of the tower is cooled to enchance the precipitation. The precipitate is then filtered and dried.

The bicarbonate obtained by this method does not comply with the requirements of I.P., so the bicarbonate is ignited to get Na_2CO_3.

$$2NaHCO_3 \longrightarrow Na_2CO_3 + CO_2 + H_2O$$

Na_2CO_3 is then dissolved in pure water and CO_2 is passed through pure solution to saturation.

$$Na_2CO_3 + H_2O + CO_2 \longrightarrow 2NaHCO_3$$

The solution is cooled and the precipitated bicarbonate is filtered and dried.

Another method, the laboratory process, is by bubbling CO_2 into solution of NaOH.

$$2NaOH + CO_2 \longrightarrow Na_2CO_3 + H_2O$$
$$Na_2CO_3 + H_2O + CO_2 \longrightarrow 2NaHCO_3$$

Description It is a white crystalline powder with saline taste. It is soluble in 10 parts of water and insoluble in alcohol; when it is ignited to a temperature of 100°C sesquicarbonate Na_2CO_3, $NaHCO_3$, $2H_2O$ is formed 1% w/v solution has pH not more than 8.6.

Tests for identity: It yields reactions characteristic of sodium and carbonates (App. I).

Tests for purity: It is tested for alkalinity; aluminium; calcium and insoluble matter; As; Fe; heavy metals; Cl; SO_4 and ammonium compounds.

Assay: Since it is an alkali it is assayed by titration with acid. The solution of the substance (about 1 g in 20 ml of water) is titrated with 0.5 N H_2SO_4, using methyl orange as an indicator.

$$2NaHCO_3 + H_2SO_4 \longrightarrow Na_2SO_4 + 2CO_2 + 2H_2O$$

1000 ml of 0.5 N H_2SO_4 is equivalent to 1/2 g $NaHCO_3$.

Or each ml of 0.5 N H_2SO_4 is equivalent to 0.042 grams of $NaHCO_3$.

Storage: Sodium bicarbonate is preserved in a well-closed container.

See also assay method in I.P. 2007, which uses 1.5 g dissolved in 50 ml water and titrating with 1 M HCl, using methyl orange as indicator.

Uses: Sodium bicarbonate is used as an antacid, which reduces acidity of gastric juice. It reacts with hydrochloric acid, producing carbon dioxide and giving rise to epigastric distress. Since it has lot of disadvantages as a gastric antacid, other gastric antacids are perferred. However, it is specific in the treatment of systemic acidosis. It is also an effective antipuritic and finds use as an ingredient in effervescent mixtures, alkaline solution and douches.

Doses: 1-4 g.

SODIUM BICARBONATE INJECTION

Sodium Bicarbonate Injection is a sterile solution of sodium bicarbonate in water for injection containing not less than 94 per cent and not more than 106 per cent of the stated amount. The label should state the percentage of w/v of sodium bicarbonate.

Tests for identity and **tests for purity** are the same as described under sodium bicarbonate above.

The injection is tested for pyrogens and is required to comply with the test for pyrogens, using a quantity containing not less than 0.25 g of sodium bicarbonate. The test for pyrogens is described in I.P. on page 1018.

Assay is performed using an accurately measured volume equivalent to about 1 g of sodium bicarbonate and titrating with 0.5 N hydrochloric acid using solution of methyl orange as indicator.

Each ml of 0.5 N hydrochloric acid is equivalent to 0.042 g $NaHCO_3$.

Usual strength of sodium bicarbonate injection is 1.4 per cent w/v.

COMPOUND SODIUM BICARBONATE TABLETS
(Co. Sod. Bicarb. Tab.)

Compound Sodium Bicarbonate tablets contain Sodium Bicarbonate and Mentha Oil. The weight of total carbonate, calculated as $NaHCO_3$, in each tablet of average weight, as determined by the assay described below, is equivalent to not less than 0.30 g and not more than 0.35 g of $NaHCO_3$.

Each tablet contains:

Sodium bicarbonate .... 0.320 g

Mentha oil .... 0.004 ml

The tablets are compressed by moist granulation method.

The tablets are tested for sodium and bicarbonate.

The tablets are assayed in similar way as described under Sodium Bicarbonate. Twenty tablets are taken, powdered and an accurate amount of the powder is assayed and the weight of $NaHCO_3$ in each tablet of average weight is calculated.

The tablets are preserved in a well-closed container and stored in a cool place.

Dose: 2 to 6 tablets. The tablets should be allowed to dissolve slowly in the mouth.

POTASSIUM BICARBONATE
(Synonym: Potassium Hydrogen Carbonate

Chem. formula: $KHCO_3$ Mol. weight: 100.1

Potassium Bicarbonate contains not less than 99.0% of $KHCO_3$. It is not official in I.P. 2007.

Preparation: It is prepared by passing CO_2 through a saturated solution of K_2CO_3. The solution is filtered and evaporated to crystallization (below 60°C).

$$K_2CO_3 + CO_2 + H_2O = 2KHCO_3$$

When the temperature exceeds 70°C it gets decomposed to K_2CO_3.

Description: It occurs as colourless, transparent, monoclinic prism or crystalline mass or white granular powder. It is odourless but has saline and feeble alkaline taste. It is soluble in water but not in alcohol.

Tests for identity: Yields reactions characteristic of potassium and bicarbonate (App. I). pH of 1.0 per cent solution is not more than 8.6 normal.

Tests for purity: It is tested for Cl, SO_4, heavy metals, carbonate, Al, Ca and insoluble matter, As and Na.

Assay: An accurately weighed quantity (1.5 g) is dissolved in water (20 ml) and titrated with 0.5 N sulphuric acid using methyl orange as indicator.

$$2KHCO_3 + H_2SO_4 \longrightarrow K_2SO_4 + 2CO_2 + 2H_2O$$

1000 ml of N/2 H_2SO_4 is equivalent to 1/2 $KHCO_3$.

Or 1 ml of 0.5 N sulphuric acid is equivalent to 0.05005 g of $KHCO_3$.

Storage: It is preserved in a well-closed container.

Uses: It is used as a pharmaceutical aid and as antacid and electrolyte replenisher. This salt is less prescribed as compared to sodium bicarbonate which is cheaper and less toxic. It has sometimes been used as a diuretic.

Dose: 1–3 g per day in divided doses.

SODIUM ACID PHOSPHATE
(Synonym: Sodium Dihydrogen Phosphate)

Chem. formula: $NaH_2PO_4.2H_2O$ Mol. weight: 156.0

Sodium acid phosphate contains not less than 98.0% and not more than the equivalent of 100.5% of $NaH_2PO_4 \cdot 2H_2O$.

Preparation:

(1) It is prepared by adding a solution of phosphoric acid to a solution of sodium phosphate in required proportions and evaporating the resulting solution to crystallization.

$$H_3PO_4 + Na_2HPO_4 \longrightarrow 2NaH_2PO_4$$

(2) It can be prepared by adding sodium carbonate gradually to hot dilute solution of phosphoric acid until the liquid is alkaline. To the resulting sodium phosphate is added a further quantity of the same volume of phosphoric acid as before and the resulting solution is crystallized.

$$H_3PO_4 + Na_2CO_3 \longrightarrow Na_2HPO_4 + H_2O + CO_2$$
$$Na_2HPO_4 + H_3PO_4 \longrightarrow 2NaH_2PO_4$$

Description: It is a white or colourless crystalline substance which is odourless with acid and saline taste, soluble in water but insoluble in alcohol.

Tests for identity: Gives reactions for sodium and phosphate (App. I). 5% w/v solution has pH 4.3 to 4.5.

Tests for purity: It is tested for As; Ca and Mg; heavy metals; Cl; SO_4; as well as for Na_2HPO_4.

For Na_2HPO_4 1 g of substance is dissolved in 50 ml of H_2O which should require not more than 1 ml of 0.1 N sulphuric acid for neutralisation.

Assay: It is assayed by acidimetry. The solution of NaH_2PO_4 (3 g in 100 ml) is titrated with 0.5 N NaOH using phenolphthalein as indicator, after adding sufficient quantity of sodium chloride (25 g):

$$NaH_2PO_4 + NaOH \longrightarrow Na_2HPO_4 + H_2O$$

1000 ml of N/2 NaOH is equivalent to 1/2 $NaH_2PO_4 \cdot 2H_2O$.

Or each ml of 0.5 N NaOH is equivalent to 0.0780 g of $NaH_2PO_4 \cdot 2H_2O$.

Storage: Sodium acid phosphate is preserved in a well-closed container.

Uses: In large doses it is used as a laxative. It is a urinary acidifier and thus it indirectly acts as a urinary antiseptic due to acidic pH which prevents the growth of microorganisms.

SODIUM CITRATE

Chem. formula: $CH_2(COONa)C(OH)(COONa).CH_2(COONa).2H_2O$ Mol. Weight: 294.1

Sodium citrate contains not less than 99.0 per cent and not more than equivalent of 101.0 per cent of $C_6H_5C_7Na_3.2H_2O$.

Preparation: Sodium citrate is prepared by adding sodium carbonate to a solution of citric acid until effervescence ceases. The solution is evaporated and granules are obtained.

$$3Na_2CO_3 + 2H_3C_6H_5O_7 \longrightarrow 2Na_3C_6H_5O_7 + 3CO_2 + 3H_2O$$

Description: Sodium citrate occurs as colourless crystals or white crystalline powder, which is stable in air. It has a cooling, saline taste and dissolves in water (1 g in 1.5 ml) and in boiling water (1 g in 0.6 ml), but is insoluble in alcohol. The aqueous solution should be neutral to phenolphthalein (though it is slightly alkaline to litmus).

Tests for identity: It gives reactions characteristic of sodium and citrates (App. I).

Tests for purity: It is tested for acidity or alkalinity; chloride; sulphate; oxalate; arsenic; tartrates; heavy metals; and readily carbonizable substances.

The aqueous solution of sodium citrate is alkaline in reaction because of the hydrolysis that takes place.

$$C_6H_5O_7Na_3 + 3H_2O \rightleftharpoons C_6H_5O_4(OH)_3 + 3NaOH$$

For oxalate: 1 g of the substance is dissolved in a mixture of 1 ml of water and 3 ml of hydrochloric acid and to the solution are added 4 ml of alcohol and 4 drops of calcium chloride. The mixture on being allowed to stand for one hour should remain clear.

Readily carbonizable substances: When 1 g of the substance is heated with 10 ml of sulphuric acid in the boiling water bath for one hour not more than a pale brown colour is produced.

Assay: It is assayed with the help of potentiometric titration method. The drug sample is acidified by using glacial acetic acid and heating to about 50°C. A blank titration must also be done.

An accurately weighed amount of about 0.25 g of the sample is dissolved in 50 ml of glacial acetic acid by heating to about 50°. The solution is cooled and titrated with 0.1 N perchloric acid ($HClO_4$), determining the end point potentiometrically. A blank determination as stated above is done and any necessary correction made.

Each ml of 0.1 N $HClO_4 \equiv 0.008602$ g of $C_6H_5O_7Na_3$ (sodium citrate).

Storage: Sodium citrate is preserved in a tight container.

Uses: It is used as an anticoagulant and systemic antacid. As an anticoagulant it is used to prevent the clotting of blood, which is stored.

Sodium citrate is also used as an expectorant and systemic alkaliser. In the body sodium citrate is oxidised and excreted in urine as bicarbonate. It can be given orally for acidoses and for overcoming excessive urinary acidity. It is also known to increase the urinary excretion of calcium. Sodium citrate is also used as a pharmaceutical aid as it prevents darkening of preparation containing tannins with iron.

Dose: 1–2 g diluted with water every two hours as expectorant and 1–4 g, 3–4 times a day as systemic antacid.

Preparations:

1. Sodium Citrate Anticoagulant Injection.
2. Sodium Citrate Tablets.

SODIUM CITRATE ANTICOAGULANT INJECTION
(Sod. Cit. Anticoag. Inj.)

Sodium Citrate Anticoagulant injection contains not less than 3.8 and not more than 4.2 per cent w/v of $C_6H_5O_7Na_3.H_2O$.

Ingredients:

Sodium citrate .... 40 g

Water for injection, sufficient to produce .... 1000 ml

Preparation: Sodium citrate is dissolved in 900 ml water for injection and the solution is filtered and its volume is made up to 1000 ml by adding sufficient water for injection. The solution is immediately sterilised by heating in an autoclave or by filtration.

The injection contains no bacteriostatic agents. A 3.02 per cent solution of Sodium Citrate Anticoagulant injection is said to be isotonic.

Description: It is a clear and colourless solution.

Tests for identity: It gives the reaction characteristic of sodium and citrate (App. I).

Reaction: The injection has pH between 6.4 and 7.5.

Test for pyrogens: It should comply with the test for pyrogens. The injection should also comply with all the other I.P. requirements for injection.

Assay: It is assayed by evaporating a known volume of injection to dryness and igniting the residue carefully and dissolving it in an excess of standardised sulphuric acid with the help of heat, and titrating the residual acid after filtration with standardised sodium hydroxide solution. The strength of sulphuric acid and sodium hydroxide solution is 0.5 N and since citric acid is a tribasic acid, the equivalent weight is 1/3 of the molecular weight.

The I.P. 85 assay is reproduced hereunder:

Measure 25 ml, evaporate to dryness and carefully ignite the residue until it is thoroughly charred. After allowing the carbonised mass to cool, disintegrate it with the aid of a stout glass rod and transfer the mass and the crucible to a beaker. Add 50 ml of water and 50 ml of 0.5 N sulphuric acid, cover the beaker with a watch glass and boil the contents for thirty minutes. Filter the solution, wash the residue with hot water, until the washings cease to redden blue litmus paper. Determine the residual acid in the cooled filtrate by titration with 0.5 N sodium hydroxide, using solution of methyl orange as indicator.

Each ml of 0 5 N sulphuric acid is equivalent to 0.04902 g of $C_6H_5O_7Na_3 \cdot 2H_2O$.

Storage: Sodium Citrate Anticoagulant injection may cause the separation of small solid particles from a glass container. A solution containing such particles must not be used. Sodium Citrate Anticoagulant injection kept in a container closed with cotton wool is used within one month after its preparation. It may be stored for a longer period in fused glass container.

Uses: As anticoagulant for plasma and for blood for fractionation.

(Also see under Sodium Citrate above.)

SODIUM CITRATE TABLETS
(Sod. Cit. Tab.)

Sodium Citrate tablets may be prepared by usual process and the weight of sodium citrate, $C_6H_5O_7Na_3 \cdot 2H_2O$, in each tablet of average weight is not less than 95.0% and not more than 105.0% of the stated amount of sodium citrate.

Tests for identity: The powder of the tablets gives the reactions characteristic of sodium and citrates.

Disintegration: The tablets should not take more than three minutes to disintegrate.

Clarity of solution: The solution is clear if a quantity of the tablet equivalent to 0.65 g of sodium citrate is dissolved in 100 ml of water.

Assay: As usual the assay is carried out by weighing 20 tablets and reducing them to a fine powder. The assay is the same as described under sodium citrate. The weight of Sodium Citrate in each tablet of average weight is then calculated.

Uses: Same as mentioned under Sodium Citrate. Since the tablets are given to infants, they should be dissolved in water and added to the feed.

Dose: 1–4 g.

Usual strength: 120 mg.

POTASSIUM CITRATE

$$\underset{\text{COOK}}{\text{HO}}\diagdown\underset{\text{COOK}}{\diagup}\underset{\text{COOK}}{\diagdown}\underset{\text{COOK}}{\diagup}\;,\;H_2O$$

Chem. formula: $C_6H_5O_7K_3, H_2O$ Mol. weight: 324.4

Potassium citrate contains not less than 99% and not more than the equivalent of 101% of potassium citrate.

Preparation: It is prepared by adding potassium bicarbonate or potassium carbonate to a solution of citric acid until effervescence ceases. The solution is filtered and evaporated.

$$C_6H_5O_7H_3 + 3KHCO_3 \longrightarrow C_6H_5O_7K_3 + 3H_2O + 3CO_2\uparrow$$
$$\text{Citric acid} \qquad\qquad\qquad \text{Pot. citrate}$$

Description: It occurs as colourless or white crystal or granular powder, odourless with saline taste. It is soluble in water and glycerol but insoluble in alcohol.

Tests for identity: Yields reactions characteristic of potassium and citrates (see App. I).

Tests for purity: It is tested for acidity or alkalinity; As; heavy metals; Na; Cl; oxalate; SO_4; and readily carbonisable matter.

Assay: To an accurately weighed amount (about 0.15 g) of potassium citrate is added 20 ml of glacial acetic acid and the vessel is heated at about 50° to effect solution. The sol. is cooled and to it is added 0.25 ml 1-naphtholbenzein sol. and titrated with 0.1 N perchloric acid, until a green colour is obtained. A blank titration is performed and any necessary correction is made.

Each ml of 0.1 N perchloric acid $\equiv 0.01021$ g of $C_6H_5K_3O_7$.

Storage: Potassium citrate is preserved in a well-closed container.

Uses: It is used as an osmotic diuretic. It is a systemic urinary alkalizer. It is sometimes used as an expectorant.

AMMONIUM CHLORIDE

Chem. formula: NH_4Cl Mol. wt.: 53

Ammonium chloride contains not less than 99.5% and not more than 100.5% of NH_4Cl, calculated with reference to the dried substance.

Preparation: Ammonium chloride is made by neutralizing hydrochloric acid with ammonia and evaporating the solution to dryness.

$$NH_3 + HCl \longrightarrow NH_4Cl$$

The product is purified by recrystallization.

Description: It is a white crystalline powder or colourless crystals, odourless with saline taste.

Tests for identity: It gives reactions of ammonium salts and chlorides (App. I).

Tests for purity: It is tested for clarity and colour of solution; reaction; arsenic; heavy metals; barium sulphate: thiocyanate and sulphated ash; and calcium.

Clarity and colour of solution: A 10% w/v solution is clear and colourless.

Reaction: A 5% w/v solution has a pH between 4.5 to 6.0.

Test for arsenic: Not more than 4 ppm.

Test for heavy metals: A solution of sample (2 g in 25 ml of water) contains not more than 10 ppm.

Test for barium: No turbidity is produced within two hours, when 0.5 g of the sample is dissolved in 10 ml of water and 1 ml of dil. H_2SO_4.

Test for sulphate: 2 g complies with the limit test for sulphates.

Test for thiocynate: 10 ml of a 10% solution is acidified with HCl, which on addition of a few drops of ferric chloride solution does not produce red colour.

Sulphated ash: Not more than 0.1%.

Loss on drying: Not more than 1% determined on 1 g by drying in an oven at 105°.

Assay: The assay is based upon the principle of **Formal Titration** which is a special modification in the direct titration of weak acids. This is done in the presence of formaldehyde.

$$NH_4Cl + HCHO \xrightarrow{H_2O} H-\overset{\displaystyle \|}{\underset{\displaystyle NH}{C}}-H + HCl + H_2O$$

Imine

$$HCl + NaOH \longrightarrow NaCl + H_2O$$

$$H-\overset{\displaystyle \|}{\underset{\displaystyle O}{C}}-H + NH_4Cl + H-\overset{\displaystyle \|}{\underset{\displaystyle O}{C}}-H \xrightarrow{H_2O} H_2N-\overset{\displaystyle \|}{\underset{\displaystyle O}{CH_2}} + H_2O$$

An accurately weighed sample (0.1 g) is dissolved in water (10 ml) to which is added a mixture of formaldehyde solution (5 ml), previously neutralised to dil. phenolphthalein solution and water (20 ml). After 2 minutes, the acid which is formed is titrated with 0.1 N NaOH using a further 0.2 ml. of dil. phenolphthalein solution.

Each ml of 0.1 N NaOH $\equiv$ 0.005349 g of NH_4Cl.

Storage: It is stored in tightly-closed containers.

Uses: It is used as an expectorant, diuretic and systemic acidifier.

AMMONIUM CHLORIDE TABLETS

These are enteric coated tablets and each tablet should contain not less than 95% and not more than 105% of the stated amount of ammonium chloride, as per assay process described hereafter. The principle of assay is the same as described under pure ammonium chloride, i.e. Volhard's method for precipitation type of titration is used. In this method an excess of standard silver nitrate is used and after filtration the excess of silver left behind unreacted is determined with standard solution of ammonium thiocyanate.

Assay: Twenty tablets are weighed and they are reduced to fine powder. From the powder an accurately weighed portion of the tablets' powder, representing about 0.2 g equivalent of ammonium chloride is transferred to a beaker containing 40 ml of water. The suspension is stirred occasionally during 30 minutes, filtered and washed until the last washing yields a clear solution when 2 drops of solution of silver nitrate and 1 ml of dilute nitric acid are added to 5 ml of the last washing. The filtrate and the washings are combined and transferred to a 500 ml glass-stoppered flask to which 50 ml of 0.1 N silver nitrate, 3 ml of nitric acid and 5 ml of nitrobenzene are added. The flask is shaken vigorously and 2 ml of solution of ferric ammonium sulphate is added and the solution is titrated for the excess of silver nitrate with 0.1 N ammonium thiocyanate.

$$NH_4Cl + AgNO_3 \longrightarrow NH_4NO_3 + AgCl\downarrow$$
$$AgNO_3 + NH_4SCN \longrightarrow \underset{\substack{\text{Silver} \\ \text{thiocyanate}}}{AgSCN} + NH_4NO_3$$

Each ml of 0.1 N silver nitrate is equivalent to 0.005349 g of ammonium chloride. The weight of ammonium chloride in each tablet is then calculated on the basis of average weight.

Note: In this assay method nitrobenzene is used to coat the precipitate of silver chloride. This coating of silver chloride decreases the solubility of silver chloride and prevents it from reacting with the ammonium thiocyanate (to silver thiocyanate). In the absence of nitrobenzene more ammonium thiocyanate will be required during titration. The nitric acid is used to prevent the precipitation of silver as silver carbonte and phosphate. Besides, nitric acid prevents hydrolysis of ferric ammonium sulphate, which is used as an indicator in this titration.

The usual strength of ammonium chloride in a tablet is 0.5 g.

Dose: 6 to 12 tablets in divided doses.

ELECTROLYTE COMBINATION THERAPY

Electrolyte combination therapy involves therapy with solutions containing a combination of electrolytes. Ideally combinations should be tailored to the needs of each individual. This is not feasible with regard to cost and sterility and hence a selection is made from a broad spectrum of commercially available electrolyte solutions. The combination products can be divided into two groups namely fluid replacement, intended to supply normal requirements for water and electrolytes for patients who cannot take it orally; and electrolyte replacement.

Official combination electrolyte infusions are Ringer's solution, lactated Ringer's injection, sodium chloride and dextrose tablets, and oral rehydration salt (ORS).

INORGANIC DIURETICS

Diuretics are drugs that increase the flow of urine. They are mainly used for the treatment of oedematous conditions and indicated in fluid overload situations such as congestive heart failure, nephritic syndrome, cirrhosis of liver, etc. They lead to renal excretion of water along with varying proportions of sodium and potassium.

Potassium Salts

Since the kidneys rapidly excrete excess potassium, potassium salts are used as diuretics, as a certain volume of urine will be excreted to keep the K salt in solution. Hypokalemia may occur with thiazide and loop diuretics and potassium supplements may be given to counteract this effect.

Potassium acetate and potassium citrate are both, as diuretics and as electrolytes, used in acid-base therapy. They have been described earlier in this chapter.

Compounds of Mercury

The diuretic action of inorganic and organic mercury salts was due to their reacting with protein sulfhydryl groups, thereby inactivating specific enzymes of the renal tubules. The resulting prevention of sodium ion reabsorption leads to sodium and water diuresis. The inorganic salts like *mercuric chloride* can be dissipated throughout the body, thereby causing undesirable toxic effects. *Chlormerodrin* N.F. XIII was the one official mercurial diuretic administered orally. Mercurial diuretics although effective are now almost never used because of their nephrotoxicity.

Ammonium Chloride

Ammonium chloride is a systemic acidifier and has diuretic effect. The actual diuresis is brought about by increase in chloride ion, resulting in its excretion with an equivalent amount of cation and an isoosmotic equivalent of water. The above mechanism therefore also causes sodium and potassium depletion, as there must be a cation excreted for each chloride ion excreted. Due to the risk of ammonia toxicity, NH_4Cl is contraindicated in patients with impaired hepatic or renal function.

Lithium

The lithium ion has diuretic action and lithium chloride was once used for this action and as a component of salt substitutes used by patients on salt-free diets. It has been discontinued because of its toxic nature.

Essential and Trace Ions

Keeping minerals in proper balance throughout the body while providing all of them in sufficient quantities needed for optimal health is complex. Balance is important to all areas of our lives and nutrition, but it is particularly crucial when it comes to essential and trace minerals. It is becoming increasingly evident when studying the relationship of minerals to human health that keeping the level of mineral in balance in every tissue, fluid, cell and organ in the human body may be the key to maintaining human health. Minerals should be ionic to be readily absorbed through transfer in the small intestine. They also have unique properties that distinguish them from each other, and allow them to freely take part in biochemical communication throughout the body.

Elements found in the body in mg/kg concentrations are called trace elements, whereas in concentrations of μg/kg or less are ultra-trace elements. Essential and trace ions are required by the body in minute concentrations for its normal functioning. Its deficiency results in impairment of certain biologic or biochemical functions, which can be corrected by the replacement of the ion. Excess concentrations may be toxic. Deficiency of trace elements can occur as a result of decreased intake as in malnutrition states, decreased absorption, conditions resulting in chronic loss, chronic disease of liver and kidney, alcoholism (ex. zinc deficiency), or as a result of genetic abnormalities. Excessive or toxic concentrations can occur as a result of accidental or deliberate ingestion of the ion-containing compound (acute toxicity), continuous use of utensils containing the element (chronic toxicity) or impaired excretion of the ion from the body.

Essential and trace mineral supplements are available orally in their salt form, as oral colloidal mineral solutions or from plant sources to enable better absorption and bioavailability.

COPPER

Copper plays an important role as a component of enzymes or proteins involved in redox reactions. Certain enzymes containing copper are cytochrome c oxidase, tyrosinase and lysyl oxidase.

The biochemical functions of ionic copper include pigmentation, bone development, oxygen transport, protein and neucleic acid synthesis. Deficiency characteristics of copper are disorders in pigmentation, retarded growth, anaemia in children, Wilson's disease and Menkes' syndrome. An early feature of copper deficiency is neutropenia. Copper deficiency causes a microcytic, hypochromic anaemia associated with low concentrations of ceruloplasmin, that can be corrected by the administration of ceruloplasmin. Severe copper deficiency affects collagen maturation and blood vessel defects.

Excess copper can cause free radical production and damage. Copper overload in brain and liver can cause cirrhosis of the liver and brain lesions. Administration of BAL (dimercaprol), penicillamine, or ammonium tetrathiomolybdate chelates copper and increases its urinary excretion. It has been reported that penicillamine and BAL treatment is associated with harmful side effects, whereas ammonium molybdate blocks copper absorption and appears to preserve neurologic functions.

There are no official preparations for the administration of copper for deficiency although solutions of copper salts are available in the market. Cupric sulphate is official as an antidote for phosphorus poisoning and is used topically as a fungicide.

ZINC

Zinc-containing enzymes are found in every enzyme class and zinc is a co-factor for more than 300 enzymes. Enzymes containing zinc include DNA polymerase, alkaline phosphatase, alcohol dehydrogenase, carbonic anhydrase etc.

Zinc enzymes are essential to growth, haemoglobin synthesis, collagen metabolism, bone development, wound healing, protection from free radical damage, reproductive function and to immune system. Symptoms of deficiency include skin lesions, diarrhea, male impotence, dwarfism, sensory alterations and susceptibility to infections.

Zinc itself is relatively non-toxic. It however competes for absorption with copper and iron, and high zinc intake can interfere with the transfer of copper to the circulation. Zinc toxicity has resulted from the ingestion of acid food kept in a galvanized metal container and from industrial workers inhaling zinc oxide.

Oral zinc sulphate has been suggested for wound healing and doses of 220 mg three times daily has been reported to increase healing following surgery. Zinc sulphate is official as a topical astringent.

CHROMIUM

Inadequate chromium intake may affect overall health. Numerous studies have demonstrated that taking extra chromium daily in the form of a supplement may improve glucose tolerance in people whose blood sugar levels range from slightly elevated to full-blown diabetes. Chromium supplementation in non-insulin-dependent diabetes mellitus has demonstrated improved glucose tolerance, reduced insulin concentrations, and decreased total cholesterol. Chromium increases the effects of insulin and decreases insulin requirements. Supplementation doses of chromium did not produce toxic effects at concentrations associated with improved glucose tolerance. However, chromium supplements won't help people who have high blood sugar inspite of getting adequate dietary chromium. Excessive intake can result in toxicity characterized by renal failure and pulmonary cancer.

The adequate intake (AI) for chromium is 35 micrograms (mcg) daily for men and 25 mcg for women. High sugar intakes, trauma and hard exercise can increase chromium excretion. Because the mineral improves insulin function, a shortfall can impair the cells' ability to remove excess sugar from the blood stream.

Chromium picolate is a well absorbed and popular chromium supplement sold today. A new formulation has also been developed as a complex of chromium and the amino acid histidine, which according to its developer, Richard Anderson, is absorbed at least 50% better than chromium picolate.

MANGANESE

The minimum daily requirement of manganese has been estimated at 3–9 mg. Manganese functions in many metalloproteins as a non-specific cation. Manganese is associated with several enzymes including pyruvate carboxylase, mitochondrial superoxide dismutase, arginase and glucokinase. It is therefore required for the biochemical functions of growth and reproduction, oxidative phosphorylation and cholesterol metabolism. Deficiency can result in disorders in spermatogenesis, bone abnormalities and bleeding disorders.

Very high doses except by inhalation are not toxic. In patients having magnetic resonance imaging using manganese agents, deposition of manganese in brain tissue has been demonstrated which may be associated with neurologic symptoms. Excessive manganese intake can lead to chronic manganism (manganese poisoning), which in many ways is similar to Parkinson's disease. Interestingly, the use of levodopa (used in the treatment of Parkinson's disease) has been successful in relieving many of the symptoms of manganism.

The rate of manganese absorption is low and is decreased by phosphate, phytate. calcium and iron. Manganese salts which were once official and used as tonics include a citrate, $Mn_3(C_6H_5O_7)_2$, a glycerphosphate, $MnC_3H_5(OH)_2PO_4$, and a hypophosphite, $Mn(PH_2O_2)_2 \cdot H_2O$.

Since the effect of manganese deficiency can be minimized by substitution of other similar ions in enzymes, symptoms of its deficiency are extremely rare and there is no current therapeutic rationale for the administration of manganese.

MOLYBDENUM

Dietary molybdenum is absorbed at a high rate. Several oxidases like xanthine dehydrogenase/xanthine oxidase, sulphate oxidase and aldehyde oxidase have molybdenum incorporated in them. Molybdenum is required in xanthine metabolism. Molybdenum has been found associated with flavin-dependent enzymes. Deficiency characteristics of molybdenum include mental disturbances and esophageal cancer. Toxicity is characterized by hyperuricemia.

Molybdenum can form complexes with copper and iron thereby inhibiting their absorption. This complex formation is the basis for the treatment of Wilson's disease, a genetically determined defect resulting in cirrhosis in liver and brain lesions, due to copper overload in the brain and liver.

Molybdenum is used as the oxide in a specially coprecipitated complex with ferrous sulphate, marketed in the ratio of 3 mg oxide/195 mg ferrous sulphate as a hematinic preparation (Mol-Iron)

SELENIUM

Selenium varies widely in its availability in the soil, which is reflected in its content in the vegetation grown. The biochemical functions of selenium include oxygen metabolism and free radical protection and has been implicated in cellular respiration and as an antioxidant in conjunction with vitamin E. Its deficiency can result in muscle degeneration and carcinogenesis. There is a report that the increase in dental cavities in children is proportional to the amount of selenium in their diet. Excessive concentrations can result in hepatotoxicity.

Toxicity or deficiency of selenium may occur as a result of the selenium concentration in food stuffs cultivated in soils with varying contents of selenium.

Selenium is official as Selenium sulfide N.F. XII as a suspension for the treatment of seborrheic dermatitis of the scalp (dandruff).

SULPHUR

Sulphur is widely distributed throughout the body as sulphydryl groups of cystine, disulphide linkages in protein, and sulphate salts and esters found in mucopolysaccharides and sulpholipids. The minimum daily requirement of sulphur is 2–3 g. This requirement is met from normal plant and animal foodstuffs in the diet. Hence currently there is no need for dietary supplements of sulphur.

Therapeutically, sulphur has been used in the following conditions and actions:

- Cathartic action.
- Parasiticide in scabies
- Stimulant in alopecia
- Fumigation
- Miscellaneous skin diseases
- Sulphides used as depilatories

IODINE

Iodine is an essential ion necessary for the biosynthesis of triiodothyronine (T_3) and thyroxine (T_4) produced by the thyroid gland. The biochemical functions of thyroid hormones include calorigenesis and oxygen consumption through regulation of carbohydrate, lipid and protein metabolism; central nervous system activity and brain development; cardiovascular stimulation: bone and tissue growth and development; gastrointestinal regulation and sexual maturation.

When the levels of thyroid hormones are insufficient to meet the metabolic needs of the body at the cellular level, hypothyroidism occurs. Symptoms of hypothyroidism include enlargement of the thyroid gland – goitre, impairment of cognition (including memory, speech and attention), fatigue, slowing of mental and physical performance, change in personality, intolerance to cold, exertional dyspnea, hoarseness, constipation, decreased sweating, easy bruising, muscle cramps and dry skin. Hypothyroidism has also been associated with increased cholesterol and risk of coronary heart disease. Severe hypothyroidism results in myxedema.

Internally iodine or iodide can be administered, since iodine is reduced to iodide in the intestinal tract. For solubility reasons, the official iodine preparations contain KI in addition to iodine which combines with iodine to form KI_3. Approximately 150 mg of iodide is absorbed in the intestine each day. The thyroid gland has a very high attraction for iodide and traps it (about 70 mg/day) by active transport.

Excessive administration of iodides may result in iodism bringing about certain irritative phenomena of the skin and mucous membrane. Iodism is exhibited by coryza (head cold), rashes. headache, conjunctivitis, etc. Hence it is not recommended to give iodides in cases of acne. Gastrointestinal effects include nausea, vomiting and diarrhoea.

IRON COMPOUNDS

Iron occurs in two forms, namely Ferrous (Fe^{++}) and Ferric (Fe^{+++}) forms. Although there are only three salts that are official in I.P. yet a large number of formulations (preparations) of these compounds are marketed. Most important compounds of iron are divalent or trivalent. Iron compounds are usually green in colour and get easily oxidised by atmospheric oxygen.

FERROUS FUMARATE

Chem. formula: $C_4H_2FeO_4$ Mol. wt. 169.9

It is a ferrous salt of fumaric acid, HCCOOH
$$\overset{\displaystyle \|}{}$$
HOOCCH

Preparation: It can be prepared by reaction between ferrous sulphate and sodium fumarate.

$$FeSO_4 + \underset{HC-COONa}{\overset{HC.COONa}{\|}} \longrightarrow C_4H_2FeO_4 + Na_2SO_4$$

Description: It occurs as a reddish-orange brown fine powder with slight odour and slightly astringent taste.

Solubility: It is slightly soluble in water and very slightly in alcohol.

According to I.P. standards, ferrous fumarate should contain not less than 93% and not more than 101.0% of $C_4H_2FeO_4$, calculated w.r.t. the dried substance.

Tests for identity:

(1) An acidic solution of the compound gives the reaction of ferrous salts.

(2) With resorcinol in presence of few drops of H_2SO_4 gives a deep-red, semisolid mass on heating. On dilution with water, it gives an orange yellow solution.

See also I.P. 2007 for tests for identity, A, B, C.

Tests for purity: It is tested for arsenic, heavy metals; sulphate; ferric iron and loss on drying.

Arsenic: Note more than 5 ppm.

Heavy metals: Not more than 20 ppm.

Sulphate: Boil a specific amount of sample (0.3 g) in dil. HCl (10 ml) and water (30 ml), after cooling with ice and filtering the filtrate complies with the limit test for sulphates.

Ferric iron: Not more than 2%. An accurately weighed specified amount of the sample (3 g) is dissolved in a mixture of water (200 ml) and HCl (20 ml) by heating to boiling point. Boil for 15 seconds rapidly and cool and add potassium iodide (3 g). Keep it in dark for 15 minutes, and titrate the liberated iodine with 0.1 N $Na_2S_2O_3$ (sodium thiosulphate) using starch as an indicator. Run a blank titration. The difference between the titrations represents the amounts of iodine liberated by the ferric iron.

Each ml of 0.1 N $Na_2S_2O_3 \equiv 0.005585$ g of ferric iron.

Loss on drying: Not more than 1% determined on 1 g by drying at 105°.

Assay: For determination of ferrous iron, the compound is titrated with 0.1 N ceric ammonium sulphate, using ferroin sulphate solution (1,10-phenanthroline) as an indicator. This indicator forms a complex with iron. The complex of 1,10-phenanthroline with ferrous iron is known as ferroin.

Ferroin

In presence of a reducing agent eeric ammo sulphate undergoes reduction to the cerous state:

$$20Ce(SO_4)_2 + 2FeSO_4 = Ce_2(SO_4)_3 + Fe_2(SO_4)_3$$

Accurately weigh the substance (0.3 g) and dissolve in dil H_2SO_4 (15 ml) and heat. Cool, add water (50 ml) and titrate with 0.1 N ceric amm. sulphate, using ferroin as indicator.

Each ml of 0.1 N Ceric Ammonium Sulphate is equivalent 0.01699 g of $C_4H_2FeO_4$.

Use: It is haematinic in dose of 0.2–0.6 g daily.

Storage: It is stored in well-closed containers.

FERROUS FUMARATE TABLETS

According to I.P. requirements it should contain between 90 to 105% of the stated amount of ferrous fumarate $C_4H_2FeO_4$.

Usual strength: 0.2 g.

Disintegration time: Maximum 1 hour.

Other particulars: Same as Ferrous Fumarate.

Dose: Prophylactic, 0.2 g daily; therapeutic, 0.4 to 0.6 daily in divided doses.

Use: It is used as a haematinic.

FERROUS GLUCONATE

Chem. formula: $C_{12}H_{22}O_{14}Fe, 2H_2O$ Mol. weight: 482.2

Ferrous gluconate is the dihydrated ferrous salt of gluconic acid, obtained by the oxidation of dextrose.

$CH_2(OH).(CHOH)_4COOH$ $[CH_2(OH) (CHOH)_4COO]_2Fe, 2H_2O$
Gluconic acid   Ferrous gluconate

Structural formula of ferrous gluconate

Ferrous Gluconate contains not less than 95.0 per cent of $C_{12}H_{22}O_{14}Fe$, calculated with reference to the substance dried at 105° for five hours.

Method of preparation of ferrous gluconate: It is prepared by double decomposition in solution between barium gluconate and ferrous sulphate. Barium sulphate precipitates out and is removed by means of filtration. The remaining solution is evaporated which is helpful in the production of ferrous gluconate.

$$FeSO_4 + [CH_2(OH)(CHOH)_4COO]_2.Ba \longrightarrow [CH_2(OH)(CHOH)_4.COO]_2Fe.2H_2O + BaSO_4$$

Description: It occurs as a yellowish grey or pale greenish yellow fine powder having slight odour resembling that of burnt sugar. It is soluble in water (10 parts) and almost insoluble in alcohol.

Tests for identity:

(1) It gives reactions characteristic of ferrous salts (App. I).

(2) It gives test for gluconate ion by forming the phenylhydrazide crystals of gluconic acid. melting at 200°-202°C with decomposition (I.P. p. 205). The reaction is given below:

$$CH_2OH(CHOH)_4COOH + C_6H_5NH.NH_2 \longrightarrow CH_2OH.(CHOH)_4CO.NH.NH.C_6H_5 + H_2O$$

Gluconic acid   Phenylhydrazine   Gluconic acid phenylhydrazide

Tests for purity: It is tested for acidity; arsenic; barium; ferric iron; heavy metals; chloride; sulphate; oxalic acid; dextrose and sucrose and loss on drying.

Note: Here ferrous gluconate is tested for ferric, because a ferrous compound if kept open is oxidised into ferric by the oxygen of air. That is why the tablets of ferrous salts are kept in a closed container.

$$Fe^{++} \xrightarrow{\text{Air}} Fe^{+++}$$

Tests for acidity is done with 5 per cent w/v solution, which should be acidic to litmus solution.

Determination of ferric iron is done by iodometric method by titrating the liberated iodine from acidic solution of potassium iodide by ferric iron against standard sodium thiosulphate.

Test for oxalate is done by precipitating oxalate as calcium oxalate from the residue of ether extract.

Dextrose and sucrose can be tested by reduction of Fehling's solution after removal of iron as Ferrous Sulphide. Sucrose gets hydrolysed to reducing sugars during the process of removal of iron.

Limit tests for Barium, Ferric iron, Oxalic acid, Dextrose and Sucrose are detailed hereunder:

Barium: Dissolve 0.1 g in 50 ml of water, add 5 ml of dilute sulphuric acid and allow to stand for five minutes; no turbidity is produced.

Ferric iron: Weigh accurately about 5 g and transfer to a glass-stoppered flask and dissolve in 100 ml of freshly boiled and cooled water and 10 ml of hydrochloric acid and add 3 g of potassium iodide. Shake well and allow to stand in the dark for five minutes. Titrate any liberated iodine with 0.1 N sodium thiosulphate, using solution of starch as indicator. Repeat the experiment with the same quantities of the same reagents in the same manner omitting Ferrous Gluconate. The difference between the titration represents the amount of 0.1 N sodium thiosulphate required by the ferric iron. Each ml of 0.1 N sodium thiosulphate is equivalent to 0.5585 g ferric iron. Ferrous Gluconate contains not more than 2 per cent of ferric iron.

Oxalic acid: Dissolve 1 g in 5 ml of water, add 2 ml of hydrochloric acid and transfer to a separator. Extract with two 20 ml portions of solvent ether, evaporate the combined ether extract to dryness on the water bath and dissolve the residue in 5 ml of water. Add 1 drop of acetic acid and 3 ml of solution of calcium chloride; no turbidity is produced.

Dextrose and sucrose: Dissolve 0.5 g in 10 ml of water, warm and make alkaline with dilute ammonia. Pass hydrogen sulphide into the solution to precipitate the iron and allow the solution to stand for thirty minutes. Filter and wash the precipitate with two 5 ml portions of water. Combine the filtrate and the washings and acidify with hydrochloric acid. Boil the solution until the vapours no longer darken lead paper and, if necessary, boil further to concentrate the solution to 10 ml. Cool and add 10 ml of solution of sodium carbonate, set aside for five minutes, filter and dilute the filtrate with water to 100 ml. To 5 ml of the filtrate add 2 ml of alkaline cupric tartrate and boil for one minute; no red precipitate is formed within one minute.

Assay: It is assayed by Redox titration, using ceric ammonium sulphate (approximate formula: $Ce(SO_4)_2 \cdot 2(NH_4)_2 \cdot SO_4 \cdot 2H_2O$ and solution of orthophenanthroline ferrous complex as indicator. In the presence of Fe salt, the indicator changes its colour from orange red to pale green.

$$Ce^{4+} \quad + \quad Fe^{2+} \quad \longrightarrow \quad Fe^{3+} \quad + \quad Ce^{3+}$$

Oxidised	Reduced	Oxidised	Reduced
form	form	form	form

Procedure: Weigh accurately about 1.5 gram of ferrous gluconate and dissolve it in 75 ml of water and 15 ml of dilute sulphuric acid in a 300 ml of conical tiask, fitted with Bunsen's valve. Add 0.25 gms of zinc dust and allow to stand for 20 minutes at room temperature or until the solution becomes colourless. Filter the solution through a Gooch crucible containing an asbestos mat coated with thin layer of zinc dust. Wash the crucible and contents with 10 ml to dilute sulphuric acid and then with 10 ml of water. Titrate the combined filtrate and washings immediately with 0.1 N ceric ammonium sulphate $Ce(NH_4)_2SO_4$, using orthophenanthroline compound as an indicator.

1 ml of N/10 ceric ammonium sulphate is equivalent to 0.04462 g of ferrous gluconate.

Uses: Like any other ferrous salt it is used as a haematinic. It is considered to cause less side effects than other ferrous salts including ferrous sulphate. It is usually given in the form of tablets or as elixirs.

Dose: 0.3 to 0 6 g.

Preparation: Ferrous Gluconate Tablets.

FERROUS GLUCONATE TABLETS

Each tablet should contain 93 per cent to 107 per cent of the stated amount of Ferrous Gluconate. The tablets are sugar-coated.

For description, tests for identity and tests for purity, the tablets of ferrous gluconate should conform to the same requirements as are stated under pure ferrous gluconate.

Assay: The assay procedure is also the same as that mentioned above for ferrous gluconate.

20 tablets are weighed and reduced to a fine powder. An accurately weighed quantity of powder equivalent to about 1.5 g of ferrous gluconate is dissolved in a mixture of 75 ml of water and 15 ml of dilute sulphuric acid, contained in a 300 ml conical flask, fitted with a Bunsen valve. The assay described under ferrous gluconate is carried out commencing with the word "add 0.25 g of zinc dust."

Each ml of 0.1 N ceric ammonium sulphate is equivalent to 0.04822 g of $C_{12}H_{22}O_{14}Fe \cdot 2H_2O$.

From the result obtained above the amount of ferrous gluconate in each tablet of average weight is calculated.

Uses: Iron in the body plays a very important role. About 5 g of iron is present in an adult body; 65% is in haemoglobin, 15% in the form of ferritin in the liver, spleen and bone marrow and the rest in other tissues. Ferritin is a protein which may contain upto 23% ferric iron. Haemoglobin has 0.34% iron. There is very little iron in blood plasma (i.e. 0.08 to 0.12 mg per cent only). Haem which is a colloidal ferric hydroxide phosphate of various iron contents upto 35% is present in small amounts in the bone marrow of individuals as iron stores. Iron is transported in the blood plasma in the form of ferric iron (Fe^{+++} ion).

FERROUS SULPHATE

Chem. formula: $FeSO_4.7H_2O$ Mol. weight: 278.0

Synonym: Green vitriol.

Ferrous sulphate contains an amount of iron equivalent to 97–103% of $FeSO_4 \cdot 7H_2O$.

Ferrous sulphate gets oxidised readily on exposure to moist air and the crystals become coated with brownish yellow ferric sulphate.

Ferrous sulphate so deteriorated should not be used.

Preparation: Ferrous sulphate is prepared by adding a slight excess of iron to dilute sulphuric acid. In commercial practice scraped iron is used.

$$Fe + H_2SO_4 \longrightarrow FeSO_4 + H_2$$

After effervescence ceases, the liquid is concentrated by boiling, filtered and allowed to cool. Green crystals separate on cooling which are removed at room temperature. (Various sulphates are called

---

The most significant iron compound of living organism is haem, which in most forms of life is a component of important oxidising enzymes such as cytochromes, cytochrome oxidase, catalase and peroxidase. The respiratory mechanisms of the body are dependent on iron, because it is an essential component of several important metalloproteins such as haemoglobin and myo-haemoglobin. It is necessary for the formation of erythrocytes. Haemoglobin in animals is a carrier of O_2 and CO_2. Hence iron is absolutely essential for the transport of O_2 to the tissues and for maintenance of oxidative systems without which life would cease within a few seconds.

Iron is indispensable for the synthesis of chlorophyll in green plants. Although iron does not enter into the chlorophyll molecule, deficiency of this element results in the development of a characteristic chlorosis. Most of the iron present in plants, in some form or the other, is a constituent of organic compounds. Physiologically iron is received in ferrous state although it is often absorbed as the ferric iron; much of it is rapidly reduced within the cell when taken orally. Ferric ions in the acid medium of the stomach are reduced to ferrous ions with simultaneous oxidation of ascorbic acid (Vit. C) and other reducing agents present in foodstuff.

Iron deficiency causes hypochromic microcytic anaemia. Repeated haemorrhages even if they are of small nature, result in anaemia due to iron loss. Iron treatment prevents or cures such type of anaemias. Reduced iron and various iron salts are used in medicines as haematinic (increasing the haemoglobin present in erythrocytes) in the treatment of iron-deficiency anaemias and as a source of iron in the mineral supplement preparations.

Ferrous sulphate is commonly used. Ferrous gluconate and fumarate salts employed as haematinics cause less gastrointestinal disturbance. Ferric iron is astringent and preparations of ferric salt for such uses were formerly recognised.

vitriols, the crystalline ferrous sulphate is known as green vitriol, crystalline copper sulphate is known as blue vitriol and the zinc sulphate is known as white vitriol.)

Properties:

1. Ferrous sulphate, on being heated, decomposes into ferric oxide, sulphur dioxide and sulphuric acid.

$$2FeSO_4, 7H_2O \xrightarrow{\text{Heat}} Fe_2O_3 + SO_2 + H_2SO_4 + 13H_2O$$

The finely divided Fe_2O_3 which is known as jewellers' rouge is used as pigment.

2. The solutions of ferrous sulphate absorb nitric oxide resulting dark brown solutions due to the formation of double compound, $FeSO_4 \cdot NO$. The reaction is utilised in the detection of nitric acid and nitrates (brown ring test). Some of the ferrous sulphate reduces the nitric acid to nitric oxide (NO) which forms the double salt.

$$2KNO_3 + 6FeSO_4 + 4H_2SO_4 \longrightarrow 3Fe_2(SO_4)_3 + K_2SO_4 + 4H_2O + 2NO$$

3. Ferrous sulphate reduces silver and gold salts to corresponding metal. Mercuric chloride is reduced to mercurous chloride in the presence of light.

$$Ag^+ + Fe^{2+} \longrightarrow Ag + Fe^{3+}$$

$$Au^{3+} + 3Fe^{2+} \longrightarrow Au + 3Fe^{3+}$$

$$2HgCl_2 + 2Fe^{2+} \longrightarrow Hg_2Cl + 2Fe^{3+} + 2Cl^-$$

Description: Ferrous sulphate occurs as pale bluish-green transparent crystals or granules. It is odourless, has a saline, styptic taste (metallic and astringent). It effloresces in dry air. Its solubility in water at 25°C is 1.5 and at 100°C is 0.5. It is insoluble in alcohol.

Tests for identity: It yields reactions characteristic of iron and sulphates (App. I).

Tests for purity: It is tested for acidity; arsenic; lead; zinc; manganese and chlorides.

Acidity: Acidity can be determined by measurement of pH or by titrating with standard alkali.

A solution of 5 g in 50 ml of water requires not more than 1.0 ml of 0.1 N NaOH using solution of methyl orange as indicator.

Arsenic: Not more than two parts per million.

Copper: It is tested by dissolving 2 g in 50 ml of water acidifying the solution with 1 ml of dilute sulphuric acid and saturating the solution with hydrogen sulphide. No darkening of the solution or precipitation should take place (see I.P. for tests for lead, zinc, manganese).

Basic sulphate (insoluble sulphates): These are detected by the presence of turbidity in the aqueous solution. Recently boiled and cooled water is used in the test as otherwise the turbidity might be due to oxidation of Fe^{++} by the dissolved oxygen in water.

Assay: This is assayed by oxidation-reduction type of assay using N/10 Potassium Permanganate solution in the presence of dilute H_2SO_4.

An accurately weighed about 1 g is dissolved in 20 ml of dilute H_2SO_4 and titrated with N/10 $KMnO_4$.

$$2FeSO_4 + 2KMnO_4 + 4H_2SO_4 \longrightarrow K_2SO_4 + 2MnSO_4 + Fe_2(SO_4)_3 + 4H_2O$$

Each ml of N/10 $KMnO_4$ is equivalent to 0.0278 g of $FeSO_4.7H_2O$.

I.P. 2007 gives a modified assay by titration with 0.1 M ceric ammonium nitrate, using ferroin solution as indicator. The assay is being given in dried ferrous sulphate (given below).

Uses: It is used as a haematinic (substance that increases the haemoglobin content). It is one of the most commonly used iron preparations used in anaemias caused due to iron-deficiency. It is also used for dyeing fabrics, tanning leather, in the manufacture of ink, in photography and also as a disinfectant.

Storage: It is to be preserved in well-closed container.

DRIED FERROUS SULPHATE

Chem. formula: $FeSO_4.2H_2O$

Dried ferrous sulphate contains not less than 80% and not more than 90% of $FeSO_4.2H_2O$. In 100 g it contains about 30 g of iron.

Preparation: This substance is prepared by drying the crystalline salt in an oven at 40° until it has lost the correct amount of water. The product is a mixture and corresponds in composition to the formula $FeSO_4.2H_2O$.

Description: Dried ferrous sulphate is a greyish-white powder which dissolves slowly but completely in water. 3.5 parts of dried ferrous sulphate may be accpeted as the equivalent of 5 parts of ferrous sulphate. In other respects it resembles $FeSO_4.7H_2O$.

Tests for identity: It yields reactions characteristic of iron and sulphate (App. I).

Tests for purity: It is tested for arsenic, basic sulphates.

Basic sulphates: Dried $FeSO_4$ is required to give with freshly boiled and cooled water and a little sulphuric acid, a solution which is not more than faintly turbid.

Assay: Similar to that used for ferrous sulphate using smaller quantity because of the higher iron content. But the result is calculated on the basis of anhydrous salt, $FeSO_4$, which should not be less than 80%.

Each ml of N/10 $KMnO_4$ is equivalent to 0.01519 g of $FeSO_4$.

The modified assay of I.P. 2007 is performed by taking accurately weighed 0.5 g dissolved in a mixture of 30 ml of water and 2 ml of 1 M sulphuric acid and titrating the solution with 0.1 M ceric ammonium sulphate using ferroin solution as indicator.

1 ml of 0.1 M ceric ammonium sulphate is equivalent to 0.01519 g of $FeSO_4$.

Uses: Same as under Ferrous Sulphate.

Dose: 60 to 200 mg.

Preparation: Ferrous Sulphate Tablets.

FERROUS SULPHATE TABLETS
(Ferr. Sulph. Tab.)

Ferrous sulphate tablets are prepared from dried sulphate and are required to contain 80–90% of $FeSO_4$. They are dispensed or supplied as sugar-coated tablets.

Assay: The ferrous sulphate tablets cannot be titrated with $KMnO_4$ because of the presence of some other reducing substances other than ferrous ion, Fe^{2+} ion. The tablets are, therefore. first digested with dilute sulphuric acid. The solution is filtered and to an aliquot volume of the filtrate strong iodine monochloride solution is added, followed by the addition of concentrated hydrochloric acid. Iodine monochloride oxidises the Ferrous to the Ferric ions with the liberation of Iodine.

$$2Fe^{2+} + 2ICl \longrightarrow 2Fe^{3+} + 2Cl + I_2$$

I_2 is titrated with the standard potassium iodate solution till the colour becomes light brown. A small quantity of chloroform is then added and the titration continued till the colour in the chloroform layer disappears, indicating complete removal of free iodine.

$$KIO_3 + 2I_2 + 6HCl \longrightarrow KCl + 5ICl + 3H_2O$$

One half of KIO_3 is equivalent to 2 moles of $FeSO_4$.

Each ml of M/20 KIO_3 is equivalent to 0.03038 g of $FeSO_4$.

Modified assay method given under dried ferrous sulphate can also be used.

Dose: Prophylactic dose 0.2 g daily. Therapeutic dose 0.6 to 1.2 g daily in divided doses.

Ferric ammonium citrate (Iron and ammonium citrate, Scale preparations of iron)

It contains 20.5–22.5 of Fe.

Preparation:

(1) The preparation is done in the following steps: First ferric hydroxide is prepared by the interaction of ferric solution with an alkali. Ferric salt solution is added to the alkali with constant stirring and not vice versa. The precipitate may contain a basic ferric salt which prevents the formation of transparent scales.

$$Fe_2(SO_4)_3 + 6NaOH \longrightarrow 2Fe(OH)_3 + 3Na_2SO_4$$

$Fe(OH)_3$ is collected and washed.

(2) Without drying $Fe(OH)_3$ is stirred with enough citric acid solution to dissolve whole of the ppt.

(3) A slight excess of NH_3 is added and a small quantity of undissolved $Fe(OH)_3$ is removed by filtration.

(4) The clear reddish brown filtrate is evaporated to a syrup and a little ammonia is added from time to time so as to maintain a slight excess of NH_3 throughout the process of evaporation.

(5) The syrupy mass is painted on glass plates and dried below 40°C and the scales are scraped off. The scales will be green if excess of citric acid is used.

Description: The scales are thin, red to dark red in colour, odourless or have ammonial odour and saline taste; very soluble in water and insoluble in alcohol.

Tests for purity: It is tested for purity for As; Zn; SO_4 and Pb.

Assay: Accurately weighed quantity is dissolved in H_2O, acidified with H_2SO_4, warmed and cooled. A solution of N/10 $KMnO_4$ is used in drops to oxidise any small quantity of Fe^{++}. It is then treated with

There are quite a few more iron salts which have been and are of considerable importance. Although they are not official in I. P., their mention here should be quiet relevant.

excess of HCl and KI. The liberated HI is oxidised by Fe^{++} salt with the liberation of I_2, which after dilution is determined by titrating with $N/10$ $Na_2S_2O_3$, using starch as indicator.

$$2FeCl_3 + 2HI \longrightarrow 2FeCl_2 + I_2 + 2HCl$$

$$Na_2S_2O_3 + I_2 \longrightarrow Na_2S_4O_6 + 2NaI$$

1000 ml of $N/10$ $Na_2S_2O_3$ is equivalent to $1/10$ Fe.

Uses: It is used as a source of iron in treating iron deficiency anaemias. It is less constipative than other inorganic forms of iron. Since it is very soluble, it can be dispensed as a solution (see also p. 127).

IRON AND QUININE CITRATE

It is a complex ammonium quinine citrate. It contains 14.5 to 15.5% quinine and 12–14% of Fe.

Preparation: The preparation is similar to Ferrous Amm. Citrate, along with quinine salt is added.

Description: Greenish yellow scales with bitter taste, deliquescent.

Tests for purity: Tested for As, heavy metals. SO_4, acidity.

Assay:

(a) **For quinine:** An accurately weighed quantity of the substance is dissolved in H_2O. A slight excess of dil. NH_3 solution is added and the solution extracted with successive quantities of ether until complete extraction of quinine is effected. Each time the etheral layer is washed with water. Ether is then separated and evaporated. The residue is then ignited to a const. wt. at 105°C. It gives the wt. of anhydrous quinine in the sample used.

(b) **For Fe:** The solution and washings obtained from the first assay for quinine is evaporated by stirring on a water bath until dissolved ether and NH_3 are expelled completely. 20 ml of this solution is treated with H_2SO_4 and is warmed till the dark brown solution turns pale yellow. The solution is cooled and to it is added $N/10$ $KMnO_4$ followed by excess of HCl and KI. The liberated I_2 is titrated with $Na_2S_2O_3$ using starch as indicator. 1000 ml of $N/10$ $Na_2S_2O_3$ is equivalent to $1/10$ Fe.

Uses: As haemitinic like other salts.

IRON AND AMMONIUM CITRATE

Synonym: Ferric Ammonium Citrate. With this nomenclature it has been described as a footnote in the last pages. It is being describd below again, in rather more detail.

It occurs in a complex form as scales and contains not less than 20.5% and not more than 22.5% of Fe. This preparation of iron is preferred to ordinary iron salts because of its comparatively non-astringent nature and also because of the fact that this form can be dispensed with ammonia or alkali carbonates without the precipitation of iron as ferric hydroxide.

Preparation: Ferric hydroxide is freshly precipitated by adding a solution of ferric sulphate with constant stirring to sodium hydroxide.

$$Fe_2(SO_4)_3 + 6NaOH \longrightarrow 2Fe(OH)_3 + 3Na_2SO_4$$

It is to be noted that the solution of ferric salt should be added to the alkali and not vice versa, otherwise precipitation of basic ferric sulphate will occur which will render the scales as non-transparent.

The ferric hydroxide precipitate is filtered, washed and treated in a wet condition with a sufficient quantity of citric acid solution to dissolve almost whole of ferric hydroxide. This solution is then neutralized with a slight solution of aqueous ammonia. This undissolved ferric hydroxide precipitate is a clear reddish brown solution, which is evaporated to a syrupy consistency. During evaporation some of the ammonia is lost which is replaced or made up by further addition of NH_3, during the process to maintain it in slight excess. The syrup is painted in thin films on glass plates and dried below 40°C in a dust-free atmosphere. The hard mass is then scraped off as glistening amorphous transparent dark scales or flakes.

Description: It is odourless and has astringent taste. Ferric ammonium citrate is freely soluble in water and insoluble in alcohol. The composition of ferric ammonium citrate is not definitely known. I.P. requires it to contain 20.5–22.5% of iron. Almost whole of the iron is present as complex ions or as colloidal ferric hydroxide. The approximate composition of ferric ammonium citrate is:

$$FeC_6H_5O_7.\ xFe(OH)_3$$

where x is greater than 1 but less than 2. This structure is stable only in the alkaline medium provided by ammonia. In the acidic solution (if NH_3 were not added during preparation) it occurs as normal ferric citrate, $FeC_6H_5O_7$, which is yellowish green. Ferric ammonium citrate also contains a certain amount of colloidal ferric oxide. Its coagulation is prevented by the basic complex present in it.

Decrease in hydrogen-ion (H+) concentration

$$FeC_6H_5O_7 \longrightarrow FeC_6H_5O_7.X\ Fe(OH)_3 \longrightarrow Fe(OH)_3$$

Normal Fe citrate	Basic complex	Colloidal hydroxide
(yellowish green)	(reddish brown)	(brown)

Tests for identity:

(1) Residue on ignition dissolved in hydrochloric acid yields reactions characteristic of ferric salts (App. I).

(2) On being warmed with the solution of sodium hydroxide evolves ammonia and the solution yields reactions characteristic of citrate.

Tests for purity: It is tested for lead (I.P. p. 1245); zinc (I.P. p. 1245); chloride; ferric compounds and sulphates.

Assay: An accurately weighed quantity (0.5 g) is dissolved in water (15 ml), acidified with H_2SO_4 and warmed till the colour of the solution becomes yellow. To the cooled solution N/10 $KMnO_4$ is added drop by drop to oxidise the small quantity of ferrous iron that may be present in the salt. The pink colour should persist for only few seconds because decolourisation of potassium permanganate may be due to oxidation of citric acid instead of ferrous ion. To the liquid is then added excess of hydrochloric acid (15 ml) and pot. iodide (2 g). The liberated hydro-iodic acid is oxidised by the ferric salt with the liberation of iodine.

The free iodine is estimated by titrating with N/10 sod. thiosulphate using starch mucilage as indicator towards the end point.

1000 ml of N/10 $Na_2S_2O_3$ is equivalent to 1/10 Fe or 1 ml of 0.1 N sodium thiosulphate is equivalent to 0.00585 g of Fe.

Uses: Ferric Ammonium Citrate is used as a source of iron in the treatment of iron deficiency anaemia. It is less constipating and less irritant than inorganic forms of iron, such as ferrous sulphate and ferrous gluconate (See uses of other iron compounds).

COPPER SULPHATE

Chem. formula: $CuSO_4.5H_2O$ Mol. weight: 249.07

Copper sulphate contains not less than 98.5% and not more than the equivalent of 101% of $CuSO_4.5H_2O$. It is not official in I.P. now.

Preparation: Copper sulphate is prepared by the action of H_2SO_4 on copper turnings:

$$Cu + 2H_2SO_4 \longrightarrow CuSO_4 + SO_2 + 2H_2O$$

On large scale it is prepared by heating copper with sulphuric acid in presence of air. The solution is filtered and evaporated to crytallisation. The oxygen of air assists the reaction. The salt crystallises as pentahydrate.

Description: It occurs as deep blue prisms or crystalline powder, freely soluble in water and slowly soluble in glycerol and almost insoluble in alcohol.

Tests for identity: It yields reactions characteristic of copper and sulphates (App. I).

Tests for purity: It is tested for acidity, As, Fe, Pb and Zn.

Tests for acidity: Copper sulphate solution is acidic to litmus and phenolphthalein.

Test for iron: It is determined by gravimetric method. A solution of the sample is first boiled with nitric acid in order to oxidise any ferrous iron to the ferric iron. The iron is precipitated as $Fe(OH)_3$ by addition of excess of ammonia. The copper remains as deep blue cupra ammonium sulphate (Cu $(NH_3)_4SO_4$). The precipitate is washed and ignited to ferric oxide and the residue weighed. The pharmacopoeial limit corresponds to less than 0.1% of iron calculated as Fe (I.P., p. 205).

Test for lead: The test depends upon the formation of PbS as is the case in the ordinary pharmacopoeial quantitative test for lead. In this test, however, considerable, more than the usual, amount of potassium cyanide must be added to prevent the precipitation of CuS.

Zinc is detected during the above test by a precipitate or opalescene due to the formation of ZnS.

Arsenic: Not more than 8 parts per million.

Assay (principle): It depends on the instability of cupric iodide which is formed in the reaction between $CuSO_4$ and KI and which decomposes to Cu_2I_2 with the liberation of free iodine.

Procedure: An accurately weighed quantity of copper sulphate is dissolved in water and a slight excess of KI is added followed by acetic acid. The liberated iodine is titrated with standard sodium thiosulphate using starch as indicator. The titration is continued till faint blue colour persists.

$$2CuSO_4 + 4KI \longrightarrow \underset{\text{Cupric iodide}}{2CuI_2} + 2K_2SO_4$$

$$2CuI_2 \longrightarrow Cu_2I_2 + I_2$$

2 g of potassium thiocyanate (KCNS) is then added and the titration continued till the blue colour disappears.

$$I_2 + 2Na_2S_2O_3 \longrightarrow Na_2S_4O_6 + 2NaI$$

$$Cu_2I_2 + KCNS \longrightarrow 2CuCNS + 2KI$$

1000 ml of 0.1 N $Na_2S_2O_3$ is equivalent to 1/10 $CuSO_4.5H_2O$.

Or each ml of 0.1 N $Na_2S_2O_3$ is equivalent to 0.02497 g of $CuSO_4.5H_2O$.

Uses: It is used as an astringent. It is considered to be an antidote for phosphorus poisoning. It is also used in routine as an emetic though its use as an emetic can be dangerous because of large and corrosive doses. Besides its medicinal uses, it is used as one of the most important salts in the industry.

Dose: 5 to 10 mg three times a day in capsules (300 mg as an emetic).

CHAPTER

7

Gastrointestinal Agents

The **Gastrointestinal Tract** (GIT) functions as a co-ordinated unit for the absorption of nutrients and the excretion of unabsorbed and waste products. The various symptoms of gastrointestinal disorders include pain, anorexia (loss of appetite), vomiting, waterbrash (the sudden filling of the mouth with saliva due to a variety of symptoms from the upper GIT e.g. peptic ulcer), indigestion, heartburn (a burning sensation due to inflammation or dysmotility of the oesophagus), flatulence, constipation and diarrhoea. The above symptoms may occur as a result of certain food habits, increased acid secretion in the stomach, inflammation of the GIT, food containing toxic material, or contaminated with pathogenic microorganisms, ulceration or due to more serious conditions like carcinoma.

Since several patients approach a pharmacist first, for over the counter preparations (OTC drugs) for several of the above symptoms, it is necessary to use discernment and advise the patient during the dispensing of drugs for the above ailments as very often they are representative of a more serious underlying disorder.

A number of inorganic agents that are used to treat some of the above disorders are discussed below. These include acidifying agents, antacids, protectives, adsorbents and saline cathartics.

ACIDIFYING AGENTS

Gastric fluid has a high content of hydrochloric acid and stomach pH can range from 1 when empty to 7 when food is present. HCl is secreted against a H^+ gradient as great as 1,00,000 times the concentration in plasma. Gastric secretion occurs in response to neurogenic impulses from the brain (in response to sight, smell, or anticipation of food), distention of the stomach with food or fluid, contact of protein breakdown products (secretagogues) and the hormone gastrin.

Gastric hydrochloric acid acts by killing of bacteria in ingested food and drink, softening fibrous foods and promoting the conversion of pepsinogen to pepsin (a proteolytic enzyme). Lack of hydrochloric acid could cause gastrointestinal disturbances which include symptoms like mild diarrhoea, frequent bowel movements, epigastric pain, fullness of stomach after meals, belching and sensitivity to spicy foods.

Approximately 10 to 15% of the population suffers from hypochlorhydria (decreased HCl secretion) or achlorhydria (absence of HCl secretion). Patients with achlorhydria include those with subtotal gastrectomy, atropic gastritis (chronic gastritis with atrophy of the mucous membranes and glands), carcinoma of the stomach, and gastric polyps. Patients with achlorhydria who respond to stimulation with histamine phosphate include those with chronic nephritis, chronic alcoholism, tuberculosis, hyperthyroidism, pellagra and parasitic infestations. It is also common in normal individuals after age 50.

Acidifying agents are agents used to relieve the gastrointestinal symptoms caused by achlorhydria. Dilute hydrochloric acid diluted with water is commonly used as an acidifying agent.

HYDROCHLORIC ACID

Chem. formula: HCl   Mol. weight: 36.46

Hydrochloric acid was commonly called spirit of salt as it was first prepared by distilling sea salt with sulphuric acid. It is an aqueous solution of hydrogen chloride in water and contains not less than 35% w/w and not more than 38% w/w of HCl.

Preparation: Hydrochloric acid is manufactured by the interaction of sodium chloride and sulphuric acid. Calculated quantities of common salt and conc. sulphuric acid are heated in the cast iron pan of a salt cake furnace. Sodium bisulphite in the reaction is mixed with more of common salt and heated strongly in the muffle to get more of HCl.

$$NaCl + H_2SO_4 \longrightarrow NaHSO_4 + HCl$$
$$NaHSO_4 + NaCl \longrightarrow Na_2SO_4 + HCl$$

Hydrochloric acid gas is passed up a tower down which cold water is sprayed, when dilute acid is collected at the bottom. This is again sprayed down the tower to absorb more HCl gas and gets concentrated. The acid so manufactured is purified.

Large quantities of hydrogen and chlorine are obtained as by-products during the manufacture of caustic soda by electrolysis of sodium chloride solution. The gases are combined to give hydrogen chloride.

$$H_2 + Cl_2 \longrightarrow 2HCl$$

Description: It is a colourless fuming liquid with pungent odour. The pungent odour and fumes disappear when it is diluted with double the quantity of water. It is very strongly acidic to litmus even in highly diluted form. Qualitatively it can be recognised by the formation of a white precipitate of silver chloride with silver nitrate. It attacks many metals with the evolution of hydrogen. It is mixable with water or alcohol. Its specific gravity is 1.18.

Tests for purity: It is tested for weight per ml; As; Pb; bromide and iodide; sulphite; sulphate; free chloride and residue on ignition.

The test for bromide and iodide is performed by diluting the acid with double amount of its water, adding chloroform (1 ml) and solution of chlorinated lime and noting the colour of chloroform layer, which should not become brown or violet.

Assay: An accurate amount, about 4 g, of HCl is taken in a stoppered flask containing 40 ml of water and the solution is titrated with 1 N sodium hydroxide, using solution of methyl orange as indicator.

$$NaOH + HCl \longrightarrow NaCl + H_2O$$

Each ml of 1 N NaOH is equivalent to 0.03646 g of HCl.

Note: The acid is weighed and not measured because the result is required as percentage of weight by weight. The acid is weighed in stoppered flask containing water, as loss of HCl on being diluted is little.

Uses: It is used as acidifier and hence it is a pharmaceutical necessity for preparing diluted hydrochloric acid.

DILUTE HYDROCHLORIC ACID

Dilute hydrochloric acid contains 10% w/w of HCl (limits 9.5 to 10%). It is prepared by mixing the following ingredients:

Hydrochloric acid .... 274.0 g

Purified water .... 726.0 g

Description: It is a colourless liquid which is strongly acidic and has about 1.05 specific gravity.

Tests for purity and assay are perfomed in the same way as for concentrated acid.

Uses: It is used as an acidifier.

Dose: 0.6 to 8 ml.

ANTACIDS

Gastric antacids are substances, which on ingestion, neutralize gastric hydrochloric acid and thereby lower the acidity of gastric contents. Another objective may be to inactivate the proteolytic enzyme pepsin. Antacids are indicated in conditions of excess gastric hydrochloric acid that may cause pain and possible ulceration, peptic ulcer, gastro-oesophageal reflux, for the neutralization of gastric acid to protect from aspiration pneumonitis during anaesthesia, preparation of endoscopy, and for the prophylaxis of stress ulceration.

Antacids include aluminium hydroxide, aluminium phosphate, dihydroxyaluminium aminoacetate, dihydroxyaluminium sodium carbonate, magnesium hydroxide, magnesium carbonate, magnesium trisilicate, calcium carbonate, tribasic calcium phosphate and sodium bicarbonate. No single antacid meets all the criteria of an ideal antacid and may produce constipative or laxative effects. Hence a combination of drugs is more satisfactory and mixtures are often used. Liquid preparations are more acceptable for frequent use and tablets are normally to be chewed or sucked. Since gastric hydrochloric acid production is continuous, the administration of antacids is also usually on a continuing basis. Due to gastric emptying, the effect of antacids lasts longer when taken an hour after meals (lasts for 2–3 hours) than on an empty stomach (where it is effective only for 20–40 minutes).

ALUMINIUM HYDROXIDE GEL

It is a colloidal aluminium hydroxide. It is a white, viscous suspension, translucent in thin layers. Small amounts of clear liquid may separate on standing.

It is an aqueous suspension of hydrated aluminium oxide with varying proportions of basic aluminium carbonate and bicarbonate. It contains not less than 3.5% w/w and not more than 4.4% w/w of Al_2O_3. It may contain glycerine, sorbitol, sucrose or saccharin as sweetening agent and peppermint oil or other suitable flavours. It may contain suitable preservatives.

Preparation: It is prepared by adding sodium carbonate to a solution of aluminium sulphate and by subsequent hydrolysis of the aluminium carbonate formed.

$$3Na_2CO_3 + Al_2(SO_4)_3 \longrightarrow 3Na_4SO + Al_2(CO_3)_3$$

$$2Al_2(CO_3)_3 \xrightarrow{6H_2O} 4Al(OH)_3 + 6CO_2$$

Tests for identity: A solution in dil. HCl gives reaction of aluminium.

Tests for purity: pH, ammonium salts; arsenic; heavy metals; chloride; sulphate; neutralising capacity and microbial limits.

pH: Between 5.5 and 8.0.

Ammonium salts: To a weighed quantity of sample (25 g) is added sodium hydroxide solution (25 ml) and water (250 ml). The mixture is distilled to collect the distillate in 25 ml 0.1 N HCl. The excess of acid is titrated with 0.1 N NaOH using methyl red solution as an indicator. Not less than 20 ml of 0.1 N NaOH is required.

Arsenic: Not more than 1 ppm.

Heavy metals: Not more than 10 ppm. The solution is prepared by dissolving sample (5 g) in dil. HCl (10 ml), filtering, if necessary, and diluting with water (25 ml).

Chloride: A weighed amount of sample (0.5 g) is dissolved in dil. HNO_3 (5 ml), boiled, cooled and diluted with water to 100 ml and filtered. 25 ml of the filtrate complies with the limit test for chlorides.

Sulphate: A weighed quantity of sample (2.5 g) is dissolved in dil. HCl (5 ml) with the aid of heat. It is cooled and diluted to 200 ml with H_2O. It is mixed well and filtered if necessary. To 10 ml of the filtrate is then added 2 ml of dil. HCl. The solution complies with the limit test for sulphates.

Neutralising capacity: A weighted quantity of sample is dissolved in water and 0.1 N HCl is also added to the soultion to get pH 1.8 at temp. 37°C. pH of the solution at 37°C after 10, 15 and 20 minutes is not less than 1.8, 2.3 and 3.0 respectively and at no time is not less than 4.0. HCl is then added and the sol. stirred at 37° C for one hour. It is titrated with 0.1 N NaOH at pH 3.5. The amount of 0.1 N NaOH used (50 ml) complies with I.P. requirement.

Microbial limits: The toal microbial count does not exceed 100 per ml. It must comply with I.P. requirement for the absence of *E. coli* and *Pseudomonas*.

Assay: It is based upon complexometric titration. Disodium ethylenediamine tetraacetate is used as chelating agent or sequestering agent.

$$Al(OH)_3 \rightleftharpoons[\text{}]{HCl} Al^{3+} + 3OH^-$$

$$[HOOC-CH_2N(CH_2COONa)CH_2]_2 + Al^{3+} \longrightarrow$$

A weighed quantity of sample (5 g) is taken and dissolved in HCl (3 ml) by warming on a water bath. The solution is cooled to below 20° and diluted with water to 100 ml. To a measured volume of this solution (20 ml) is added 0.05 M disodium edetate (40 ml), water (80 ml) and methyl red solution (0.15 ml). It is neutralised by the dropwise addition of 1 N NaOH, warmed on a water bath for 30 minutes and to it is added hexamine (3 g). The solution is titrated with lead nitrate (0.05 M) using xylenol orange (0.5 ml) solution as indicator.

$$2Al + 6HCl \longrightarrow 2AlCl_3 + 3H_2$$
$$2AlCl_3 + 6H_2O \longrightarrow Al_2O_3 + 6HCl + 3H_2O$$
$$Al(OH)_3 + 3HCl \longrightarrow AlCl_3 + 3H_2O$$

Each ml of 0.05 M disodium edetate is equivalent to 0.002549 g of Al_2O_3.

Uses: As an antacid in the management of peptic ulcer, gastritis, peptic esophagitis, gastric hyperacidity and hiatal hernia. It reacts chemically to neutralise the gastric contents. It is a non-systemic antacid but significant amounts are absorbed in patients with renal failure. It is excreted as the phosphate.

Aluminium compounds decrease the absorption of certain drugs, such as the tetracycline antibiotics. These compounds are also constipating.

Storage: It is stored in tightly closed containers in a cool place but avoid freezing.

Dose: 5 to 30 ml upto 12 times daily. Usual adult dose of oral suspension is 15 ml four to six times a day between meals and at bed time.

DRIED ALUMINIUM HYDROXIDE GEL

Synonyms: Aluminium Hydroxide Powder, Aluminium Hydrate Powder.

It contains not less than 47% Al_2O_3. U.S.P. requirement is 50% Al_2O_3. It also contains varying small quantities of basic aluminium carbonate and bicarbonate.

Preparation: It is prepared in the same way as is described under Aluminium hydroxide gel. It is dried at a temperature until it has the required amount of Al_2O_3.

Description: It is a white, light, amorphous powder, odourless and tasteless. The filterate from the aqueous suspension (1 in 25) is neutral to litmus.

Solubility: It is not soluble in water and alcohol but is soluble in dilute mineral acids and in large volume of caustic alkali solution.

Tests for identity: A solution in dil. HCl gives the reactions of aluminium (App. I).

pH: A solution of 40% of it in O_2-free water gives pH not more than 10.

Tests for purity: Ammonium salts, arsenic, heavy metals, chloride, sulphate, neutralising capacity and microbial limits.

Neutralising capacity: A sufficient quantity is passed through a sieve of nominal mesh aperture of 150. G.m. 0.5 g of the sifted material is taken and is added to 200 ml of 0.05 N HCl previously heated to 37° and the test is completed in the same way as is described under test for neutralising capacity under Aluminium hydroxide gel. Not more than 35 ml of 0.1 N NaOH is required.

Microbial limits: The total microbial count does not exceed 100 per ml. It must comply with I.P. 85 requirement for the absence of *E. coli* and *Pseudomonas*.

Assay: An accurately weighed quantity of about 0.4 g is dissolved in a mixture of 3 ml of HCl and 3 ml of water by warming on a water bath and the assay is completed as per procedure described under Al. hydro. gel beginning at the words "cooled to below 20° ....".

Use: Same as Al hydr. gel. (Antacid).

Dose: 0.5–1 g four to six times daily.

ALUMINIUM HYDROXIDE TABLETS

Aluminium hydroxide tablets contain not less than 45% Al_2O_3. It may contain a flavouring agent.

Test for identity: Same as in Al hydr. gel.

Neutralising capacity: Same as Al. hydr. gel, using 1 g of sample. The volume of 0.1 N HCl consumed is not less than 230 ml for each 1 g of dried Al hydr. gel.

Disintegration: Does not apply to Al. hydr. gel. tablets.

Other requirements: Should comply with the requirements stated under Tablets in I.P. 1985.

Assay: 20 tablets are weighed and powdered (avoid frictional heat). An accurately weighed quantity of the powder equivalent to an amount 0.4 g of dried Al hydr. gel is dissolved as completely as possible in a mixture of 3 ml of HCl and 3 ml of water. The assay is continued in the same way as given in Al hydr. gel.

Each ml of 0.05 M disodium edetate is equivalent to 0.002549 g of Al_2O_3.

Storage: It is stored in well-closed containers in a cool place.

Dose: 0.5 to 1 g of Al hydr. tablets should be masticated before being swallowed.

Use: It is used as an antacid.

Lebelling: Tablet should be chewed or masticated before swallowing.

HEAVY MAGNESIUM CARBONATE

Approx. chem. formula: $3MgCO_3Mg(OH)_2.4H_2O$.

Magnesium carbonate is a heavy basic carbonate and its composition is approximately $3MgCO_3(OH)_2.4H_2O$. It contains equivalent of not less than 40.0% and not more than 45.0% of MgO.

Preparation of heavy magnesium carbonate: Magnesium carbonate is prepared from $MgSO_4$ (125 parts) and Na_2CO_3 (150 parts). $MgSO_4$ and crystalline Na_2CO_3 are dissolved separately, each in 25 parts of boiling water. The solutions are mixed and evaporated to dryness and the residue is digested with boiling water (500 parts) for half an hour. The insoluble carbonate is then collected on a calico filter, washed until freed from SO_4^- ions and dried in an oven.

$$Na_2CO_3 + MgSO_4 \longrightarrow Na_2SO_4 + MgCO_3$$

Description: Heavy $MgCO_3$ is a white granular tasteless powder which is insoluble in water. When heated to redness it loses CO_2 and H_2O leaving a residue of MgO.

Tests for purity: It is tested for As; Ca; Fe; Cu; Pb; Cl; SO_4; heavy metals; residue on ignition; soluble substances; substances insoluble in acetic acid.

Residue on ignition: Leaves not less than 42% and not more than 45% of residue when ignited to a constant weight at a temperature above 900°C.

Tests for soluble substances: Boil 1 g in 50 ml of water for five minutes, and filter. Evaporate the filtrate and dry to constant weight at 105°C. The residue weighs not more than 10 mg.

Assay: An accurately weighed amount (0.15 g) is dissolved in a mixture of water (20 ml) and 2 M hydrochloric acid (2 ml), to which is added water (50 ml) and strong ammonia-ammonium chloride solution. The mixture is titrated with 0.05 M disodium edetate, using 0.1 g of mordant black II mixture as indicator until a blue colour is obtained.

1 ml of 0.05 M sodium edetate $\equiv$ 0.002015 g of MgO.

Uses: It is used as an antacid and laxative. Its pharmacological properties are similar to magnesium oxide.

It is comparatively a weak antacid. It is also used as a cathartic.

Dose: 0.3 to 0.6 gm as antacid and 2 to 4 gm as laxative.

LIGHT MAGNESIUM CARBONATE

Approx chem. formula: $3MgCO_3Mg(OH)_2.3H_2O$.

Light $MgCO_3$ is a hydrated basic carbonate which differs only slightly in its composition from that of heavy carbonate, in spite of great difference in its bulk density. The composition of light $MgCO_3$ seems to be most satisfactorily represented by the formula $3MgCO_3Mg(OH)_2.3H_2O$.

Preparation: Light $MgCO_3$ is prepared by Na_2CO_3 and $MgSO_4.MgSO_4$ (125 parts) and Na_2CO_3 (150 parts) are dissolved separately, each in 1000 parts of cold water. The solutions are mixed and boiled for 15 minutes; the precipitate is then collected on a calico filter, washed until it gives a slight reaction for SO_4 with $BaCl_2$ and dried in oven.

From the above it is to be noted that the differences in the methods of preparation of light and heavy magnesium carbonates lie only in the concentration and temperature of the reacting solutions and in the subsequent treatment of the precipitates.

It is to be tested and assayed like heavy magnesium carbonate.

Uses: It is used as an antacid and laxative similar to Heavy Magnesium Carbonate.

Dose: 0.3 to 0.6 g and 2 to 4.0 g.

MAGNESIUM OXIDE HEAVY
(Synonym: Heavy Magnesia)

Chem. formula: MgO   Mol. weight: 40.30

Preparation: The heavy magnesium oxide is prepared by heating the heavy magnesium carbonate to red hot when carbon dioxide and water are expelled and magnesium oxide remains behind.

$$3MgCO_3Mg(OH)_2.3H_2O \longrightarrow 4MgO + 3CO_2\uparrow + 4H_2O$$

Description: It is a white odourless powder with alkaline taste. It absorbs moisture and carbon dioxide when exposed to air.

It is almost insoluble in water and alcohol but soluble in dilute acids.

Tests for purity: Same as for Magnesium Oxide Light (mentioned below).

Uses: It is used as an antacid and laxative.

As an antacid it is quite effective and given as a non-systemic gastric antacid. In water, it is converted to the hydroxide and hence its biological properties are similar to hydroxide. Compared to Heavy Magnesium Carbonate, it does not liberate carbon dioxide and is fairly long-acting. Sometimes it is also administered as a cathartic.

MAGNESIUM OXIDE LIGHT
(Synonym: Light Magnesia)

Chem. formula: MgO   Mol. weight: 40.30

Preparation: The light MgO is prepared by heating light $MgCO_3$ to dull red until CO_2 is no longer evolved.

$$3MgCO_3Mg(OH)_2.3H_2O \longrightarrow 6MgO + 12H_2O + 3CO_2\uparrow$$

Description: Magnesium oxide is a white powder which slowly absorbs water and CO_2 from the atmosphere forming basic carbonates. It is only very slightly soluble in water but enough of it dissolves in water to form a solution which is clearly alkaline to phenolphthalein and contains Magnesium Hydroxide. It differs from heavy Magnesium Carbonate only in its bulk density.

Tests for purity: It is tested for As; Ca; Cu; Fe; Cl; SO_4 and soluble matter and also Pb and loss on ignition. Also for heavy metals, substances soluble in acetic acid.

Assay: Similar as in other magnesium compounds, using 0.05 M sodium edetate using about 50 mg of mordant black II mixture as indicator.

1 ml of 0.05 M disodium edetate $\equiv$ 0.002015 g of MgO.

Uses: It is used as an antacid and laxative. It is preferred over heavy magnesium oxide, otherwise its uses are similar as an antacid and as a laxative (see Heavy Magnesium oxide).

Dose: 0.3 to 0.6 gms.

MILK OF MAGNESIA

Milk of Magnesia is a suspension of 8.5% w/w of magnesium hydroxide in purified water and contains not less than 7.0% w/w and not more than 8.5% w/w of $Mg(OH)_2$. It is also called Magnesium Hydroxide Mixture or Cream of Magnesia. It has been official in I.P., B.P., U.S.P. etc.

Preparation: It is prepared from sodium hydroxide and magnesium sulphate. Light magnesium oxide is mixed with a solution of NaOH and the suspension is diluted with water. It is then poured slowly in a solution of magnesium sulphate with constant stirring. The precipitate is allowed to settle down and the upper clear liquid is decanted off. The residue is collected on a calico filter, washed with water until free from sulphate and mixed with the required quantity of purified water.

$$2NaOH + MgSO_4 \longrightarrow Mg(OH)_2 + Na_2SO_4$$

As shown in the above reaction the Sodium Hydroxide and Magnesium Sulphate interact to form Magnesium Hydroxide. If Magnesium Oxide is not used, the hydroxide would form gelatinous translucent aqueous suspension. With the addition of Magnesium Oxide the suspension is white and of a creamy consistency.

Tests for purity: It is tested for alkalinity; microbial limit; soluble alkalies; soluble salts; carbonates and acid insoluble matter; As; calcium oxides and heavy metals.

Assay: After thoroughly shaking about 5.0 g in a stoppered flask is taken and weighed accurately. 25 ml of 1 N H_2SO_4 is added and the solution is titrated for the excess of acid with 1 N NaOH using methyl red as indicator. The result is calculated as $Mg(OH)_2$.

$$H_2SO_4 + Mg(OH)_2 = MgSO_4 + 2H_2O$$

1 ml of 1 N H_2SO_4 is equivalent to 0.02917 g of $Mg(OH)_2$.

Uses: It is used as a laxative and antacid.

Doses: 8–16 ml as a laxative and 1–4 ml as an antacid.

Note: To minimise the action of glass container on milk of magnesia 0.1% of citric acid may be added (because glass gives some alkalis which will affect the alkalinity of $Mg(OH)_2$). Not more than 0.5 ml of volatile oils or a blend of volatile oils suitable for flavouring purposes may be added to one litre of milk of magnesia.

Preservatives like methyl paraben 0.2% or sodium benzoate 0.125% may be added to the milk of magnesia.

MAGNESIUM TRISILICATE
(Synonym: Epson Salt, Hydrated Magnesium Trisilicate)

Chem. formula: $2MgO_23SiO_2.3H_2O$ (or $4H_2O$)

Magnesium Trisilicate is a compound of magnesium oxide and silicon dioxide with varying proportion of water of crystallisation. It contains not less than 29.0% and not more than 32.0% of MgO, and not less than 66% and not more than 69.5% of SiO_2, both calculated with reference to the substance ignited to constant weight at a temperature above 1000°.

Preparation: When a solution of sodium silicate of the proper composition is precipitated by running into it an equimolar solution of magnesium sulphate or chloride, magnesium trisilicate is obtained which is filtered, washed and dried at low temperature. It is powdered, if required.

Description: Magnesium trisilicate is a white or nearly white fine powder, odourless and tasteless and free from grittiness. It is slightly hygroscopic. It is almost insoluble in water and alcohol. It is readily decomposed by mineral acids.

Tests for purity: It is tested for As; Fe; heavy metals; chloride; sulphate; acid absorption and loss on ignition, free alkali and soluble salts (I.P. 2007).

Assay for MgO: Accurately weighed sample (1 g) is dissolved in water (50 ml) by adding HCl (35 ml). The solution is boiled on a water bath for 15 mins, cooled, filtered, the residue washed with water and the filtrate and washings diluted with water (to 250 ml). A specified volume of the solution (50 ml) is neutralised with 10 N NaOH (8 ml). The resulting solution is titrated with 0.05 M disodium EDTA using ammonia buffer (10 ml, pH 10) and 50 mg of mordant black II mixture at 40°. The end point is noted in change in colour from violet to full blue.

Each ml of 0.05 M disodium EDTA = 0.002015 g MgO.

Assays for SiO$_2$: 0.7 g of the substance is taken in 10 ml of NH$_2$SO$_4$ and 10 ml of H$_2$O, and heated for one and a half hour on a water bath with frequent shaking replacing the water lost through evaporation. The contents are allowed to cool and then decanted on to an ashless filter paper (7 cm in diameter). The ppt. is washed by decantation with three quantities, each of 5 ml of hot water until 1 ml of the filtrate remains clear on the addition of 2 ml of 0.25 M barium chloride and 0.05 ml of 2 N HCl. The filter paper and its contents are ignited in a tared platinum crucible at 1000° to constant weight; the residue being SiO$_2$.

Uses: Magnesium trisilicate is a nonsystemic antacid and adsorbent. As an antacid it is slow-acting and weak. It is regarded as totally harmless when taken orally. It is liable to cause diarrhoea in large doses.

Dose: 0.3 to 2 g.

PROTECTIVES AND ADSORBENTS

Protectives and adsorbents are gastrointestinal agents commonly used for the treatment of mild diarrhoea. Diarrhoea may occur as a result of impaired digestion and/or absorption. It is a symptom and not a disease and may be caused by bacterial toxins, chemical poisons, drugs, allergy, disease, gastrointestinal surgery, carcinomas, chronic inflammatory conditions and various absorptive defects. Products used in the treatment of diarrhea may include an adsorbent-protective, an antispasmodic and possibly an antibacterial agent.

The adsorbent-protectives adsorb toxins, bacteria, and viruses along with providing a protective coating of the intestinal mucosa. They include bismuth salts, special clays and activated charcoal. The reader is advised to refer to the topic of 'Adsorbents' in the chapter on 'Pharmaceutical Aids and Necessities'.

BISMUTH SUBCARBONATE
(Synonym: Bismuth Carbonate)

Chem. formula: $(BiO)_2CO_3$ (?)

Bismuth subcarbonate is a basic salt which, upon ignition, yields not less than 80% and not more than 82.5% Bi, calculated with reference to the substance dried at 105° for three hours.

Preparation: Bismuth subcarbonate with its approximate composition is prepared by dissolving metallic bismuth in 50 per cent nitric acid and evaporating the solution to small volume and adding this solution gradually and with constant stirring to a cold solution of sodium carbonate.

$$2Bi + 8HNO_3 \longrightarrow 2Bi(NO_3)_3 + 2NO + 4H_2O$$

$$4Bi(NO_3)_3 + 6Na_2CO_3 + H_2O \longrightarrow [(BiO)_2CO_3]_2.H_2O + 12NaNO_3 + 4CO_2$$

The precipitate of bismuth subcarbonate is filtered and washed with cold water till the washings are neutral and dried at 55°.

Description: Bismuth subcarbonate is a white or pale yellowish, odourless and tasteless powder, which though stable in air is slowly affected by light.

The powder is insoluble in water and alochol; with hydrochloric acid and nitric acid it gives copuous effervescence and forms corresponding salts.

Tests for identity: It yields reactions characteristic of bismuth and carbonates (App. I).

Tests for purity: It is tested for loss on drying; arsenic; copper; lead and silver; sulphide; alkalis and alkaline earths; chloride and nitrate.

Tests for copper, lead, silver and sulphate are carried out by preparing a test solution by dissolving 3 g of bismuth subcarbonate in 4 ml of nitric acid, pouring the solution in 100 ml of water, collecting and washing the white precipitate so obtained with nitric acid and evaporating the filtrate and washing on a water bath to about 30 ml, filtering again and applying the following tests to the filtrate (Test solution).

Copper: To 5 ml of test solution is added dilute ammonia solution in slight excess. A white precipitate is produced and the supernatant liquid does not show a bluish tint, if copper is absent.

Lead: To 5 ml of test solution is added 5 ml of dilute H_2SO_4. No cloudiness is produced, if lead is absent.

Silver: To 5 ml test solution are added 10 drops of HCl. No precipitate is produced, if silver is absent.

Sulphate: To 5 ml of test solution are added a few drops of solution of barium nitrate. No immediate turbidity is produced if sulphate is absent.

Nitrate: The test depends upon comparing the colour produced by bismuth subcarbonate with that produced by a control in the following way: 0.5 g of bismuth subcarbonate is gently mixed with 5 ml of solution of phenoldisulphonic acid. To the mixture is added water to make 100 ml followed by the addition of dilute ammonia solution with constant stirring to obtain the maximum yellow colour. More water to make 500 ml is added and the solution is mixed and set aside for four hours. The solution is filtered and the first 50 ml of filtrate is rejected. The next 50 ml of filtrate is taken in a colour comparison tube and yellow colour in this tube is compared with that produced by control, containing in a volume of 50 ml, 10 ml of the filtrate, 5 ml of dilute ammonia solution and 60 ml of a solution prepared by grinding 81.5 mg of potassium nitrate with 4 ml of solution of phenoldisulphonic acid and dissolving the resolution in sufficient water to make 100 ml.

The yellow colour in the first solution is not darker than that produced in control.

Alkalis and alkaline earths: 1 g of bismuth subcarbonate is boiled with 20 ml of equal volume of acetic acid and water. The solution is cooled, filtered and washed. To the filtrate is added 2 ml of dilute HCl and 20 ml of water. The solution is boiled and hydrogen sulphide is passed through the solution, till no further precipitate is produced. The solution is filtered, precipitate is washed and the filtrate and the washings are evaporated to dryness. The dried residue is ignited gently with a drop of sulphuric acid. The residue after ignition weighs not more than 10 mg.

Assay: It is assayed by gravimetric method. An accurately weighed amount (1 g) in a tared crucible is ignited to constant weight. Yield on ignition should not be less than 90% of Bi_2O_3.

In I.P. 2007 assay is carried out by taking an accurately weighed (0.5 g) dissolved in nitric acid (3 ml), diluting to 250 ml with water, adding strong ammonia solution until appearance of cloudiness. More nitric acid (0.5 ml) is added and the mixture heated to 70°C till the solution becomes completely clear. After adding about 50 mg of xylol orange mixture, the solution is titrated with 0.1 M disodium acetate until the colour changes from pinkish violet to lemon yellow.

Each ml of 1 M disodium edetate ≡ 0.02090 g of Bi.

Uses: Bismuth subcarbonate is used as an astringent and absorbent. As an antacid it is very mild. In lotions and ointments, it is used topically as a protective. It is given in varying doses in the treatment of diarrhoea, dysentery and ulcerative colitis.

Dose: 1–3 g in divided doses.

BISMUTH SUBGALLATE
(Synonyms: Bismuth Oxygallate, Basic Bismuth Gallate)

Chem. formula: $(BiOH)_2 C_7H_5O_5$ (approx) or $C_7H_7BiO_7$ Mol. wt. : 412.13 (Approx.)

Bismuth subgallate is a basic salt of bismuth and contains not less than 50% and not more than 57% of Bi_2O_3, calculated with reference to the substance dried to constant weight at 105°.

Bismuth subgallate

The structure of bismuth subgallate, like many other bismuth compounds is not fully established. Basic bismuth gallate is not deemed as an oxy oxide salt, because it dissolves in alkalis, forms disodium compound and less only at 170° a molecule of water.

Preparation: It is prepared by dissolving Bismuth Subnitrate in dilute acetic acid and precipitating the solution with gallic acid.

Description: It occurs as an amorphous bright yellow powder. It is effected by light. It is insoluble in water, alcohol and ether. It dissolves in hot mineral acids and in solutions of alkali hydroxide.

Tests for purity: It is tested for arsenic; copper; lead; silver; nitrate; alkalis and alkaline earths; loss on drying and gallic acid.

All the tests, except for gallic acid, can be performed with little modifications mentioned in I.P. (page 108) in the same way as described in Bismuth subcarbonate.

Free gallic acid test: 1 g accurately weighed substance is shaken with 20 ml of alcohol for one minute. The solution is filtered and the residue is washed with 5 ml of alcohol. The filtrate and washing are combined and evaporated to dryness on a water bath. The residue is dried to constant weight at 105°. The residue should not weigh more than 0.25% of the weight of the substance taken.

Assay: It is assayed by gravimetric procedure. It is no more official in I.P.

About 1 g of bismuth subgallate is dried at 105° to constant weight and it is then weighed accurately. The substance is ignited in a porcelain crucible and allowed to cool. Nitric acid is added dropwise and the crucible warmed until solution is evaporated. The residue is ignited carefully to constant weight. The residue represents quantity of Bi_2O_3 in the weight of bismuth subgallate taken.

Uses: Like bismuth subcarbonate, it is used as astringent and antacid.

Dose: 1 g.

SALINE CATHARTICS

Saline cathartics (purgatives) are salts of poorly absorbable anions and sometimes cations that quicken and increase evacuation from the bowels. Laxatives are mild cathartics. Diminished intake of water and indigestible residue can lead to constipation. A large number of drugs cause constipation as one of the adverse effects.

Cathartics are used for the following conditions:

- To ease defecation in patients with painful hemorrhoids, rectal disorders and hernias.
- To avoid straining during defecation, and resultant potentially hazardous rises in blood pressure in patients with hypertension, cerebral, coronary or other arterial diseases.
- To relieve acute constipation.
- To remove solid material from the intestinal tract prior to certain roentgenographic studies.

Laxatives may be stimulant, bulk forming, emollient and saline. Saline cathartics act by increasing the osmotic load on the GIT. To relieve the hypertonicity of the gut, the body secretes additional fluids into the intestinal tract. The increased bulk stimulates peristalsis. Saline cathartics are water soluble and taken with large amounts of water, thereby preventing excessive loss of body fluids and preventing nausea and vomiting when too hypertonic a solution reaches the stomach.

Poorly absorbed ions used as saline cathartics are biphosphate ($H_2PO_4^-$), phosphate (HPO_4^{2-}), tartarate, sulphate and magnesium. Official saline cathartics include sodium biphosphate, sodium phosphate, potassium sodium tartrate, magnesium hydroxide, magnesium citrate and magnesium sulphate. Non-official saline cathartics include sodium sulphate, potassium phosphate potassium bitartrate, and calomel (Hg_2Cl_2).

SODIUM PHOSPHATE
(Synonym: Disodium Hydrogen Phosphate)

Chem. formula: $Na_2HPO_4.12H_2O$ Mol. weight: 358.2

Sodium phosphate contains not less than 98.0% and more than the equivalent of 101.0% of Na_2HPO_4 calculated with reference to the substance dried to constant weight at 130°C.

Preparation:

(1) It is prepared by adding Na_2CO_3 to a hot solution of phosphoric acid which are in equal amounts.

$$Na_2CO_3 + H_3PO_4 \longrightarrow Na_2HPO_4 + H_2O + CO_2$$

The solution should be just alkaline to litmus and then concentrated at the room temperature. The crystals are separated by centrifuging, washed and dried.

(2) It can also be prepared from calcium phosphate which on being treated in correct proportions with sulphuric acid yields calcium sulphate and monobasic calcium phosphate, the former gets precipitated, while the latter goes in solution.

$$Ca_3(PO_4)_2 + 2H_2SO_4 \longrightarrow Ca(H_2PO_4)_2 + 2CaSO_4\downarrow$$

The above mixture after the addition of boiling water is filtered and the filtrate is treated with sodium carbonate. Dibasic calcium phosphate gets deposited leaving sodium phosphate (disodium hydrogen phosphate) in solution. The reaction is as follows:

$$Ca(H_2PO_4)_2 + Na_2CO_3 \longrightarrow CaHPO_4 + Na_2HPO_4 + CO_2 + H_2O$$

The solution is filtered and the crystals of sodium phosphate are obtained by concentrating the solution and ultimate crystallisation.

Description: It occurs as odourless, colourless, monoclinic crystal which slowly effloresces. It has a saline taste. It is converted into sodium pyrophosphate on being heated at 300°C.

$$2Na_2HPO_4 \xrightarrow{\ 300°C\ } Na_4P_2O_7 + H_2O$$

It is soluble in water but almost insoluble in alcohol.

Tests for identity: The solution yields reactions characteristic of sodium and phosphate.

Reaction: A 2% w/v solution has pH between 9 to 9.2.

Tests for purity: It is tested for alkalinity; As; calcium and magnesium; heavy metals; Cl; SO_4 and loss on drying.

Test for calcium and magnesium: It is performed by dissolving 2 g of sodium phosphate in 50 ml of water, adding 3 ml of dilute ammonia solution and setting aside the solution for five minutes. No turbidity is produced.

In this test sodium phosphate itself acts as a precipitant, i.e. calcium is precipitated as calcium phosphate and magnesium as magnesium ammonium phosphate, as follows:

$$3Ca^{++} + 2NH_3 + 2HPO_4^{2-} \longrightarrow Ca_3(PO_4)_2 + 2NH_4^+$$

$$3Mg^{++} + 2NH_3 + 2HPO_4^{2-} \longrightarrow Mg_3(PO_4)_2 + 2NH_4^+$$

For heavy metals: A solution containing 2 g in 10 ml water is prepared and to this is added 4 ml of dilute HCl and water to make 25 ml. The limit for heavy metals is 10 parts per million.

Loss on drying: It is not less than 57% and not more than 66% at 130°.

Assay: It is determined by using basic principle of potentiometric type of titration. In this assay, a pH range of 4.4 to 9.2 is taken into consideration.

An accurately weighed amount of about 4 g of the sample is taken in 25 ml of N hydrochloric acid and diluted to 100 ml with water. 10 ml of the above solution is titrated potentiometrically with 0.1 N sodium hydroxide until pH 4.4 is reached (V_1). To the titrated solution is added 4 g of sodium chloride and titration is continued with 0.1 N sodium hydroxide to pH 9.2 (V_2). The percentage content of Na_2HPO_4 is determined by using the following formula:

$$\text{Percentage content of } Na_2HPO_4 = \frac{1420\,(V_2 - V_1)}{W(100 - D)}$$

where,

V_1 = Volume of NaOH used in first titration.

V_2 = Volume of NaOH used in second titration.

W = Weight of the sample taken.

D = The percentage loss on drying.

I.P. 2007 gives a modified method, but based on the same type of potentiometric titration.

Storage: It is preserved in a well-closed container.

Uses: It is used as a saline laxative and cathartic.

Dose: 2 to 16 g.

DRIED SODIUM PHOSPHATE
(Synonym: Anhydrous Sodium Phosphate)

Chem. formula: Na_2HPO_4 Mol. weight: 142.0

Dried sodium phosphate contains not less than 99.0% of Na_2HPO_4 calculated with reference to the substance dried to constant weight at 105°.

Description: It is a white hygroscopic powder which is odourless but has a saline taste. Like sodium phosphate it is soluble in water (8 parts) and insoluble in alcohol.

Tests for identity: It gives reaction characteristic of sodium and phosphates (App. I).

Reaction: A 5% w/v solution is alkaline to solution of litmus (limit test for alkalinity).

Tests for purity: It should comply with all the limit tests as mentioned under sodium phosphate. In the test for calcium and magnesium only 0.8 g of the substance is taken, dissolved in 50 ml of water and followed by the addition of 3 ml dilute solution of ammonia. After setting aside for five minutes, turbidity is noticed.

Test for heavy metals is performed in the same way and with the same quantities as mentioned under sodium sulphate.

Test for loss on drying is done at 105° and the substance loses not more than 2.5% of the weight taken.

Assay: The assay is carried out in the same way as for sodium phosphate. The substance taken is about 2.5 g accurately weighed.

Each ml of 0.5 N sulphuric acid is equivalent to 0.07098 g of Na_2HPO_4.

Storage: Anhydrous sodium phosphate is preserved in a tightly-closed container.

Uses: Same as reported under sodium phosphate.

Dose: 0.6 to 5 g.

POTASSIUM SODIUM TARTRATE
(Synonym: Rochelle Salt)

Chem. formula: CH(OH).COONa   Mol. weight: 282.2
$$CH(OH).COOK.4H_2O$$

Potassium sodium tartrate contains not less than 99.0% and not more than the equivalent of 104% of $C_4H_4O_6NaK, 4H_2O$. It is no more official.

Preparation: It can be prepared from a solution of Na_2CO_3 and potassium bitartrate. The solution is boiled for short time and then allowed to stand at 60°C for completion of reaction. Carbon dioxide is slowly evolved. The solution is filtered and evaporated to crystallisation.

$$Na_2CO_3 + 2C_4H_4O_6KH \longrightarrow 2C_4H_4O_6NaK + CO_2 + H_2O$$

Description: Rochelle salt occurs as colourless, odourless crystals or as white crystalline powder having saline taste. It is soluble in water and insoluble in alcohol. The crystals melt at 74°C; when they are ignited they become red and leave a residue of Na_2CO_3 and K_2CO_3.

$$2C_4H_4O_6KNa + 5O_2 \longrightarrow K_2CO_3 + Na_2CO_3 + 4H_2O + 6CO_2$$

Tests for identity:
  (1) Salt on being ignited emits an odour of burning sugar and leaves a residue which is alkaline to litmus paper and gives effervescence with acids.
  (2) Salt gives reactions characteristic of sodium and potassium and tartrates (App. I).

Tests for purity: It is tested for acidity and alkalinity; As; Fe; heavy metals; Cl; SO_4 and loss on drying.

For acidity and alkalinity: 1 g of the substance is dissolved in the recently boiled and cooled water and tested as under:
  (a) The solution is not alkaline to solution of phenolphthalein.
  (b) The solution does not require more than 0.1 ml of 0.1 N sodium hydroxide to produce a pink colour.

Assay: An accurately weighed quantity of substance (about 2 g) is ignited until it is fully carbonised. The cooled residue is extracted with water (50 ml) and excess of 0.5 N sulphuric acid (15 ml) is added. The solution is filtered to remove any insoluble impurities, the residue washed with water and the excess of acid with washings is titrated with 0.5 N sodium hydroxide using methyl orange as indicator.

Each ml of 0.5 N H_2SO_4 is equivalent to 0.07055 g of $C_4H_4O_6NaK.4H_2O$.

Uses: Rochelle salt is an important saline purgative.

Dose: 8 to 16 g.

MAGNESIUM SULPHATE
(Synonym: Epsom salt)

Chem. formula: $MaSO_4 \cdot 7H_2O$ Mol. weight: 246.47

Magnesium sulphate contains not less than 99.5% and not more than the equivalent of 100.5% of $MgSO_4$ calculated with reference to the substance dried to constant weight at 300°C.

Preparation:

(1) Magnesium sulphate can be prepared on the laboratory scale by neutralising hot, dilute sulphuric acid with magnesium or its oxide or carbonate and evaporating the filtered solution to crystallisation.

$$MgCO_3 + H_2SO_4 \longrightarrow MgSO_4 + H_4O + CO_2\uparrow$$

(2) It is manufactured by the action of sulphuric acid on the native carbonate (magnesite) or on previously powdered and calcined dolomite. When dolomite is used magnesium sulphate passes into solution and sparingly soluble calcium sulphate is deposited.

$$MgCO_3.CaCO_3 + 2H_2SO_4 \longrightarrow MgSO_4 + CaSO_4 + 2H_2O + 2CO_2\uparrow$$

The liquid is filtered and the filtrate is evaporated to crystallization.

The crystals have the composition $MgSO_4.7H_2O$.

It is also produced in large quantities from magnesium salt occurring in brine, used for the extraction of bromine. The liquors after removal of bromine are treated with milk of lime, thus precipitating magnesium salt as magnesium hydroxide. Sulphur dioxide and air are passed through the suspension of magnesium hydroxide.

$$Mg(OH)_2 + SO_2 + O \longrightarrow MgSO_4 + H_2O$$

Description: It occurs as colourless crystals which are usually needlelike. It is odourless and has cool, saline and bitter taste. It effloresces in warm dry air. It is soluble in one part of water, sparingly soluble in alcohol and dissolves slowly in one part of glycerin.

Tests for purity: It is tested for arsenic; iron, heavy metals; loss on drying and chloride.

Assay: An accurately weighed amount of about 0.3 g of the sample is taken in water (50 ml) and strong ammonia-ammonium chloride solution (10 ml) and titrated with 0.05 M disodium EDTA using mordant black II mixture (0.1 g) as indicator. The end point is achieved when the pink colour changes to blue.

Each ml of 0.05 M disodium EDTA $\equiv$ 0.00602 g $MgSO_4$.

Uses: It is used as cathartic.

Storage: It is stored in well-closed containers.

Dose: 2 to 16 g.

DRIED MAGNESIUM SULPHATE
(Synonym: Dried Epsom Salt)

Dried magnesium sulphate contains not less than 62 per cent and not more than 70 per cent of $MgSO_4$.

Description: It is a white powder, odourless with saline and bitter taste, freely soluble in water and more rapidly soluble in hot water.

Assay: An accurately weighed amount about 0.4 g is used and the assay is performed as described in Magnesium Sulphate.

Uses: It is used as a cathartic.

Dose: 2-12 g.

SODIUM SULPHATE
(Synonym: Glauber's Salt)

Chem. formula: $Na_2SO_4.10H_2O$ Mol. weight: 322.2

Sodium sulphate contains not less than 99% and not more than the equivalent of 100.5% of Na_2SO_4, calculated with reference to the substance dried to constant weight at 105°. It is not official now.

Preparation: It is manufactured by heating sodium chloride with concentrated sulphuric acid. The product, sodium bisulphate, is again treated with NaCl to get sodium sulphate. The decahydrate is obtained from sodium sulphate cake by crystallisation from water.

$$NaCl + H_2SO_4 \longrightarrow NaHSO_4 + HCl$$

$$NaHSO_4 + NaCl \longrightarrow Na_2SO_4 + HCl$$

Sodium sulphate can also be obtained by heating sodium nitrate with sulphuric acid with the production of nitric acid as follows:

$$2NaNO_3 + H_2SO_4 \longrightarrow NaHSO_4 + 2HNO_3$$

As a matter of fact here the production of sodium sulphate can be deemed as a by-product during the manufacture of hydrochloric acid and nitric acid.

Sodium sulphate also occurs as such in nature, dried or hydrated sodium sulphate. In India it was found in Rajasthan, but now this source of natural salt is exhausted. It is said to be occurring as natural deposits in Italy, Spain, Germany and Siberia.

Description: It occurs as colourless, odourless, transparent crystals or as a granular powder. It is bitter and saline in taste. It effloresces rapidly in air, liquefies in its water of hydration and fuses at about 886° and loses all its water at 100°. It is soluble in water (2.5 parts) and insoluble in alcohol.

Tests for identity: It gives reactions characteristic of sodium and sulphates (App. I).

Tests for purity: Acidity and alkalinity; arsenic; iron and zinc; heavy metals; magnesium; chloride and loss on drying.

Acidity and alkalinity: It is tested by dissolving 10 g of salt in 100 ml of recently boiled and cooled water and titrating the solution for neutralisation to the given colour of solution of bromothymol blue. Not more than 0.5 ml of 1 N sulphuric acid is required. Sodium sulphate should give a neutral reaction (pH 7).

Iron and zinc: They are tested by acidifying a 10 per cent solution (2 g in 20 ml of H_2O) with acetic acid (1 ml), adding a few drops of solution of potassium ferrocyanide and noting the turbidity or blue colour; which should be absent. Turbidity, if produced, will be due to the white precipitate of zinc ferrocyanide, while blue colour, if produced, will be due to the formation of prussian blue of iron salt.

Heavy metals: The test is performed by dissolving 2 g in 10 ml of water adding 2 ml of 0.1 N hydrochloric acid and diluting the solution with more water to make 25 ml volume. The limit for heavy metals is 10 parts per million.

Magnesium: It is tested by taking 10% solution (2 g in 20 ml), adding to it 1 ml of dilute ammonia solution and 1 ml of solution of sodium phosphate and setting aside for five minutes. No turbidity should be produced.

Test for loss on drying is carried out by drying the salt at 105° to constant weight. The loss should not be less than 51.5 per cent and not more than 57.0 per cent. The loss corresponds to the total amount of water of crystallisation.

Assay: The assay is carried out by gravimetric method. An accurately weighed quantity of salt (about 0.5 g) is dissolved in water (100 ml) and after adding 1 ml of HCl the solution is heated to boiling. A slight excess of hot solution of barium chloride is added slowly and the solution heated, digested for half an hour on water bath (to get larger crystals of $BaSO_4$). The solution is then cooled and the precipitate collected and washed on Gooch crucible (collected and washed on a Gooch). The ppt. is then ignited to constant weight.

$$Na_2SO_4 + BaCl \longrightarrow 2NaCl + BaSO_4\downarrow$$

1 gm of residue is equivalent to 0.6085 gms of Na_2SO_4.

In the above assay sulphate ion of sodium sulphate is precipitated as barium sulphate. An excess of barium chloride is added drop by drop and not at once and the precipitation is carried out in boiling solution. Heating on water bath is continued for half an hour to allow the precipitated barium sulphate to separate as larger crystals (digestion helps in forming larger particles and this helps in filtration) which can be collected on a Gooch filter or on an ashless filter paper and igniting the precipitate carefully.

Each g of the residue is equivalent to 0.6085 g of Na_2SO_4.

Uses: It is an effective cathartic and is used as a saline purgative. Its unpleasant taste and drastic action bring it discredit. However it is used commonly in veterinary practice. It is also sometimes used as a diuretic in the form of an intravenous drip for which about 4.0% sterilised solution is used.

Dose: 5 to 15 g.

Storage: Sodium sulphate is preserved in a well-closed container not above 60°.

DRIED SODIUM SULPHATE

(Synonym: Exsiccated Slamber's Salt or Exsiccated Sodium Sulphates)

Chem. formula: Na_2SO_4 Mol. weight: 142

Here there is no water of crystallization and the salt is dried.

Dried sodium sulphate contains not less than 97.5 per cent of sodium sulphate (Na_2SO_4) calculated with reference to the substance dried to constant weight at 105°.

Preparation: Same as described under Sodium Sulphate. The salt is heated at 100°C to drive off all the water.

Description: It is a white hygroscopic powder which is odourless, having bitter and saline taste. It is soluble in water.

Tests for identity: Same as under Sodium Sulphate.

Tests for purity: Acidity or alkalinity (4 g of the powder is taken for the test and the test is performed in the same way as described under sodium sulphate).

Arsenic: Not more than two parts per million.

Iron and zinc: 0.8 g of the substance is taken and test performed in the same way as in Sodium Sulphate above.

Heavy metals: Same test as in Sodium Sulphate above.

Magnesium: 0.8 g of the substance is taken and the test is performed in the same way as under Sodium Sulphate.

Chloride: 0.4 g complies with the limit test for chlorides.

Loss on drying: Loses not more than 5% of its weight when dried to constant weight at 105°C.

Assay: Assay is carried out in the same way as described under Sodium Sulphate using about 0.3 g of the substance, weighed accurately.

Storage: Dried Sodium Sulphate is stored in a well-closed container.

Uses: See under Sodium Sulphate above.

Dose: 1 to 8 g.

POTASSIUM ACID TARTRATE
(Synonym: Potassium Hydrogen Tartrate)

Formula: CH(OH)COOK   Mol. weight: 188.2

       |

    CH(OH)COOH

Potassium acid tartrate contains not less than 79.5% of $C_4H_5O_6K$ calculated with reference to the substance dried to constant weight at 105°. It is not official now.

Preparation: It is prepared from Argol (residue of wine) which consists of potassium acid tartrate, calcium tartrate, colouring matter and other impurities.

Argol is first dissolved in hot water and neutralised with Na_2CO_3. The solution is filtered and passed through soda-ash and through charcoal to remove colouring impurities. The solution is filtered which contains sodium potassium tartrate. Sod. pot. tartrate is then decomposed by adding acetic acid. Pot. bitartrate settles down as a fine precipitate while sodium acetate remains in the solution.

$$KNaC_4H_4O_6 + CH_3COOH \longrightarrow CH_3COONa + C_4H_5O_6K$$

Description: It occurs as colourless or slightly opaque or gritty, white crystalline powder, slightly soluble in water, soluble in hot water and practically insoluble in alcohol.

Tests for identity:

  (1) Filtered dilute hydrochloric acid solution of carbonised residue yields reactions characteristic of potassium.

  (2) Gives reactions characteristic of tartrates.

Tests for purity: It is tested for As; Cu; Fe; Cl; SO_4; free tartaric acid and loss on drying.

Free tartaric acid is tested by shaking and evaporating the solution to dryness. The residue should not be more than 1 mg.

Assay: An accurately weighed quantity (1.5 g) of the substance is dissolved in boiling water (100 ml) and titrated with 0.2 N NaOH while hot, using phenolphthalein as indicator.

$$KHC_4H_5O_6 + NaOH \longrightarrow KNaC_4H_4O_6 + H_2O$$

1000 ml of 0.2 N NaOH is equivalent to 1/5 $KHC_4H_4O_6$.

Or Each ml of 0.2 N NaOH is equivalent to 0.03764 g of $KHC_4H_4O_6$.

Storage: It is preserved in a well-closed container.

Uses: It is used as a purgative.

MERCUROUS CHLORIDE
(Synonym: Calomel)

Chem. formula: Hg_2Cl_2 Mol. Weight: 236.1

It contains not less than 99.6% of Hg_2Cl_2. It is no more official.

Preparation:

(1) It is obtained by heating mercury with mercuric chloride and subliming the product. The sublimate is washed with water until free from mercuric chloride.

$$Hg + HgCl_2 \longrightarrow Hg_2Cl_2$$

(2) Earlier HgCl was obtained by heating mercurous sulphate with sodium chloride and subliming the product. Mercurous sulphate was prepared by heating sulphuric acid with mercury until the dry product, mercuric sulphate, was obtained.

$$Hg + 2H_2SO_4 \longrightarrow HgSO_4 + SO_2 + 2H_2O$$

The metallic mercury which is just sufficient to convert mercuric sulphate to mercurous sulphate is mixed intimately with the dried salt and triturated, until Hg is no more visible. It is mixed with the calculated amount of sodium chloride and the mixture is sublimed in such a way that a fine, amorphous product is obtained. This is done either by mixing cold air or steam with the vapours of mercurous chloride before they reach the condensing chamber. The product so obtained is freed from any mercuric chloride by thoroughly agitating it with water and finally washing it with dilute nitric acid to remove any traces of unchanged mercury. The acid is removed by washing it out with water. The product is sublimed.

$$HgSO_4 + Hg \longrightarrow Hg_2SO_4$$
$$Hg_2SO_4 + 2NaCl \longrightarrow Hg_2Cl_2 + Na_2SO_4$$

(3) It is also prepared by adding a solution containing chloride ion to a solution of soluble mercurous salt.

Since the precipitate formed is finer, it is more active and hence is given in about 1/3rd the dose of calomel.

$$Hg_2(NO_3)_2 + 2NaCl \longrightarrow Hg_2Cl_2 + 2NaNO_3$$

Description: Mercurous chloride occurs as a dull white heavy powder, odourless and almost tasteless. It is insoluble in water, alcohol, solvent ether and in cold sulphuric acid.

It becomes yellow when triturated or compressed. It volatilises when strongly heated. It is stable in air but gradually darkens, turning slightly grey when exposed to light, due to its decomposition into mercury and mercuric chloride.

Tests for purity: It is tested for ammoniated mercury; mercuric chloride and non-volatile matter.

Assay: The assay method is based on the oxidation of mercurous to mercuric mercury with excess of standard iodine. Iodine is solubilised with KI with the formation of the complex salt, $K_2(HgI_4)$. The excess of iodine is back titrated with 0.1 N $Na_2S_2O_3$ solution, using starch solution as indicator.

$$Hg_2Cl_2 + I_2 + 6KI_2 \longrightarrow 2K_2(HgI_4) + 2KCl$$

An accurately weighed about 0.7 g of mercurous chloride is mixed with 10 ml of water in a glass-stoppered flask and to it is added 50 ml of 0.1 N iodine and 2 g of potassium iodide dissolved in 10 ml of water. The flask is closed and set aside, shaking occasionally until solution is complete. The excess of iodine is titrated with 0.1 N sodium thiosulphate using solution of starch as indicator.

$$2HgCl + I_2 \longrightarrow HgI_2 + HgCl_2$$

or

$$2HgCl + 2KI + I_2 \longrightarrow 2HgI_2 + 2KCl$$

$$2Na_2S_2O_3 + I_2 \longrightarrow Na_2S_4O_6 + 2NaI$$

Each ml of 0.1 N iodine is equivalent to 0.02361 g of HgCl.

Uses: Calomel has been used for centuries as a cathartic but in recent years it has lost importance due to cases of mercury poisoning; ointments containing calomel are sometimes used in the treatment of eczema and as a prophylactic syptulls.

Calomel is insoluble in gastric juice and is not absorbed from the stomach. It is absorbed in the intestine by the alkaline pancreatic juice where it is slowly dissociated into mercury and irritant mercuric compounds which exert a cathartic action. When calomel is administered internally, it is usually given at night and is followed by a saline purgative in the morning. If it is retained in the intestine, it may give rise to systemic mercury poisoning.

Topical Agents

Topical agents are substances/compounds used on body surfaces. Topical application of drugs may also be accomplished within body cavities (oral, vaginal and colonic). The pharmacological effects may be either localized to the area applied, or systemic depending on the degree of absorption of the drug. The systemic effect may be intended as in the case of formulations like transdermal patches, sublingual tablets, suppositories etc. On the other hand, systemic effects of some of the compounds that are absorbed may elicit toxic or allergic manifestations depending on the degree of absorption.

Topical inorganic agents intended for their localized action may be broadly categorized based on their use as protective, antimicrobial and astringent compounds. The particular use will also depend on the area of application, the concentration of the agent, the presence of other compounds in the preparation, and the solubility (e.g., insoluble zinc oxide is a protective and soluble zinc sulphate is an astringent).

PROTECTIVES

Protectives are substances applied to protect areas of the skin which are subject to constant irritation due to moisture and/or friction, or areas that have become irritated or inflamed due to friction, allergy, and the like. Many protectives are also adsorbents that adsorb moisture from the surface of the skin. Protectives are not applied to areas that are abraded and exuding fluid as the likelihood of systemic absorption is enhanced and they may mix with the exudates and form a crust, which adheres to the open tissue.

The compounds of substances most suitable as protectives have the following properties:

- Insoluble (minimizes systemic absorption).
- Chemically inert (to prevent interactions with the tissue).

The adsorbent and protective action is maximized with small particle size. A fine state of subdivision of particles possesses good adhering properties, enhances the soothing effect and minimizes irritation.

Topical inorganic protectives include formulations containing talc, zinc oxide, calamine, zinc stearate, basic aluminium carbonate and titanium dioxide.

The use of protectives and adsorbents for use internally has been dealt within the chapters on 'Gastrointestinal Agents' and 'Pharmaceutical Aids and Necessities'.

TALC, PURIFIED TALC, TALCUM

Approx. formula : $Mg_6(Si_2O_5)_4(OH)_4$

Purified Talc is natural purified magnesium silicate corresponding approximately to the formula $Mg_6(Si_2O_5)_4(OH)_4$.

It is a naturally occurring hydrous magnesium silicate (sometimes containing a small proportion of aluminium silicate) and is called soapstone or French chalk. It is said to be the softest mineral and has more free flow property than kaolin. It may contain varying amount of iron.

Preparation: Pharmaceutically required product is purified from native talc by boiling the finely powdered talc with dilute hydrochloric acid and then washing the insoluble talc well and drying.

Description: Purified talc is a very fine, white or greyish-white powder, which is odourless and tasteless. It is free from grittyness, readily adheres to skin and is unctuous to the touch. Its solution is neutral to litmus.

Tests for identity: The I.P. now gives the following two tests for identification.

Mix 0.5 g with about 0.2 g of anhydrous sodium carbonate and 2 g of anhydrous potassium carbonate and heat the mixture in a platinum crucible until fusion is complete. Cool and transfer the fused mixture to a dish or beaker with the aid of about 50 ml of hot water. Add hydrochloric acid to the liquid until it ceases to cause effervescence then add 10 ml more of the acid and evaporate the mixture to dryness on a water bath. Cool, add 20 ml of water, boil and filter the mixture. Dissolve in the filtrate about 2 g of ammonium chloride and add 5 ml of dilute ammonia solution. Remove by filtration any precipitate which may form and add solution of sodium phosphate to the filtrate; a white, crystalline precipitate of magnesium ammonium phosphate separates.

Tests for purity: It is tested for acid-soluble substance; reaction; water-soluble substances, water-soluble iron salts, carbonates and loss on drying.

Test for acid-soluble substances: It is performed by digesting 2 g with 40 ml dilute hydrochloric acid for fifteen minutes, filtering the solution and evaporating the filtrate. The residue obtained is ignited, after the addition of 0.1 ml of dilute sulphuric acid to constant weight. The residue weight not more than 20 mg.

Test for water-soluble substances: It is performed by evaporating 25 ml of the filtrate obtained by boiling 10 g with 50 ml of water for 30 minutes to constant weight at 105°. The residue does not weigh more than 10 mg.

Test for water-soluble iron: It is done by preparing a solution (as given below) which should comply with the limit test for iron. The test solution is prepared by boiling 4 g of purified talc with 25 ml of water for thirty minutes, replacing the water lost during evaporation and filtering the solution. The solution after the addition of 5 ml of nitric acid is diluted to 50 ml with water and used for the test.

Carbonates are tested by adding 1 g to 20 ml of dilute hydrochloric acid and noting the absence of effervecsence.

Loss on ignition: The substance loses not more than 6 per cent of its weight when ignited to constant weight at 1000°C, or not more than 1.0% by drying 1.0 g at 180° for 1 hour.

Storage: Purified talc is stored in a well-closed container, protected from moisture.

Uses: It is an important pharmaceutical aid. It is used in a dusting powder under the name talcum powder. It is perfumed or medicated. It is used in a stering medium for all classes of preparations as it does not absorb and retain active principles.

ZINC GELATIN
(Synonym: Unna's Paste)

Zinc gelatin contains 15 per cent w/w of zinc oxide (limit 4.10 to 16 per cent of ZnO).

Ingredients:

Zinc oxide, finely sifted	150 g
Gelatin, cut small	150 g
Glycerin	350 g
Purified water	350 ml or sufficient quantity

Preparation: The gelatin is softened thoroughly in purified water and heated with glycerin on water bath till it is dissolved. The weight of the mixture, if necessary, is adjusted to 850 g by adding more of purified water. Zinc oxide is then incorporated and the contents stirred until about to set.

Assay: An accurately weighed amount, 4 g, of zinc gelatin is warmed with 25 ml of water until the basis is dissolved. The mixture is cooled and shaken well with 25 ml of 1 N sulphuric acid. 0.1 g of ammonium chloride is added and the excess of acid is titrated with 1 N sodium hydroxide, using solution of methyl orange as indicator.

Each ml of 1 N sulphuric acid is equivalent to 0.04069 g of ZnO.

Storage: Zinc gelatin is preserved in a well-closed container.

Uses: It is used as a protective and is applied in the molten state between two layers of bandage for protective purpose and for supporting varicosities and lesions of the legs. The dressing is removed after about a fortnight on being soaked with warm water.

ZINC OXIDE

Chem. formula: ZnO Mol. wt.: 81.4

Zinc oxide contains not less than 99% of ZnO, calculated with reference to the substance ignited to constant weight.

Preparation:

(1) Zinc oxide is manufactured on a large scale by heating metallic zinc to bright redness in a current of air. The vapour of the metal burns to form the oxide, which is collected as a fine white powder, but zinc oxide so prepared is not used for pharmaceutical purposes.

$$2Zn + O_2 \longrightarrow 2ZnO$$

(2) A purer product can be obtained from zinc sulphate. A solution of zinc sulphate is added to a boiling solution of sodium carbonate. The precipitated basic carbonate of zinc is collected, washed until freed from sulphate, dried and gently ignited. It loses carbon dioxide and water, leaving the oxide.

$$ZnSO_4 + Na_2CO_3 \longrightarrow ZnCO_3 + Na_2SO_4$$
$$ZnCO_3 \longrightarrow ZnO + CO_2$$

Description: It occurs as a soft, white or faintly white, very fine powder, free from grittyness. It is odourless and tasteless. When exposed to air, it slowly absorbs carbon dioxide from the air.

Solubility: Zinc oxide is insoluble in water and alcohol but since it is amphoteric, it is soluble in solution of alkali hydroxides and in dilute mineral acids.

Tests for identity:

(1) On being strongly heated, zinc oxide assumes a yellow colour, which disappears on cooling.

(2) A solution of zinc oxide in dilute hydrochloric acid, after neutralisation of the acid, yields reactions characteristic of zinc (App. I).

Tests for purity: It is tested for alkalinity; carbonate and insoluble impurities; arsenic; iron; metallic zinc and loss on drying.

Alkalinity: It is tested by mixing 1 g of the substance with 10 ml of hot water, adding 2 drops of solution of phenolphthalein and noting the colour. In case a red colour is produced, the amount of 0.1 N hydrochloric acid required to discharge the red colour should be more than 0.3 ml.

Test for carbonate and insoluble impurities: It is carried out by mixing 2 g of the substance with 10 ml of water, adding 30 ml of dilute sulphuric acid and heating the solution on a water bath with constant stirring. No effervescence should occur and the solution should remain clear and colourless.

Arsenic as tested by the general method described is not more than 8 parts per million.

Iron is tested by dissolving 0.1 g of ZnO in a mixture of 5 ml of water and 0.5 ml of iron free hydrochloric acid and diluting the solution to 40 ml with water. The solution with 6 drops of thioglycollic acid should comply with limit test for iron.

Lead is tested by dissolving 2 g of ZnO in a mixture of 20 ml of water and 5 ml of glacial acetic acid and adding 5 drops of solution of potassium chromate. The solution should remain clear. In the test, precipitate of yellow lead chromate is expected to be formed in the presence of acetic acid; zinc chromate remains in solution.

Metallic zinc: It is tested by dissolving 2 g of ZnO in a mixture of 30 ml of dilute hydrochloric acid and 10 ml of water to which one drop of solution of lead acetate has been added. The solution should be clear and colourless.

Assay: It is titrated acidimetrically. Zinc oxide and ammonium chloride are dissolved in an excess of standard sulphuric acid, with the help of heat, if ecessary. The excess of acid is titrated with standard sodium hydroxide using methyl orange as indicator.

Ammonium chloride is used for preventing the preci tion of zinc hydroxide during the titration (due to local difference in concentration) as also at the e int. The precipitation of zinc hydroxide, if allowed to take place, would give a poor end point. The procedure is as follows:

An accurately weighed amount, about 1.5 g of ZnO, is dissolved with 2.5 g of ammonium chloride in 50 ml of 1 N sulphuric acid. The excess of acid is titrated with 1 N sodium hydroxide using methyl orange as indicator.

$$ZnO + H_2SO_4 \longrightarrow ZrSO_4 + H_2O$$

Each ml of 1 N sulphuric acid is equivalent to 0.04069 g of ZnO.

I.P. 2007 has given the modified assay, consisting of dissolving the substance (0.15 g) in acetic acid

2 M (10 ml) and water (50 ml). Adding to the solution 50 mg of xylol orange triturate and sufficient hexamine to produce violet-pink colour, adding more (2 g) of hexamine and titrating with 0.1 M disodium edetate until the solution becomes yellow.

1 ml of 0.1 M sodium edetate $\equiv$ 0.008138 g of ZnO.

Storage: Zinc oxide is preserved in a well-closed container.

Uses: Zinc oxide is used for its mild astringent antiseptic and protective action on the skin. It is widely employed in the treatment of skin diseases in the form of ointment and pastes, which are official in various pharmacopoeias. It is used for treating eczema, impetigo, psoriasis, ringworm etc. It is also used in bandages and adhesives. Dentists use it as a dental cement and for temporary fillings.

ZINC OXIDE COMPOUND PASTE
(Synonym: Zinc Paste)

Zinc oxide compound paste contains 25% of zinc oxide (limits 23.5–26.5% of zinc oxide).

Ingredients:

Zinc oxide, finely sifted	250 g
Starch, finely sifted	250 g
White soft paraffin	500 g

The white soft paraffin is melted and the zinc oxide and the starch is incorporated and paste stirred until cold.

Assay: Same as described under zinc oxide ointment. I.P. 2007's assay can be used also.

Uses: See under zinc oxide.

HYDROUS ZINC OXIDE OINTMENT

Hydrous zinc oxide ointment contains 15% ZnO (Limit 14.0 to 15.5).

Ingredients:

Zinc oxide, finely sifted	150 g
Hydrous ointment	850 g

Preparation: The zinc oxide is triturated with a portion of the hydrous ointment until smooth. The remainder of the ointment is added gradually with thorough mixing.

Tests for identity: The residue obtained in the assay gives the tests (1) and (2) described under zinc oxide.

Tests for purity: It is tested for calcium; magnesium; and other foreign substances.

The test is carried out by taking the residue obtained in the assay and adding to it 6 ml of dilute hydrochloride acid. When no effervescence should occur upon heating the mixture on a water bath for fifteen minutes, no more than trace of insoluble residue should remain. The solution is filtered and diluted to 10 rnl with water and to this is then added dilute ammonia solution, until the precepitate first formed is dissolved, followed by the addition of 2 ml of equal volumes of solutions of ammonium oxalate and sodium phosphate. The solution is observed for five minutes, during which time not more than slight turbidity is produced.

Assay: The assay is carried out in the similar way as described under zinc oxide ointment.

Uses: See under Zinc Oxide.

ZINC OXIDE OINTMENT *
(Zinc Ox. Oint.)
(Synonym: Zinc Ointment)

Zinc oxide ointment contains 15 per cent of ZnO (limit 14 to 15.5%).

Ingredients:

Zinc oxide, finely sifted	150 g
Simple ointment	850 g

The zinc oxide is triturated with a portion of the simple ointment until smoothed. The remainder of simple ointment is added gradually and then mixed thoroughly.

Tests for identity: The tests are performed in the same way as described under Hydrous Zinc Oxide Ointment.

Tests for purity: It is tested for calcium; magnesium and other foreign substances and the test carried out the same way as described under Hydrous Zinc Oxide ointment (see above).

Assay: An accurately weighed amount, about 2 g, of ointment is taken in a tared porcelain crucible and melted gently. The heating is continued, gradually raising the temperature, until the mass is thoroughly charred. The charred mass is ignited until the residue becomes uniformly yellow. The residue is of ZnO and ignited to a constant weight.

Storage: The zinc oxide ointment is preserved in a well-closed container and is not allowed to be exposed to prolonged temperature exceeding 30°C.

Uses: See under zinc oxide.

In I.P. 2007 Zinc Oxide Cream is made official.

CALAMINE
(Synonym: Prepared Calamine)

Calamine is a zinc oxide with small amount of ferric oxide and contains, after ignition, 98% to 100.5% of zinc oxide, ZnO.

Preparation: Calamine is prepared by thoroughly mixing zinc oxide with ferric oxide (0.5 to 1%). It used to be prepared earlier by roasting zinc carbonate, which alone used to be known as calamine.

Description: Calamine is a pink powder, passing through a No. 100 mesh sieve. It is odourless and tasteless.

It is insoluble in water, but dissolves completely in mineral acids.

Tests for identity:

(1) The filtrate, obtained after dissolving 1 g of calamine in 10 ml of dilute hydrochloric acid, yields reactions characteristic of zinc.

(2) A reddish-brown colour is obtained if solution of ammonium thiocyanate is added to the filtrate, obtained after boiling 1 g of calamine with 10 ml of dilute hydrochloric acid and filtering the solution.

Tests for purity: It is tested for acid-insoluble substances; alkaline substances; arsenic; calcium; magnesium; lead; water-soluble dyes; alcohol-soluble dyes and loss on ignition.

Acid-insoluble substances are tested dyes; by dissolving 1 g in 25 ml of warm dil. hydrochloric acid. The insoluble residue, if any, is collected on a tared filter, washed with water, dried to constant weight at 105°, cooled and weighed. The residue on cooling should not weigh more than 20 mg.

Alkaline substances are tested by digesting 1 g with 20 ml of warm water, filtering the solution and adding 2 drops of the solution of phenolphthalein to the filtrate. The red colour, if produced, should not require more than 0.2 ml of 0.1 N sulphuric acid to discharge it.

Arsenic: Not more than 8 ppm.

Calcium: A weighed quantity of sample (0.5 g) is dissolved in water (10 ml), made acidic with glacial acetic acid (2.5 ml) and warmed on a water bath to effect complete dissolution. The solution is filtered and to the filtrate (0.5 ml) is added 5 N ammonia (15 ml) and a 2.5% w/v solution of ammonium oxalate (2 ml).

The solution remains clear on standing for 2 minutes.

Calcium and magnesium: The test is performed by taking 10 ml of solution prepared in the test for calcium above. To the solution is added 2 ml of solution of sodium phosphate. The turbidity produced should not be more than slight.

Lead: A weighed quantity of the sample (2 g) is dissolved in a mixture of water and glacial acetic acid (20 ml : 5 ml), filtered and to the filtrate is added solution of potassium chromate (0.25 ml). The solution remains clear for 5 minutes.

Water-soluble dyes: A weighed quantity of the sample (1 g) is shaken with water (10 ml) and filtered. The filtrate is colourless (I.P. App. 6.2).

Ethanol-soluble dyes: Same as "Water-soluble dyes test." Alcohol (90%) is used instead of water. The filtrate is colourless (I.P. App. 6.2).

Loss on ignition: The sample (2 g) is ignited at temp. not less than 90°C. Not more than 2% of the sample is lost on ignition.

Storage: It is stored in a well-closed container.

Assay: The assay procedure is based on the principle of volumetric titration.

A weighed quantity of the sample is dissolved in a measured volume of 1 N H_2SO_4 and the excess of H_2SO_4 is then determined by titration with 1 N NaOH using methyl orange as an indicator. Zinc sulphate ($ZnSO_4$) may react with NaOH to give Zinc hydroxide $Zn(OH)_2$.

$$ZnSO_4 + 2NaOH \longrightarrow Zn(OH)_2\downarrow + Na_2SO_4$$

The $Zn(OH)_2$ gets precipitated and it leads to a poor end point, both during the titration (by local differences in concentration) and at the finish. In order to present a poor end-point, ammonium chloride is used.

If more amount of NaOH is used, it is possible to dissolve the precipitate but the end-point is not correct because NaOH with $Zn(OH)_2$ forms sodium zincate (ZnO_2Na_2).

$$Zn(OH)_2 + Excess\ 2NaOH \longrightarrow ZnO_2Na_2 + 2H_2O$$

An accurately weighed sample (1.5 g) from freshly ignited calamine is dissolved in 1 N sulphuric acid (50 ml) and warmed gently, if required. The solution is filtered and the residue on filter is washed with hot water till the washings are not acidic to litmus paper. To the combined filtrate and washing is added ammonium chloride (2.5 g) (to prevent precipitation of zinc hydroxide) and the solution is titrated with 1 N NaOH, using solution of methyl red as indicator.

$$ZnO + H_2SO_4 \longrightarrow ZnSO_4 + H_2O$$

1 ml of 1 N H_2SO_4 is equivalent to 0.04069 g of ZnO.

Uses: Calamine is used as an astringent and protective. It is used for soothing purposes in ointments and lotions for sunburns etc.

Dose: In lotion and ointments in different concentrations.

CALAMINE LOTION
(Calam. Lot.)

Ingredients:

Calamine	150. g
Zinc oxide	50. g
Bentonite	30. g
Sodium citrate	5. g
Liquefied phenol	5. ml
Glycerin	50. ml
Rose water of commerce sufficient to produce	1000. ml

Preparation: Calamine lotion is prepared as per the composition given above. The preparation is included in the general pharmacy syllabus and is prepared by triturating the first three ingredients with a solution of the sodium citrate in about 700 ml of rose water to which are added liquefied phenol and glycerin and sufficient rose water to make the volume to 1000 ml.

Storage: Calamine lotion is preserved in a well-closed container.

Uses: It is used as a protective.

I.P. 2007 also includes the preparations: Aqueous Calamine Cream and Calamine Ointment.

ZINC STEARATE
(Zinc Stear.)

Chem. formula $(CH_3CH_2)_{16}COO)_2Zn$ Mol. weight: 632.34

Zinc stearate consists of zinc stearate $(CH_3(CH_2)_{16}COO)_2Zn$, together with variable proportion of zinc palmitate $(CH_3(CH_2)_{14}COO)_2Zn$. It contains not less than 13% and not more than 15.5 per cent of ZnO.

Preparation: Zinc stearate is prepared by adding an aqueous solution of zinc sulphate to a solution of sodium stearate and washing the precipitate with water, until freed from sulphide and drying it.

The commercial stearic acid, used for preparing sodium stearate is always available mixed with different proportions of palmitic acid. It is prepared by hydrolysis of fats and is subjected to partial purification to separate other fatty acids of low melting points, which are produced along with the stearic acid.

In order to prepare zinc stearate, first sodium stearate is prepared by adding gradually with constant mixing, calculated quantity of stearic acid to a hot solution of sodium hydroxide or sodium carbonate.

$$NaOH + C_{17}H_{35}COOH \longrightarrow C_{17}H_{35}COONa + H_2O$$

$$NaCO_3 + 2C_{17}H_{35}COOH \longrightarrow 2C_{17}H_{35}COONa + H_2O + CO_2$$

The above solution of sodium stearate is allowed to cool and a solution of zinc sulphate is added to it. The precipitated zinc stearate is collected, washed and dried.

$$2C_{17}H_{35}COONa + ZnSO_4 \longrightarrow (C_{17}H_{35}COO)_2Zn + Na_2SO_4$$

Sod. stearate   Zinc sulph.   Zinc stearate   Sod. sulphate

Description: Zinc stearate is a light, fine, white, impalpable, amorphous powder. It is free from grittyness and has faint characteristic odour. It is unctuous to touch and adheres to the skin readily.

Zinc stearate is insoluble in water, alcohol and ether. A suspension is neutral to moistened litmus paper.

Tests for identity:

(1) Zinc stearate is easily hydrolysed by heating with dilute mineral acid to give soluble zinc salt and an insoluble oily layer of stearic acid (as also palmitic acid).

$$2(C_{17}H_{35}COO)_2Zn + H_2SO_4 \longrightarrow 2C_{17}H_{35}COOH + ZnSO_4$$

$$(C_{17}H_{35}COO)_2Zn + 2HCl \longrightarrow 2C_{17}H_{35}COOH + ZnCl_2$$

1 g of stearic acid is added to a mixture of 25 ml of water and 5 ml of sulphuric acid and the mixture is boiled.

The solution separates into an upper oily layer of stearic acid and an aqueous lower layer containing zinc salt which after neutralisation yields the reaction characteristic of zinc.

(2) The oily layer consisting of stearic acid in the above test is separated and placed on a filter wetted with water and washed with boiling water to free it from sulphate or chloride. The stearic acid is collected in a small beaker and cooled. The supematant water, if any, is poured off, the acid melted, filtered while hot in a dry beaker and dried at 105°C for twenty minutes. The melted stearic acid congeals at a temperature not below 54°.

Tests for purity: It is tested for reaction; alkalis and alkaline earths and free fatty acids.

Tests for alkalis and alkaline earths: It is performed by boiling 1 g of the substance with a mixture of 25 ml of water and 5 ml of hydrochloric acid, filtering the fatty acids formed and washing the precipitate with 25 ml of hot water. From the filtrate, after making it alkaline with dilute solution of ammonia, zinc sulphide is completely precipitated by using a solution of ammonium sulphide. The precipitate is filtered off and the filtrate evaporated to dryness after the addition of 0.5 ml of sulphuric acid. The residue, on being ignited to constant weight, should not weigh more than 20 mg.

Test for free fatty acids: It is carried out by mixing 5 g of the substance with 100 ml of solvent ether, shaking the mixture for half an hour. The mixture (suspension) is filtered and 50 ml of the filtrate is evaporated to dryness. The residue weighs not more than 50 mg.

Assay: In this assay the basic concept of complexometric titration is used. As per I.P. standards the presence of Zinc Oxide (ZnO) should be determined.

Method: An accurately weighed amount of about 1 g of sample is boiled with 50 ml of 0.1 N sulphuric acid until the fatty acid layer is clearly separated. More water is added to maintain the original volume. It is cooled and filtered. The residue is washed with water to remove all acids and then 15 ml of strong ammonia-ammonium chloride solution is added to the combined filtrate and washings. The resulting solution is heated to about 40° and is titrated with 0.05 M disodium EDTA using 0.2 ml eriochrome black T solution as indicator. The end point is of blue colour.

Each ml of 0.05 M disodium EDTA $\equiv$ 0.004069 g of ZnO.

I.P. 2007 gives a modified assay method though the principle of titration method with disodium edetate remains the same.

Uses: It is an important pharmaceutical aid and is widely used like magnesium stearate as a lubricant in tablet making. Zinc stearate is a mild astringent and possesses antimicrobial properties. It is used in water-repellent ointments and in dusting powders. It is very popularly used in dermatological practice because of its desiccating and protective properties. Its use as a routine dusting powder for children should be discouraged, as its inhalation is said to cause pulmonary inflammation.

TITANIUM DIOXIDE

Chem. formula: TiO_2 Mol. wt.: 79.90

Titanium (Ti, atomic weight 47.90) largely occurs as the dioxide in some minerals, like brookite, rutile and anastase. Ilmenite, ferrous titanate, is yet another mineral which is used to obtain titanium (Ti) as follows

$$2FeTiO_3 + 4HCl + Cl_2 = 2TiO_2 + 2FeCl_3 + 2H_2O$$

The precipitate is filtered, washed and calcined to obtain anhydrous oxide. It is not official now.

I.P. requires it to contain not less than 8% of TiO_2 calculated with reference to the dried substance.

Description: It is a white powder without odour and taste.

Solubility: It is insoluble in water and in dilute mineral acids. It can be dissolved slowly in hot sulphuric acid.

Tests for identity:

(1) Dissolve specified amount of sample (0.5 g) along with anhydrous sodium sulphate (5 g) in water (10 ml). To this solution add H_2SO_4 (10 ml) and boil until a clear solution is obtained. Cool the sol. and add more H_2SO_4 (30 ml of 25% w/v) and dilute with water (to 100 ml). Name this solution as A. To a specified volume of solution A (5 ml) add strong H_2O_2 (0.1 ml). It should develop an orange red colour.

(2) To a specified volume of solution A (5 ml) add one piece of granulated zinc. The sol. should develop a violet-blue colour after about 45 min.

Tests for purity: It is tested for clarity and colour of solution; acidity or alkalinity; water-soluble matter; As; Ba; heavy metals; iron; loss on drying and loss on ignition (I.P. 85, p. 522).

Assay: An accurately weighed amount of titanium dioxide about 0.3 g is transferred to a beaker to which is added 20 ml of H_2SO_4 and 8 g of ammonium sulphate. The contents are mixed and heated till white fumes appear. The heating is continued over a strong flame until solution is effected. It is cooled and carefully diluted with 100 ml of water. The diluted solution is heated gently and boiled with continuous stirring. It is cooled, filtered and washed with several quantities each of 10 ml of water. To the combined filtrate and washings, 10 ml of strong ammonia solution is added and the solution cooled and diluted to 200 ml with water. 50 ml of the resulting solution is pipetted into a flask to which 100 ml of water and 4 ml of strong hydrogen peroxide solution are added. 50 ml of 0.05 M disodium EDTA is added to the flask which is allowed to stand for five min. The pH of the sol. is adjusted to 5.0 with NaOH solution to which 5 g of hexamine is added. The contents are titrated with 0.05 M zinc chloride using xylenol orange sol. as indicator.

Each ml of 0.05 M disodium EDTA ≡ 0.003995 g of TiO_2.

Storage: Titanium dioxide is stored in well-closed containers. Its contact with aluminium should be avoided.

Uses: TiO_2 is used as a pharmaceutical aid and as a topical protectant in ointments and creams.
The officials compounds are:

(1) Aluminium hydroxide gel, B.P., U.S.P., I.P.
(2) Aluminium sulphate, I.P., U.S.P.
(3) Aluminium hydroxide tablets, I.P.
(4) Aluminium, U.S.P.

ALUMINIUM: AI

Atomic wt.: 26.98

Aluminium is a trivalent and strongly electropositive metal. Its hydroxide, $Al(OH)_3$, is amphoteric in character with weak basic properties. Aluminium is the third most abundant element in the earth's crust and is the most abundant metal. The most important ore of aluminium is bauxite, $Al_2O_3.H_2O$, but aluminium also occurs in many aluminosilicate rocks and clays.

ALUMINIUM U.S.P.

It is finely divided aluminium powder, oleic or stearic acid may be present as a lubricant.

Properties: Free following, very fine, silvery powder and free from gritty or discoloured particles.

Solubility: Insoluble in water or ethanol but soluble in hydrochloric acid.

Tests for purity: Tests for acid-insoluble substances; arsenic; alkalis and alkaline earths; heavy metals; iron and suitability.

Acid-insoluble substances: A weighed sample is dissolved (as far as possible) in hydrochloric acid; the solution is filtered and the filtrate used in the test for alkalis and alkaline earth etc. The residue is washed and the lubricant extracted from it by means of acetone. The filtrate is evaporated to dryness and the residue weighed. The residue left in the crucible is washed, dried and weighed. The combined weight of the residue must not exceed 5% of the total weight of the sample taken.

Test for suitability: Rubbing a sample between the fingers the powder must be smooth and unctuous, showing the absence of gritty particulate.

Assay: It is based upon the complexometric titration. Aluminium is only slowly complexed with edetate. Hence excess edetate is added and the mixture is heated to ensure complete complexation. Dithizone is used as an indicator.

A weighed sample is dissolved in HCl and the solution is heated and filtered from lubricant. To an aliquat of the filtrate and washing is added a known excess of M/20 sodium edetate and acetic acid-ammonium acetate buffer and the mixture is heated to complete complexation. Dithizone is added and the excess edetate is back titrated with M/20 zinc sulphate.

The difference in blank and back titration is equal to the amount of edetate consumed. Amoun of Al is calculated from the amount of edetate consumed.

$$\text{Edetate} \equiv \text{Aluminium}$$
$$1000 \text{ ml of M/20} \equiv 1/20 \text{ g Al}$$

ALUMINIUM PASTE U.S.P.

Aluminum paste consists of aluminium, mineral oil and zinc oxide ointment.

Assay: Sufficient quantity of dil. HCl is added to the preparation in order to extract Al and Zn as their chloride.

$$Al \xrightarrow{\text{HCl}} AlCl_3$$
$$Zn \xrightarrow{\text{HCl}} ZnCl_2$$

After adjustment of **pH, Al and Zn** are determined in a portion of the extract by the procedure described under Aluminium above.

Zinc is determined in another portion of the extract after addition of ammonia-ammoniun chloride buffer. The mixture is cooled to below 5° (in order to prevent complexation of Al), mordan black is added and the zinc is titrated with M/20 sodium edetate. The difference between the titration represents the volume of ecetate equivalent to the aluminium present.

ANTIMICROBIAL AGENTS

Antimicrobial agents are agents that are effective against microorganisms. With reference to their specific activity, antimicrobial agents may be

- Antiseptic: An agent that kills or inhibits the growth of microorganisms when applied to the tissues.
- Germicidal: This refers specifically to agents that kill microorganisms. Depending on the various classes or organisms they may be bactericidal, fungicidal, amoebicidal, etc.
- Disinfectant: An agent used to destroy microorganisms that cause disease in man, animals or plants, commonly applied to inanimate objects (e.g., instruments, equipments, rooms, etc.)

Those agents which kill microorganisms are called are germicidal, while those which do not kill the microbes, but function by inhibiting their growth, are suffixed '*stat*', specifically they an bacteriostat, fungistat, etc.

The mechanism of action of inorganic antimicrobial agents is by oxidation, halogenation or protein precipitation.

Antimicrobial agents that function through oxidative mechanisms are hydrogen peroxide, metal peroxides, permanganates, halogens (i.e. chlorine and iodine) and certain oxohalogen anions. They act on the –SH group in cysteine present in most proteins to form a disulphide bridge between two –SH groups. This alters the specific function of the protein in the microorganism. This overall change is responsible for the ultimate destruction of the microorganism.

Inorganic compounds like hypochlorite (OCl^-) chlorinate primary and secondary amides present in the peptide linkage between amino acid groups comprising the protein molecule. This ultimately results in the destruction of the function of the microbial protein.

Metal ions of copper, silver, zinc and aluminium, due to their charge and small ionic radius, precipitate microbial protein through a complexation interaction. Certain metals like mercury, arsenic and antimony show enzyme specificity forming covalent bonds. The protein precipitant property of metal cations depends upon the concentration in which used. By increasing concentrations, antimicrobial, astringent, irritant and corrosive properties are successively available.

HYDROGEN PEROXIDE SOLUTION

Chem. formula: H_2O_2 Mol. weight: 34.016

Hydrogen peroxide solution is an aqueous solution of hydrogen peroxide and contains not less than 6% w/v of H_2O_2, corresponding to about 20 times its volume of available oxygen.

Hydrogen peroxide solution is a colourless, odourless liquid. It has slight acidic taste. It is rapidly decomposed on coming in contact with oxidiable organic matter and with certain metals and also if allowed to become alkaline.

Preparation: It can be prepared by the following methods.

(1) **From Barium Peroxide:** This is an original method for the industrial manufacture of Hydrogen Peroxide. Barium Peroxide is made into a thick paste in ice cold water. A calculated quantity of dilute sulphuric acid is also cooled in ice. The barium peroxide paste is then added to the well cooled dilute acid. Hydrogen peroxide H_2O_2 and insoluble barium sulphate are formed. $BaSO_4$ is filtered off.

$$BaO_2 + H_2SO_4 \longrightarrow BaSO_4 + H_2O_2$$

The yield of H_2O_2 is 10–20%.

(2) H_2O_2 can also be prepared by decomposing barium peroxide with phosphoric acid or by passing carbon dioxide through a suspension of barium peroxide in water.

$$3BaO_2 + 2H_3PO_4 \longrightarrow Ba_3(PO_4)_2 + 3H_2O_2$$

(3) **From Sodium Peroxide:** By treating sodium peroxide with dilute H_2SO_4 at low temperature. Sodium sulphate crystallises and H_2O_2 is distilled under 10 mm pressure.

$$Na_2O_2 + H_2SO_4 \longrightarrow Na_2SO_4 + H_2O_2$$

(4) **Manufacture of H_2O_2:** Nowadays H_2O_2 is manufactured by electrolysis of 50% ice cold sulphuric acid. Persulphuric acid is obtained first, which on distillation under reduced pressure gives H_2O_2 with 30% yield.

$$2H_2SO_4 \xrightarrow{\text{Electrolysis}} \underset{\text{Persulphuric acid}}{H_2S_2O_8} + H_2$$

$$H_2S_2O_8 \xrightarrow[\text{reduced pressure}]{\text{Distilled under}} 2H_2SO_4 + H_2O_2$$

Description Pure H_2O_2 is a colourless and odourless liquid. It slowly decomposes at ordinary temperature and readily when heated.

$$2H_2O_2 \longrightarrow 2H_2O + O_2$$

The decomposition is promoted by a catalyst like Cu, Fe, Mn etc., while small quantity of acid H_2SO_4, H_3PO_4 and alcohol, if added, retards the decomposition of H_2O_2. They act as negative catalysts and are, therefore, used as preservatives or stabilizers in commercial preparations. Some of them are boric acid, urea, acetanilide or hexamine. Hydrogen peroxide which is available in commerce is usually adjusted to pH 2–3. It is a strong oxidising agent and it attacks many organic materials very violently. Hydrogen peroxide solution is miscible with any amount of water from which it can be extracted with solvent ether.

Tests for identity:

(1) When made alkaline and heated it is decomposed with effervescence, evolving oxygen.

(2) The ethereal layer gets coloured blue, if shaken with H_2O_2 in presence of dilute H_2SO_4 and solution of potassium chromate.

Tests for purity: It is tested for acidity; preservative; loss on evaporation; barium and stability.

Acidity is tested by using 0.1 N Sodium Hydroxide using methyl red as indicator. For 10 ml no less than 0.2 ml and not more than 1 ml of 0.1 N NaOH is required.

Tests for preservative is performed by extracting 100 ml of H_2O_2 with a mixture of chloroform and solvent ether (in 3 : 2 ratio) and evaporating the extract to dryness at room temperature. For 100 ml of solution of H_2O_2 the residue does not weigh more than 50 mg.

Test for barium depends upon treating the H_2O_2 with dilute H_2SO_4. No turbidity should be produced. (Barium's presence in H_2O_2 is considered a possibility, if it is manufactured from BaO_2.)

Loss on evaporation is tested by evaporating on water bath in a platinum dish. It should leave not more than 0.2% of residue.

Stability is tested as per the I.P. test reproduced hereunder:

The solution should not lose more than 3% of its strength by weight. 100 ml of hydrogen peroxide (of 20 volume strength) is taken in a 250 ml round bottom neutral glass flask to which is attached a neutral glass condenser and the solution is refluxed for 30 minutes. The flask and condenser are then cooled, cleaned and kept exclusively for the following test; but before the test the flask and condenser are cleaned with nitric acid and thoroughly rinsed with purified water.

Test: 100 ml of the sample (hydrogen peroxide solution) is pipetted in the flask to which is attached the condenser by a ground-glass joint. The flask is covered up to the shoulder in a liquid bath of a mixture of glycerin and water in the ratio of 55 : 45 and maintained at a temperature of about 110°C. The sample is refluxed for exactly three hours and the time period is counted from the commencement of the boiling. After three hours the boiling is discontinued and the flask is disconnected and covered with a clear paper cap and cooled rapidly under running water to attain room temperature, taking care to avoid any contamination with extraneous matter. The contents of hydrogen peroxide solution are determined by the usual assay for hydrogen peroxide (describe below).

Assay: 10 ml of H_2O_2 is diluted to 250 ml in a volumetric flask. To 25 ml of the diluted solution is added 10 ml 5 N H_2SO_4 and the solution titrated with 0.1 N potassium permanganate till pink colour appears and persists.

Each ml of 0.1 N potassium permanganate is equivalent to 0.001701 g of H_2O_2.

Storage: Hydrogen peroxide is preserved in a light-resistant container with stopper resistant to hydrogen peroxide. It is stored in a dark and cool place.

Uses: It is used as a germicide and deodorant. The liberation of gaseous oxygen provides an additional cleansing action on cuts and wounds. It is used for bleaching the hair. It is considered as an effective oxidizing antidote for phosphorus and cyanide poisonings. It is used for cleaning ears and removing the surgical dressings.

It is a very strong oxidizing agent, because it yields nascent oxygen. The medicinal as well as industrial use of hydrogen peroxide is based on the liberation of nascent oxygen.

Preparations: I.P. refers to two solutions of hydrogen peroxide as of 20 vol. and 100 vol.

SODIUM PERBORATE
(Sod. Perbor.)

Chem. formula: $NaBO_3.4H_2O$ Mol. weight: 153

Sodium perborate contains not less than 96.0 per cent and not more than the equivalent of 103.0 per cent of $NaBO_3 \cdot 4H_2O$.

Description: It is white, crystalline granules or a white powder. It is odourless and has saline taste.

Solubility: It is soluble in 40 parts of water. It is more soluble in boric, tartaric or citric acids and in glycerin. Its solubility is also increased by the presence of magnesium or ammonium sulphate.

Tests for identity:

(1) An acidified solution of the substance discharges the colour of potassium permanganate and produces a violet colour with a solution of potassium iodide.

(2) 1 ml saturated solution is mixed with 1 ml of dilute sulphuric acid and 0.2 ml of solution potassium dichromate and shaken with 2 ml of solvent ether. On being separated, the solvent ether layer imparts a blue colour.

(3) A saturated solution of the substance is alkaline to solution of phenolphthalein and when acidified with hydrochloric acid, it yields reactions characteristic of sodium and borate (App. I).

Tests for purity: It is tested for alkalinity and heavy metals.

Test for alkalinity is performed by noting the reaction. A 1% solution is alkaline to litmus solution.

Test for heavy metals: It is performed by dissolving 1 g in 10 ml of water and 5 ml dilute hydrochloric acid. The solution is evaporated to dryness on a water bath with frequent stirring. The residue is dissolved in 10 ml of water and again evaporated to dryness on a water bath.

The residue is then dissolved in 23 ml of water and to the solution is added 2 ml of 0.1 N hydrochloric acid and the test for heavy metals applied. The limit of heavy metals is 20 parts per million.

Assay: An accurately weighed about 0.3 g of substance is dissolved in 50 ml of water and to the solution is added 10 ml of dilute sulphuric acid and solution titrated with 0.1 N potassium permanganate.

Each ml of 0.1 potassium permanganate is equivalent to 0.007695 g of $NaBO_3 \cdot 4H_2O$.

Storage: Sodium perborate is preserved in a tight container and stored in a cool place.

Uses: It is an oxidant and local anti-infective.

POTASSIUM PERMANGANATE

Formula: $KMnO_4$ Mol. Weight: 158.0

It contains not less than 99.0% $KMnO_4$.

Preparation: It is prepared by heating a solution of KOH with MnO_2 and potassium chlorate.

$$6KOH + 3MnO_2 + KClO_3 \longrightarrow 3K_2MnO_4 + KCl + 3H_2O$$
$$\text{Pot. manganate}$$

The solution is then evaporated to a green mass of K_2MnO_4. The green mass is extracted with boiling water and a current of chlorine is passed through the solution until all the potassium manganate is converted to $KMnO_4$.

$$2K_2MnO_4 + Cl_2 \longrightarrow 2KCl + 2KMnO_4$$

Carbon dioxide can also be passed through the solution in place of chlorine, when two-thirds of manganate is converted as follows:

$$3K_2MnO_4 + 2CO_2 \longrightarrow 2KMnO_4 + MnO_2 + 2K_2CO_3$$

The solution is evaporated to crystallisation.

Description: It occurs as a dark purple, slender, prismatic crystals with metallic lustre. It has no odour but sweet astringent taste. It is soluble in 15 parts of water and 3.5 parts of boiling water. It decomposes in presence of traces of organic matters.

Tests for purity: It is tested for Cl and SO_4. Since the purple colour of $KMnO_4$ may interfe with the test of purity, the colour is destroyed by boiling with 95% alcohol which does not interfere with the test.

$$2KMnO_4 + 3C_2H_2OH \longrightarrow 2MnO_2 + 2KOH + 2H_2O + 3CH_2CHO$$

The precipitated MnO_2 is removed by filtration.

Test for Cl and SO_4 is carried out in the usual manner.

Assay: The assay involves an oxidation reduction type of reaction. A solution of weighed sample is titrated with standard N/10 oxalic acid. Here $KMnO_4$ is taken in the burette. Excess of dilute H_2SO_4 is added to the $H_2C_2O_4$ before commencing the titration and the temperature is maintained at 70°C throughout the titration, otherwise the reaction is slow (I.P. 2007 has given a modified assay method in which the liberated iodine is titrated with sodium thiosulphate using starch solution.

$$2KMnO_4 + 3H_2SO_4 \longrightarrow K_2SO_4 + 2MnSO_4 + 3H_2O + 5(O)$$
$$5H_2C_2O_4 + 5(O) \longrightarrow 10CO_2 + 5H_2O$$

1000 ml of N/10 $H_2C_2O_4$ is equivalent to 1/50 $KMnO_4$.

Or 1 ml of 0.1 N oxalic acid is equivalent to 0.00316 g of $KMnO_4$.

Storage: It is preserved in a well-closed container. While handling potassium permanganate care must be taken as dangerous explosions may take place if it is brought in contact with organic or other readily oxidised substances, either in solution or dry state.

Uses: It is used as an antiseptic in mouth wash and in cleaning ulcers or abscesses. As anti-infective it is considered of immense value. It is used in the treatment of urethritis. It is capable of oxidising some drugs and venoms and hence it is used in case of poisonings by barbiturates, chloral hydrate, many alkaloids etc. A solution of potassium permanganate destroys the poison and prevents absorption. The solution of pot. permanganate should not be left in the stomach. In veterinary practice it is very much used as an antiseptic.

IODINE

Formula: I_2 Mol. weight: 253.8

Iodine of I.P. standard contains not less than 99.5 per cent of I_2.

Iodine compounds are quite common in nature. Sea water also contains traces of combined iodine, which is absorbed by some specific plants and sea weeds, like _Laminaria digitata, Fucus vesiculosus._ Iodine is also present in the form of sodium iodate in crude Chile saltpetre ($NaNO_3$).

Preparation: Iodine is manufactured from Kelp (Sea-weed's ash) which is extracted with water. The solution is concentrated when the sulphates and chlorides of sodium and potassium crystallize out, leaving freely soluble sodium and potassium iodides in solution.

The solution after the addition of sulphuric acid is decanted. The decanted mother liquid is treated with MnO_2 and warmed to collect iodine which distills over.

$$2NaI + 2H_2SO_4 + MnO_2 \longrightarrow MnSO_4 + NaSO_4 + I_2 + 2H_2O$$

Alternatively the solution containing freely soluble iodides (see above) is treated with required proportion of chlorine and the precipitated iodine is collected and purified by sublimation.

More recently iodine has been found in the brine of oil wells and this source is utilised now-a-days for obtaining iodine in U.S.A. and Russia.

Description: Iodine is heavy, bluish black, brittle and occurs in rhombic prisms or plates with a metallic lustre. It has a characteristic odour and it volatilises at ordinary temperature. It melts at 114° and at or below 700° it gives rise to one of the heaviest vapours. At higher temperature the density of iodine decreases as it dissociates.

$$I_2 \rightleftharpoons 2I^-$$

Iodine is present in thyroid glands. Its deficiency causes serious diseases, the outstanding iodine deficiency disease being Goiter.

Children, who have iodine deficiency show depressed growth and their sexual development is retarded. The skin becomes rough and hair becomes thin. If the deficiency is severe cretinism, feeble mindedness and deafness may occur. The reproductivity in the female is impaired while fertility in the male decreases. Goiter usually occurs in children. Iodized salt is marketed whieh reduces the incidence of Goiter. Iodine is said to be helpful for the production of thyroid hormones.

Iodine is almost insoluble in water (one part in 3,000) but is soluble in 12 parts of alcohol, 4 parts of carbon disulphide. It is more freely soluble in chloroform, carbon tetrachlorides, solvent ether and carbon and in aqueous solutions of iodides.

Tests for identity:
(1) Gives off violet vapour upon heating.
(2) Gives a deep blue colour with solution of potassium iodide in presence of starch.

Tests for purity: It is tested for chloride and bromide; cyanogen; and non-volatile matter.

Chloride and Bromide are tested by triturating thoroughly 3.5 g with 35 ml of water and decolourising the filtrate by a little zinc powder. To 25 ml of the decolourised filtrate is added 5 ml of dilute ammonia solution, followed by 5 ml of silver nitrate and diluting the filtrate to 50 ml and acidifying it with 4 ml of nitric acid. The opalescence produced should not be more than the opalescence produced in the limit test for chlorides (p. 4).

Cyanogen is tested by taking 5 ml of the above filtrate and adding to it few drops of solution of ferrous sulphate and 1 ml of solution of sodium hydroxide, warming the solution gently and acidifying with hydrochloric acid. No blue colour should be produced.

Non-volatile matter: Not more than 0.5% residue on being volatilised on water bath.

Assay: An accurately weighed amount (about 0.5 g) dissolved in a solution of potassium iodide (1 g in 5 ml of H_2O) is slightly acidified with dilute acetic acid (1 ml) and titrated with N/10 sodium thiosulphate using starch mucilage as indicator. Because iodine volatises, it should be weighed in a stoppered vessel (weighing bottle).

$$2Na_2S_2O_3 + I_2 \longrightarrow Na_2S_4O_6 + 2NaI$$

1,000 ml of N/10 $Na_2S_2O_3$ is equivalent to 1/10 I_2.

Or 1 ml of N/10 $Na_2S_2O_3$ is equivalent to 0.01269 g of I_2,

Storage: Iodine is to be preserved in a glass-stoppered bottle.

Uses: Iodine is anti-infective and is used as local germicide, For proper thyroid functioning iodine is to be supplied to the body, to be utilized physiologically either in elemental form or in the form of iodine ion as in sodium or potassium iodide.

Elementary iodine is highly toxic and the starch and sodium thiosulphate are useful antidotes.

Preparations: Aqueous Iodine Solution, Strong Iodine Solution and Weak Iodine Solution (these preparations, though important, are not included in I.P.).

AQUEOUS IODINE SOLUTION
(Synonym: Lugol's solution)

Aqueous iodine solution contains 5 per cent w/w of Iodine. I_2 (limits 4.9 to 5.1) and 10 per cent w/w of potassium iodide, KI (limits 9.8 to 10.2).

Ingredients:

Iodine	50 g
Potassium iodide	100 g
Purified water, sufficient to produce	1000 ml

Preparation: Potassium iodide and iodine are dissolved in 100 ml of H_2O and the volume is made up to 1000 ml.

Description: Lugol's solution is a transparent liquid, having brown colour and odour of iodine.

Tests for identity:

(1) Diluted solution gives blue colour with the solution of starch.

(2) The residue left after evaporation of solution and after ignition (evaporation of I_2) yields reactions characteristic of potassium and iodide (App. I).

Assay: The assay is carried out for iodine and potassium iodide. 25 ml of the solution is diluted to 100 ml with water and this dilute solution is used for the following assays:

For iodine: To 20 ml of the diluted solution is added 10 ml of H_2O and the solution is titrated with N/10 $Na_2S_2O_3$.

1000 ml of N/10 $Na_2S_2O_3$ is equivalent to 1/10 I_2.

Or 1 ml of N/l0 $Na_2S_2O_3$ is equivalent to 0.01269 g of I_2.

For potassium iodide: To 10 ml of the diluted solution is added 20 ml of H_2O followed by 40 ml of HCl and the solution is titrated with 0.05 M potassium iodate, shaking vigorously until the dark brown colour becomes light brown. Then 5 ml chloroform is added and the titration is continued till chloroform becomes colourless and the supernatant liquid is clear yellow. From the number of ml of potassium iodate required is subtracted one-quarter of the number of ml 0.1 N sodium thiosulphate used in the assay for iodine.

$$KIO_3 + 6HCl + 2KI \longrightarrow 3KCl + 3ICl + 3H_2O$$
$$\text{Iodine}$$
$$\text{monochloride}$$

1000 ml 0.05 M KIO_3 is equivalent to 1/10 KI.

Or each ml of 0.05 M potassium iodate is equivalent to 0.0166 g of KI or 0.01499 g of NaI, if sodium iodide has been used for preparing solution.

Storage: The Lugol's solution is preserved in a well-closed container, the materials of which are resistant to iodine, e.g. glass, plastic etc.

Uses: It is a good source of iodine and is taken internally. It is a germicide and fungicide and does not cause irritation to cuts like tincture of iodine.

WEAK IODINE SOLUTION
(Synonym: Iodine Tincture)

Iodine Tincture contains 2 per cent w/v of Iodine and 2.5 per cent w/v of Potassium Iodide.

Ingredients:

Iodine	20 . g
Potassium iodide	25 . g
Alcohol 50%, sufficient to produce	1000 . ml

Preparation: Potassium iodide and iodine are dissolved in sufficient alcohol (50%) and more alcohol is added to produce the required volume.

Alcohol content 45–58 per cent w/v.

Description and tests for identity are similar to those described under Aqueous Iodine Solution.

Assay: For Iodine: 10 ml of the solution diluted with 20 ml of water is titrated with 0.1 N sodium thiosulphate.

1000 ml of N/10 $Na_2S_2O_3$ is equivalent to 1/10 I_2.

Or each ml of 0.1 N sodium thiosulphate is equivalent to 0.01269 g of I_2.

For Potassium iodide: To 10 ml is added 40 ml of water, 16 ml of HCl and 10 ml of solution of potassium cyanide and the solution is titrated with 0.05 M potassium iodate until dark brown solution turns pale yellow. 5 ml of solution of starch is then added and the titration is continued until the liquid becomes colourless.

From the number of ml of 0.05 M KIO_3 is subtracted 1/2 the number of ml of 0.1 N sodium thiosulphate required for assay of iodine.

1000 ml of KIO_3 is equivalent to 1/10 KI.

Or each ml of the remainder 0.05 M potassium iodate is equivalent to 0.0166 g of KI (or 0.01499 g of NaI).

Storage: It is stored under conditions similar to Aqueous Iodine Solution.

Uses: It is a very well known and popular antiseptic.

STRONG IODINE SOLUTION

It contains 10 per cent of I_2 and 6 per cent of KI.

Ingredients:

Iodine	100 g
Pot. iodide	60 g
Purified water	100 ml
Alcohol 50%, sufficient to produce	1000 ml

Preparation: Potassium Iodide and Iodine are dissolved in purified water and sufficient alcohol is added to produce 1000 ml.

Description and tests for identity are same as reported under aqueous iodine solution. Alcohol content 74 to 79 per cent w/v.

Storage: It is stored under conditions as described for Aqueous Iodine Solution.

Uses: It is used as an antiseptic. In making all the above solutions, Potassium Iodide may be replaced by Sodium Iodide.

POTASSIUM IODIDE

Mol. formula: KI   Mol. weight: 166.0

It contains not less than 99% of KI calculated with reference to the substance dried to constant weight at 105°C.

Preparation:

(1) Potassium iodide is prepared by treating a hot aqueous solution of potassium hydroxide with iodine in slight excess to form a mixture of potassium iodide and potassium iodate.

$$6KOH + 3I_2 \longrightarrow 5KI + KIO_3 + 3H_2O$$

$$KIO_3 + 3C \longrightarrow KI + 3CO$$

The solution after concentrating is treated with excess of charcoal powder; evaporating the mixture to dryness followed by ignition. The charcoal (carbon) reduces the iodate to iodine, utilising thus the total iodine to obtain the potassium iodide. The product is lixivated with water, filtered and potassium iodide is obtained by crystallisation (see method of preparation for potassium bromide as well).

(2) Potassium iodide is also prepared from ferrosoferric iodide in the same way as described under potassium bromide (see potassium bromide).

$$Fe_3I_8 + 4K_2CO_3 \longrightarrow 8KI + Fe_2O_4 + 4CO_2$$

Description: It occurs as colourless, transparent or some white opaque crystals or a white granular powder. It is odourless, but has, sometimes, slightly bitter taste. It is soluble in water (1 g in 0.7 ml), glycerin (1 g in 2 ml), alcohol (1 g in 23 ml) and in acetone (1 g in 75 ml).

Tests for purity: It is tested for As; Ca; SO_4; alkalinity; iodate; loss on drying; cyanide and heavy metals; thiosulphate; barium and clarity and colour of solution.

Assay: An accurately weighed quantity (0.5 g) of potassium iodide is dissolved in water (50 ml) acidified with HCl (15 ml) and treated with a solution of KCN (6 ml) maintaining the temperature at 15°C. The solution is titrated with 0.05 M KIO_3 until the dark brown coloured solution becomes pale yellow. 5 ml of starch solution is added and the solution titrated slowly further until the liquid becomes colourless.

$$KIO_3 + 2KI + 3KCN + 6HCl \longrightarrow 6KCl + 3ICN + 3H_2O$$

1000 ml of M/20 KIO_3 is equivalent to 1/10 KI.

Or 1 ml of 0.05 M potassium iodide is equivalent to 0.0166 g of KI.

Note: Molar solution is used because normality varies depending on the nature of reaction, and uniform reduction of iodate to iodide is not feasible in direct titrimetric method. I.P. 2007 has just a little modified the assay method.

Storage: It is preserved in well-closed container.

Uses: It is used as an expectorant and a source of iodine. It can be used in the form of an iodised salts (one in 1,00,000 parts of salt) to prevent goiter, in places, where iodine in the diet is not in sufficient supply. It is also used in some kinds of antifungal therapy and in veterinary practice.

SODIUM IODIDE

Chem. formula: NaI   Mol. weight: 149.9

Sodium iodide contains not less than 99% of NaI calculated with reference to the substance dried to constant weight at 105°. It is not official, although potassium iodide is.

Preparation: The methods of preparation of sodium iodide are similar to those described under potassium iodide, the difference being in the use of iodine in place of bromine. The methods are repeated here:

(1) **By action of iodine on sodium hydroxide:** In this process when excess of iodine is added to the solution of sodium hydroxide, sodium iodate is formed, which is reduced with carbon to sodium iodide as follows:

$$6NaOH + 3I_2 \longrightarrow 5NaI + NaIO_3 + 3H_2O$$
$$NaIO_3 + 3C \longrightarrow NaI + 3CO\uparrow$$

(2) **By metathesis between ferrosoferric iodide and sodium carbonate:** In this method iodide is allowed to react with iron filings and the ferrous iodide formed is decomposed with Na_2CO).

$$Fe + I_2 \longrightarrow FeI_2$$
$$3FeI_2 + I_2 \longrightarrow FeI_2.2FeI_2$$
$$FeI_2.2FeI_3 + 4Na_2CO_3 \longrightarrow \underset{\substack{\text{Sodium} \\ \text{iodide}}}{8NaI} + \underset{\substack{\text{Ferrosoferric} \\ \text{oxide}}}{FeO.Fe_2O_3} + 4CO_2$$

The precipitated ferrosoferric oxide is removed by filtration and from the filtrate sodium iodide is obtained and recrystallised.

Description: It occurs as colourless, odourless crystals or as a white crystalline powder. In moist air it tends to cake and then deliquesce, undergoing often decomposition and developing a brown tint. An aqueous solution of sodium iodide is neutral or faintly alkaline to litmus and on keeping it becomes yellow due to the formation of free iodine. Sodium iodide on being dissolved in water liberates heat due to the formation of dihydrate ($NaI \cdot 2H_2O$) (distinction from potassium iodide).

Sodium iodide is soluble in water (1 g in 0.6 ml), in alcohol (1 g in 2 ml) and glycerin (1 g in 1 ml).

Tests for identity: It gives reaction characteristic of sodium and iodides (App. I).

Tests for purity: It is tested for arsenic; barium; heavy metals; cyanide; iodate; sulphate and loss on drying (see also potassium iodide).

Assay: The assay procedure is similar to that of potassium iodide. Here potassium cyanide is used. It is added in excess to the solution of the substance containing HCl. To the acidified solution is added potassium cyanide solution. maintaining the temperature at 15°C and titrating with 0.05 M potassium iodate, using starch mucilage as indicator towards the end-point (see also potassium iodide).

$$KIO_3 + 2NaI + 3KCN + 6HCl \longrightarrow 2NaCl + 4KCl + 3ICN + 3H_2O$$

Each ml of 0.05 M potassium iodate is equivalent to 0.01499 g of NaI.

Storage: Sodium iodide is preserved in a well-closed container as its contact with moisture and light help in liberation of iodine. An aqueous solution, if alkaline, is preserved better than an acidic solution.

Uses: Its uses are similar to potassium iodide for its therapeutic action easily interchanged with potassium iodide for its therapeutic action (see also potassium iodide).

Dose: 0.3 to 0.5 g.

SILVER NITRATE

Formula: $AgNO_3$ Mol. weight: 169.0

Silver nitrate when powdered and dried in the dark over sulphuric acid for four hours, contain not less than 99.8% of $AgNO_3$.

Preparation: It is prepared by the action of hot Nitric Acid on silver metal. Nitric acid should be nearly concentrated.

$$Ag + 2HNO_3 \longrightarrow AgNO_3 + NO_2 + H_2O$$

The solution is evaporated to dryness and the residue is heated to expel nitric acid. Silver nitrate is crystallised.

Description: It is colourless or white crystals, which are odourless, but have bitter and metallic taste. It darkens when exposed to atmospheric air due to reduction to metallic silver. It melts at 209°C and is soluble in water (0.4 parts), alcohol (30 parts) and only slightly in solvent ether.

Tests for identity: Yields reactions for silver and nitrates (App. I).

Tests for purity: It is tested for bismuth; copper and lead.

A solution in water is neutral to litmus. A solution of 2 g in 20 ml of water should be clear and colourless.

Assay: It is assayed by titration with standard N/10 ammonium thiocyanate solution, using solution of ferric ammonium sulphate as indicator (about 0.50 g is accurately weighed, dissolved in 50 ml of water and to the solution 2 ml of acetic acid is added before titration).

$$AgNO_3 + NH_4SCN \longrightarrow AgSCN + NH_4NO_3$$

1000 ml of 1/10 N NH_4SCN is equivalent to 1/10 $AgNO_3$.

Or each ml of 1/10 N NH_4SCN is equivalent to 0.01699 of $AgNO_3$.

Storage: It is stored and preserved in a well-closed container, protected from light.

Uses: It is used as an anti-infective or antibacterial agent. It is also used as a pharmaceutical aid in the preparation of silver proteins. As an antiseptic, silver nitrate has a very broad spectrum activity. It is very successfully used to manage severely burnt patients. Silver ion combines readily with protein and due to this the astringent, caustic and perhaps the germicidal properties are attributed to it. It is also used to prevent gonococcal eye infections of newborns.

MILD SILVER PROTEIN

It is a silver rendered colloidal by the presence of protein or in combination with it. It contains not less than 19.0 per cent and not more than 23.0 per cent of Ag.

Mild silver protein should be freshly prepared and dispensed in amber-coloured bottles.

Description: It is dark brown or almost black shining scales or granules, odourless, hygroscopic. It is affected by light. It is freely soluble in water, forming a dark-coloured solution, practically insoluble in alcohol, chloroform and ether.

Tests for identity: It is identified by the following three tests:

(1) Heat 1 g of mild silver protein, charring will take place. Incinerate completely, a greyish white residue is obtained, which after solution in nitric acid and neutralisation, yields the reactions characteristic of silver (App. I).

(2) To a 1 per cent w/v solution is added solution of ferric chloride, the dark colour is discharged and the solution becomes opalescent on standing.

(3) To a 1 per cent w/v solution is added solution of mercuric chloride, no white precipitate is produced and the liquid is not decolorised (distinction from strong silver protein).

Test for silver salts: This is done by shaking 1 g of mild silver protein with 10 ml of alcohol (90 per cent) and adding to the filtrate 2 ml of dilute hydrochloride acid. No opalescene should be produced.

Distinction from strong silver protein: Dissolve 1 g in 10 ml of water. Add all at once, 7 g of ammonium sulphate and stir occasionally for thirty minutes. Filter through a quantitative filter paper into a 50 ml Nessler tube, returning the first portion of the filtrate to the filter, if necessary, to secure a clear filtrate and allow the filter and precipitate to drain. Add to the clear filtrate, 25 ml of a 1 per cent w/v solution of Indian gum. In a second 50 ml Nessler tube dissolve 7 g of ammonium sulphate in 10 ml of water and add to this solution 25 ml of the solution of Indian gum and 1.6 ml of 0.01 N silver nitrate. To each tube add 2 ml of nitric acid, 2 ml of dilute hydrochloric acid and enough of the solution of Indian gum to make the volume of each solution 50 ml. Mix the contents of each tube thoroughly and allow to stand for five minutes. The turbidity of the mixture containing the mild silver protein is not greater than that to which no mild silver protein has been added (strong silver protein yields a much greater turbidity than the control).

Assay: Weigh accurately about 2 g and ignite at first gently and afterwards strongly until all carbonaceous matter is destroyed. Dissolve the residue in 15 ml of nitric acid, heat until no more nitrous fumes are evolved, dilute with water to 100 ml and titrate with 0.1 N ammonium thiocyanate using solution of ferric ammonium sulphate as indicator and shaking vigorously as the end point is neared.

Each ml of 0.1 N ammonium thiocyanate is equivalent to 0.01079 g of Ag.

Storage: It is preserved in a well-closed container and protected from light.

Uses: It is used as a local antibacterial agent.

STRONG SILVER PROTEIN

Strong silver protein is a compound of silver and protein. It contains not less than 7.5 per cent and not more than 8.5 per cent of Ag.

Description: A brown powder, odourless, somewhat hygroscopic.

Solubility: Slowly soluble in water forming a dark brown solution, almost insoluble in alcohol, solvent ether and chloroform.

Tests for identity: It complies with the test Nos. 1 and 2 as mentioned under Mild Silver Protein (p. 159) and give the following additional tests:

(3) On adding solution of mercuric chloride to a 1 per cent w/v solution a white precipitate is formed and the liquid becomes colourless or almost colourless (distinction from mild silver protein).

(4) To 5 ml of a 2 per cent w/v solution, add 5 ml of solution of sodium hydroxide, 10 ml of water and 2 ml of a 2 per cent w/v solution of copper sulphate, allow to stand for a few minutes; a violet colour is produced.

Silver salts test: Shake 1 g with 10 ml of alcohol (90 per cent) and filter. To the filtrate add 2 ml of dilute hydrochloric acid; no opalescence is produced.

Tests for foreign protein:

(1) A 10 per cent solution shows no deposit within ten minutes.

(2) A 2 per cent w/v solution shows no turbidity on the addition of an equal volume of solution of sodium chloride.

Assay: Weigh accurately about 2 g and ignite at first gently and afterwards strongly until all carbonaceous matter is destroyed. Dissolve the residue in 10 ml of nitric acid, heat until no more nitrous fumes are evolved, dilute with water to 100 ml, and titrate with 0.1 N ammonium thiocyanate, using solution of ferric ammonium sulphate as indicator, and shaking vigorously as the end-point is neared.

Each ml of 0.1 N ammonium thiocyanate is equivalent to 0.01079 g of Ag.

Storage: It is preserved in a well-closed container and protected from light.

Uses: It is used as a local antibacterial agent.

Note: Solution of strong silver protein should be freshly prepared and dispensed in amber-coloured bottles.

MERCURY

Formula: Hg   Atomic wt. : 200.6

Mercury contains not less than 99.5 per cent of Hg.

Preparation: It is found in a free state. The chief ore of mercury is cinnabar (HgS).

The ore is roasted first in air; sulphide is converted into sulphur oxide.

$$HgS + O_2 \longrightarrow Hg + SO_2$$

The free mercury is liberated. It is either purified by volatilisation or chemically dropping mercury into a column of dilute nitric acid to remove basic impurities.

Description: A shining, silver-white, heavy liquid, easily divisible into globules and extremely mobile, easily volatilises on heating.

Practically insoluble in water, in alcohol and in hydrochloric acid, readily and completely soluble in nitric acid and in boiling sulphuric acid with evolution of SO_2 and formation of mercuric sulphate.

$$Hg + 2H_2SO_4 \longrightarrow HgSO_4 + SO_2 + 2H_2O$$

Density: 13.5 g/ml at 25°.

Assay: An accurately weighed quantity (0.49 g) is dissolved in equal parts (20 ml) of water and nitric acid, heated gently until the solution is colourless. The solution is then diluted with water (150 ml) and sufficient quantity of potassium permanganate is added to produce permanent pink colour. A trace of Ferrous Sulphate to discharge pink colour is added and the solution is then titrated with standard 0.1 N ammonium thiocyanate, using ferric ammonium sulphate as indicator. The temperature during the titration should not be allowed to exceed above 20°C.

$$3Hg + 8HNO_3 \longrightarrow 3Hg(NO_3)_2 + 4H_2O + 2NO\uparrow$$

$$Hg(NO_3)_2 + 2NH_4SCN \longrightarrow 2NH_4NO_3 + Hg(SCN)_2$$

Each ml of 0.1 N ammonium thiocyanate is equivalent to 0.01003 g of Hg.

Uses: It is used as a pharmaceutical aid. Formerly metallic mercury was used as such therapeutically as a cathartic and parasiticide. But it is no more used as such, because it is extremely poisonous and prolonged inhalation of even very minute amounts of mercury prove fatal. Almost all the salts of mercury, with the exception of the sulphide, are poisonous. Compounds of mercury now-a-days are used as diacitic, germicidal, anti-bacterial and anti-infectious.[*]

MERCURY WITH CHALK

Synonym: Grey powder.

Mercury w th chalk contains 33% of mercury and 66% of chalk, $CaCO_3$.

Ingredients:

Mercury	33 g
Dextrose	1 g
Chalk	66 g

These ingredients are triturated together in a porcelain mortar until the mixture acquires a uniform pale colour and no metallic globules are visible when examined under a magnifying lens of 4 diameters.

Tests for identity:

(1) With dil. hydrochloric acid gives effervescences due to the production of carban dioxide, which turns lime water milky.

(2) If a mixture of mercury with chalk and sodium carbonate, in equal proportions, is heated gently in a test-tube for ten minutes and after cooling emptied on a piece of white paper, globules of mercury separate and are seen.

(3) On being triturated (1 g) with precipitated sulphur (0.5 g) in a porcelain mortar, the powder turns black due to the formation of mercuric sulphide.

(4) It gives test for dextrose, when a filtered aqueous solution is made alkaline and treated with Fehling's solution by forming a brick-red precipitate.

Test for purity: It is tested for As.

Assay: For mercury: An accurately weighed amount (about 1.2 g) is boiled gently under a reflex condenser for five minutes with 10 ml of nitric acid and 25 ml of water and cooled. The condenser is washed with 25 ml of water and sufficient solution of Potassium Permanganate is added to produce a permanent pink colour and rest of the assay is the same as described under Mercury.

For chalk: An accurately weighed amount (about 1 g) is dissolved in 100 ml of water and 50 ml of 1 N hydrochloric acid in a 250 ml conical flask. The solution is set aside till the reaction ceases and the excess of acid is titrated with 1 N sodium hydroxide using solution of phenolphthalein as indicator.

$$CaCO_3 + 2HCl \longrightarrow CaCl_2 + H_2O + CO_2\uparrow$$

---

[*] Mercury accord ng to the alphabetic classification should not find place here. But since it is a metal whose salts, compounds and preparations are to be discussed in the next few pages, it is not only desirable but quite natural to first include Mercury here and then its compounds and preparations. In I.P., however, it is described as per the alphabetic classification in its place. Ammoniated mercury has been described earlier under ammonium compounds. There are many more compounds of mercury but they are organic compounds with mercury attached to carbon. Since the students at this stage have very scanty knowledge about organic chemistry it is considered to be appropriate to include organic mercury compounds in organic chemistry section. Such compounds are mersalyl acid, mercurophylline etc.

Each ml of 1 N HCl is equivalent to 0.05005 g of $CaCO_3$.

Uses: It is used as a purgative.

Dose: 60 to 300 mg.

YELLOW MERCURIC OXIDE

Chem. Form: HgO   Mol. Weight: 216.6

It contains not less than 99.5% of HgO, calculated with reference to the substance dried at 105° for one hour.

Preparation: Since the yellow variety is affected by light, all operations are carried out in the dark, so that a uniformly orange yellow product is obtained. The reaction between a concentrated solution of mercuric chloride and a dilute solution of sodium hydroxide is brought about at room temperature by pouring the former slowly into the latter. After allowing the reaction mixture to stand for about an hour to bring about complete precipitation of yellow mercuric oxide, the supernatant liquid is poured off, the precipitate is washed with water until free from alkali, drained from calico filter and dried in a dark place, at a temperature not exceeding 30°C.

$$HgCl_2 + 2NaOH \longrightarrow Hg(OH)_2 + 2NaCl$$
$$Hg(OH)_2 \longrightarrow HgO + H_2O$$

Description: An orange yellow, heavy amorphous powder, odourless, stable in air, but becomes discoloured on exposure to light.

Practically insoluble in water and alcohol, readily soluble in dilute HCl and in dilute nitric acid forming colourless solution.

Tests for purity: It is tested for reaction, mercurous salts, Cl, loss on drying and sulphated ash.

Assay: Mercuric oxide is assayed by dissolving it in dilute nitric acid and carrying out the assay by titrating with 0.1 N NH_4SCN using ferric alum as indicator as in the case of mercury.

$$HgO + 2HNO_3 \longrightarrow Hg(NO_3)_2 + H_2O$$

1 ml of N/10 ammonium thiocyanate is equivalent to 0.01083 g of HgO.

Uses: It is used as a local anti-infective and antibacterial and is used in ointments.

Preparations: Mercuric oxide Eye Ointment and Oleated Mercury.

MERCURIC OXIDE EYE OINTMENT

Preparation: It is prepared under aseptic conditions by triturating very finely powdered yellow oxide of mercury with a small portion of the melted base until the mixture is smooth, and then adding gradually sufficient quantity of the melted base to produce the required weight, trituration being continued until the eye ointment attains room temperature.

The amount of mercuric oxide, HgO, is not less than 95% and not more than 105% of the stated amount of yellow mercuric oxide.

Assay: To an accurately weighed quantity, equivalent to about 0.1 gm of yellow mercuric oxide, is added 10 ml of dilute nitric acid and 20 ml of water and the mixture shaken until mercuric oxide is dissolved. 50 ml of water is added to the solution and it is titrated with 0.1 N ammonium thiocyanate at a temperature not exceeding 20° using solution of ferric alum as indicator.

Each ml of N/10 ammonium thiocyanate is equivalent to 0.01083 g of HgO.

Uses: It is used in ophthalmology; 1% ointment is used for treating mild inflammatory conditions for the treatment of blepharitis and conjunctivitis.

A 2% HgO ointment is used for eczema and other skin affections.

OLEATED MERCURY

Oleated mercury contains the equivalent of 20% of yellow mercuric oxide (limits 19.0 to 21.0).

Ingredients:

Yellow mercuric oxide ....200 g
Liquid paraffin.. 50 g
Oleic acid ....750 g

The mercuric oxide is triturated with the liquid paraffin until it is thoroughly subdivided. Oleic acid is then added and contents mixed thoroughly. The mixture is heated at 50°, triturating occasionally until combination is effected. On being cooled, a yellowish preparation is obtained.

Assay: An accurately weighed amount about 0.75 g is dissolved in a mixture of 65 ml of benzene, 10 ml of glacial acetic acid and 25 ml of alcohol and warmed on a water bath to about 50°. Hydrogen sulphide is passed in for ten minutes, and the contents filtered through asbestos in a Gooch crucible; precipitate washed first with hot benzene and then with a little alcohol and dried to constant weight at 120°.

Each g of residue is equivalent to 0.9309 g of HgO.

Uses: It is used as an anti-infective and as a pharmaceutical necessity.

SULPHUR

Sulphur is an important element as it is an important component of a large number of natural and synthetic pharmaceutical aids and medicinal compounds. It is available in nature in a free state or in combined forms and geographically it is distributed in volcanic areas, especially in Sicily and United States, where it is found in free state. Iron pyrite, FeS_2, Gypsum, $CaSO_4.2H_2O$ and baryte, $BaSO_4$ are some of the important natural sources. Sulphur is obtained by mining operations. Sulphate ores afford good sources for some valuable metals like antimony, mercury, bismuth, lead, zinc and molybdenum. India imports sulphur for its requirement, but recently iron pyrites deposits have been found.

Sulphur as such, i.e. in its elementary form, is of great pharmaceutical value. It is an old and proven germicide and fungicide and for the same purpose, it has been and is being used in various dosage forms like dusting powders, ointments, creams, lotions etc. In the form of soluble sulphides, it is used in many skin affections, being perhaps the most beloved material for dermatologists.

A large number of sulphur salts, which may look as of insignificant value perhaps because they are cheap and easily available like sodium bisulphite, sodium metabisulphite find their utility in pharmaceutical preparations as antioxidants, preservatives and stabilizers. Sodium thiosulphate is an important antidote to iodine and cyanide, besides being useful in different parasitic skin diseases. The importance of sulphur and its compounds will be known when the compounds (sulpha drugs to mention an important group) are studied both in inorganic and organic pharmaceutical chemistry.

The following inorganic materials/preparations with sulphur, as such or in combination, are included in the following text. They were official in I.P. earlier.

1. Precipitated sulphur   S   At. wt. 32.06
2. Sublimed sulphur   S   At. wt. 32.06
3. Sulphur ointment

PRECIPITATED SULPHUR
(Precip. Sulp.)

At. weight: 32.06

Precipitated Sulphur is expected to contain 99.5% of S, calculated on the basis of anhydrous sulphur.

Preparation : A method, which is of theoretical interest, consists in acidifying a solution of thiosulphate with a mineral acid, when the unstable thiosulphuric acid, first liberated, gets rapidly decomposed to give precipitated sulphur. This method is costly for industrial manufacture, but can be conveniently tried on small scale in the laboratory. The reactions taking place are given below:

$$Na_2S_2O_3 + 2HCl \longrightarrow H_2S_2O_3 + 2NaCl$$
$$H_2S_2O_3 \longrightarrow S + SO_2 + H_2O$$

The I.P. 85 itself mentions the method of preparation of precipitated sulphur under its monograph, which, though unusual, is reproduced here. Precipitated sulphur may be obtained by adding hydrochloric acid to a solution prepared by boiling sulphur, lime acid water. In actual process a slurry of slaked lime (1 part) with water (10 parts) is prepared. To this slurry is added sublimed or powdered roll sulphur (2 parts) contained in water (20 parts) and the mixture is mixed and boiled for an hour, with occasional shaking, till sulphur is dissolved. The liquid is cooled and filtered. It contains a mixture of thiosulphates and polysulphides of calcium. It is treated with calculated quantity of hydrochloric acid to leave the supernatant liquid slightly alkaline. The precipitated sulphur is collected on a filter, washed until the washings are free from calcium and dried. The chemical reactions taking place during the process involved are complex, but they can be represented as under:

$$3Ca(OH)_2 + 12S \longrightarrow 2CaS_5 + CaS_2O_3 + 3H_2O$$

       Lime   Sulphur   Polysulphide Thiosulphate

$$2CaS_5 + CaS_2O_3 + 6HCl \longrightarrow 3CaCl_2 + 12S + 3H_2O$$

The yield of precipitated sulphur is about two-thirds of the theoretical yield as much of sulphur is lost as a result of escape of gases H_2S and SO_2, which are formed in the initial stages of the process.

Description: It is an odourless and tasteless pale greyish-yellow or pale greenish yellow, soft powder, free from grittyness. It burns with a blue flame with the production of sulphur dioxide. It is insoluble in water and alcohol, but soluble in carbon disulphide.

Tests for identity: 1. It melts at about 115° to a yellow mobile liquid which becomes dark and visible on further heating at about 160°.

2. When viewed under microscope, it is seen to consist of grouped amorphous subglabular particles without any admixture of crystals.

Tests for purity: As; acidity; matter insoluble in carbon disulphide and sulphated ash.

Acidity: It is tested by thoroughly agitating 5 g with 50 ml of purely boiled and cooled water and titrating with 0.1 N sodium hydroxide, using solution of phenolphthalein as indicator. Not more than 0.5 ml of alkali is required.

Test for matter insoluble in carbon disulphide is done by dissolving 1 g in 5 ml of carbon disulphide. Almost all the precipitated sulphur should be completely dissolved.

Sulphated ash should not be more than 0.25 per cent.

Uses: See also general remarks for sulphur. It is a good scabicide and may be used as constituent in sulphur ointment. It is also used in the form of lotions or ointments in the treatment of acne. Precipitated sulphur is preferred in liquid mixtures, because its particles are lighter and thus they get easily suspended. Its ointment is also more smooth and preferred. Sulphur, being an active parasiticide, is used in the treatment of many infections and skin disorders, such as ringworm infection, pediculosis, psoriasis, eczema etc.

Dose: 1 to 4 g.

SUBLIMED SULPHUR
(Sub. Sulph.)

At. weight: 32.06

I.P. does not prescribe any percentage content pertaining to purity. However, the limit tests ensure its percentage as not less than 99.5%, which is a requirement in some pharmacopoeias including U.S.P.

Preparation: I.P. mentions that sublimed sulphur may be obtained from native sulphur or from sulphides. In fact, sublimed sulphur is obtained when sulphur is heated and its vapours are lead to a chamber, which is suitably cooled. The vapours get condensed and solidified and fall on the walls and on the bottom of the chamber in the form of a crystalline powder or friable masses. This yellowish powder is sublimed sulphur or flowers of sulphur. This sulphur after collection can be sieved.

Description: Sublimed sulphur occurs as a fine, yellow, slightly gritty, powder. It has a faint characteristic odour, but is devoid of any taste.

It burns with a blue flame, producing sulphur dioxide. It is almost insoluble in water and alcohol but dissolves (1 g in 2 ml) slowly and incompletely in carbon disulphide.

Tests for identity:
(1) It melts to yellow mobile liquid on being heated at about 115°. The liquid becomes dark and visible on further heating at about 160°.
(2) Under the microscope it is seen consisting of opaque rounded amorphous panicles or aggregates.

Tests for purity: As; acidity; matter insoluble in carbon disulphide and sulphated ash.

Tests for acidity: It is performed by thoroughly agitating 2 g of sublimed sulphur with 50 ml of freshly boiled and cooled water and titrating the liquid with 0.1 N sodium hydroxide, using solution of phenolphthalein as indicator. Not more than 1 ml of 0.1 N sodium hydroxide is required. Acidity is due to the presence of traces of sulphurous and sulphuric acids; which may get formed due to oxidation of sulphur during its conversion into sublimed sulphur.

Test for matter insoluble in carbon disulphide: It is carried out by agitating 1 g of sublimed sulphur in 20 ml of carbon disulphide and allowing the liquid to stand for ten minutes. The liquid is filtered and the residue on filter is washed with carbon disulphide and dried. The residue should not weigh less than 0.2 g, i.e. not less than 20% of sublimed sulphur should be insoluble.

Sulphated ash: It should not be more than 0.2 per cent.

Uses: It is utilised for the same therapeutic uses as those mentioned under precipitated sulphur.

Dose: 1 to 4 g.

Preparation: Sulphur ointment; sublimed sulphur is one of the ingredients of Liquorice Compound Powder.

SULPHUR OINTMENT

Sulphur ointment contains 10 per cent of sulphur (limit 9.5 to 10.5 per cent of S).

Ingredients:

Sublimed sulphur, finely sifted .... 100 g

Simple ointment prepared with white soft paraffin .... 900 g

Preparation: Sublimed sulphur is triturated with a portion of the simple ointment until the mixture is smooth. The remainder of the simple ointment is then added and mixed thoroughly.

Tests for identity: The tests can only be applied by first extracting sulphur from the ointment with the help of light petroleum and then applying the same tests for identification given under sublimed sulphur (p. 205).

20 g of the ointment is refluxed with 25 ml of light petroleum in 250 ml conical flask for one hour and the petroleum layer is rejected. The residue in the flask is again refluxed with 25 ml of light petroleum for one hour. The petroleum layer is decanted and the dried residue, i.e. sulphur is used for identification tests given below:

(1) It melts at about 115° to a yellow mobile liquid, which becomes darker and viscid on heating at about 160°C.

(2) The substance from test (1) above is further heated strongly. It burns strongly with a blue fume, forming sulphur dioxide, which can be recognised by its characteristic colour.

(3) To 1 mg of the residue dissolved in 2 ml of hot pyridine is added 0.2 ml of solution of sodium bicarbonate and the mixture is boiled. A blue or green colour is produced.

Assay: The assay is carried out by converting sulphur into sodium thiosulphate by refluxing the ointment with a solution of sodium sulphite.

$$Na_2SO_3 + S \longrightarrow Na_2S_2O_3$$

The solution after cooling is filtered and the filtrate along with the washings from the residual fat on the filter is treated with formaldehyde and acetic acid to fix sodium sulphite as formaldehyde sodium bisulphite, which in cold solution is unreactive with iodine.

$$Na_2SO_3 \ + \ HCHO \ + \ H_2O \ \rightleftharpoons \ CH_2OH.OSO_2Na \ + \ NaOH$$

Sod. sulphite   Formaldehyde   Fixed Formaldehyde

Sodium bisulphite compound

The acetic acid present in the reaction mixture neutralises the sodium hydroxide.

$$CH_3COOH + NaOH \longrightarrow CH_3COONa.H_2O$$

Sodium thiosulphate is titrated as usual with standard solution of iodine and the amount of sulphur in the ointment is estimated.

$$I_2 + 2Na_2S_2O_3 \longrightarrow Na_2S_4O_6 + 2NaI$$

The assay procedure as given in I.P. is outlined hereunder:

An accurately weighed amount about 1 g of sulphur ointment is boiled with a solution of 2 g of sodium sulphite in 40 ml of water under a reflux condenser until the sulphur is completely dissolved. The mixture is cooled and the aqueous solution is filtered and the residue of fat on the filter paper is washed with hot water. The residue is again cooled and again washed with hot water. The washings are added to the filtered aqueous solution to which is added 10 ml of formaldehyde solution and 6 ml of acetic acid. The solution is diluted to 150 ml with water and titrated with 0.1 N iodine using solution of starch as indicator.

Each ml of 0.1 N iodine is equivalent to 0.003206 g of S.

Storage: The sulphur ointment is preserved in a well closed-container, preferably in a cool place.

Uses: See under precipitated and sublimed sulphur.

BORON

Boron is a metal of the aluminium group. It is available in crystalline, amorphous and adamentine forms. Boron is a trivalent element. Metallic boron is used as an industrial catalyst in metallurgy to give hardness and because it absorbs neutrons in atomic reactors.

The body weight is reduced if boric acid is given orally for longer duration, which is attributed to loss of water from cells and tissues. It was, therefore, used in obesity but now-a-days it is no more used because of its toxicity. It gets accumulated because of slow rate of excretion. The sign of poisoning is seen through vomiting, loss of appetite, dryness of skin, itching and from confused state of mind. The lethal oral dose is 10 to 20 g.

BORAX
(Synonym: Sodium borate)

Chem. formula: $Na_2B_4O_7.10H_2O$ $\qquad\qquad$ Mol. weight: 381.4

It occurs as sodium salt of pyroboric acid in the dried lakes of Tibet and India and contains not less than 99% and not more than 103% of $Na_2B_4O_7 \cdot 10H_2O$. It is not official as such now.

Preparation: Large quantities of borax are obtained from Kunite, $Na_2B_4O_7.4H_2O$, by simple crystallization from water. Borax crystallises as decahydrate, $Na_2B_4O_7.10H_2O$.

Description: It is a colourless crystalline or white crystalline powder, without any odour but saline and alkaline taste. It effloresces in dry air and loses all its water of crystallisation on ignition. It is soluble in 16 parts of cold water, in 1 part of boiling water, 1 part of glycerol and insoluble in alcohol. An aqueous solution of borax is alkaline due to hydrolysis.

$$Na_2B_4O_7 + 3H_2O \longrightarrow 2NaBO_2 + 2H_3BO_3$$

If the solution is diluted further, the sodium metaborate is further hydrolysed giving rise to alkali and boric acid.

$$NaBO_2 + 2H_2O \longrightarrow NaOH + H_3BO_3$$

Tests for identity: See under Boric acid. Also gives reaction for sodium (App. I).

Tests for purity: It is tested for arsenic; heavy metals; iron chloride and sulphate.

Assay: An accurately weighed amount (3 g) of borax is dissolved in water (76 ml) and the solution is titrated with N/2 HCl using solution of methyl red as indicator.

$$2HCl + Na_2B_4O_7 + 5H_2O = 2NaCl + 4H_3BO_3$$

Each ml of N/2 HCl is equivalent to 0.09536 g of $Na_2B_4O_7.10H_2O$.

Uses: Borax is used as a bacteriostatic and as a pharmaceutical aid. The emulsifying action of borax on oils is attributed to the formation of free alkali (NaOH) on hydrolysis (see reaction above).

BORAX GLYCERIN

Borax glycerin contains borax equivalent to 12% w/w of $Na_2B_4O_7 \cdot 10H_2O$ and is prepared by triturating the powdered borax (120 g) with glycerin (880 g) and warming slowly with constant stirring till the solution is effected.

Assay: An accurately weighed amount of borax glycerin is diluted with water and the solution is neutralised with N/2 sulphuric acid using sol. of methyl orange as indicator. To the boiled and cooled solution 20 ml of glycerin is added and it is titrated with N/2 NaOH using solution of phenolphthalein as indicator.

Uses: The borax glycerin is also used as bacteriostatic.

ANTIMONY SODIUM TARTRATE

Chem. formua: $C_4H_4O_7.Sb.Na$ Mol. weight: 308.8

Preparation: Antimony Sodium Tartrate, known as tartar emetic, is an example of certain closely related substances which are formed by the interaction of an oxide of an element (antimony, bismuth etc.) with organic hydroxy acids or their salts. Thus antimony sodium tartrate is prepared by making a paste of 5 parts of antimonious oxide and 6 parts of finely powdered sodium acid tartrate with water and setting aside the paste for a day. The paste is boiled with 40 parts of water for 15 minutes with frequent stirring. The hot liquid is filtered and the filtrate is kept aside for crystallization. The crystals of antimony sodium tartrate are collected on filter paper and dried at atmospheric temperature. The mother liquid can still be concentrated to yield another crop of tartar emetic. The I.P. requires antimony sodium tartrate to contain not less than 96% of $C_4H_4O_7.Sb.Na$, calculated with reference to the substance dried to constant weight at 105°. It is not official now.

Description: It is a colourless and transparent or white scaly powder, which is odourless, sweetish and hygroscopic. It is freely soluble in water but practically insoluble in alcohol.

Tests for identity: The substance yields reactions characteristic of sodium and antimony. After antimony is removed, tests for reactions characteristic of tartrates are carried out (App. I).

Tests for purity: It is tested for As; acidity or alkalinity; heavy metals and loss on drying.

Acidity or alkalinity is measured by the volume of N/100 acid or alkali required to neutralise a solution of definite concentration to the green colour of bromocresol green, indicative of pH 4.5. 1 g of the substance is taken and dissolved in 50 ml of water. N/100 alkali or acid used should not be more than 20 ml for neutralisation.

Loss on drying should not be more than 6 per cent, when dried to constant weight at 105° C. (The salt is hygroscopic, but the official salt is anhydrous.)

Assay: An accurately weighed amount (0.5 g) is dissolved in water (50 ml) and to the solution is added sodium bicarbonate (2 g) and is titrated with N/10 iodine, using solution of starch as indicator.

The above assay is carried out iodometrically and is an oxidation and reduction type of titration. The following reaction which is reversible takes place. The acid which is liberated in the reaction is neutralised with sodium bicarbonate to enable the reaction to go to completion.

$$2C_4H_4O_7.Sb.Na + 3H_2O + 2I_2 \rightleftharpoons 2NaHC_4H_4O_6 + Sb_2O_5 + 4HI$$

Each ml of N/10 I_2 is equivalent to 0.01544 g of $C_4H_4O_7.Sb.Na$.

Uses: It is used as an antischistosomal drug in schistosomiasis and as an emetic. Its emetic action is due to the irritant action on the gastrointestinal mucosa. It is given by intravenous injection only. Orally it is used as a reflex expectorant.

ANTIMONY SODIUM TARTRATE INJECTION

The injection is sterile solution of antimony sodium tartrate in water for injection and it contains not less than 95 per cent and not more than 105% of antimony sodium tartrate, $C_4H_4.O_7.Sb.Na$, corresponding to the amount stated on the label. The injection is sterilised by heating in an autoclave or by filtration.

Tests for identity: The injection is tested by evaporating 5 ml to dryness and testing the residue for reaction characteristic of sodium and antimony. Reaction characteristics of tartrate are given after antimony is removed (App. I).

Assay: It is assayed in the same way as described under antimony sodium tartrate, using an accurately measured volume equivalent to about 0.5 g of antimony sodium tartrate.

Uses: Injection is used intravenously in the treatment of schistosomiasis in divided doses until the total quantity administered is 1.5 g.

AMMONIATED MERCURY
(Synonym: Aminochloride of mercury)

Chem. formula: $NH_2.HgCl$ Mol. weight: 252.1

Ammoniated mercury is called aminochloride of mercury, as an amino group $(-NH_2)$ replaces an atom of chlorine from mercuric chloride. It is not official in new I.P. 2007.

$$Cl-Hg-Cl \xrightarrow[+NH_2]{-Cl} NH_2-Hg-Cl$$

Preparation: Ammon. mercury is prepared by adding a solution of mercuric chloride (3 parts) in water (60 parts) to a mixture of dilute solution of ammonia (4 parts) and water (20 parts) with constant stirring.

Reaction:

$$HgCl_2 + 2NH_3 \longrightarrow HN_2HgCl + NH_4Cl$$

The precipitate of NH_2HgCl is collected on the filter paper, washed with cold water and dried at a temperature not exceeding 30°. The washing of the precipitate is not done for a long time in an effort to remove NH_4Cl, as long washing will only give yellowish product. I.P. requires ammoniated mercury to contain not less than 98.0% of NH_2HgCl.

Description: Ammoniated mercury is a heavy, odourless, white, amorphous powder, which is stable in air, but darkens on exposure to light. It is insoluble in water and alcohol but soluble in warm acetic acid. It gradually decomposes in cold water and in boiling water it gets hydrolysed to yellow basic compound: NH_2HgCl; HgO. In boiling alkalies it gets completely decomposed as under:

$$NH_2HgCl + NaOH \longrightarrow NH_3 + HgO + NaCl$$

This reaction is also used for identification.

Tests for identity:
  (1) On being heated it volatilises without fusion.
  (2) On being heated with sodium hydroxide, it gives yellow mercuric oxide and ammonia.
  (3) Solution in acetic acid yields reactions characteristic of mercuric salts and chlorides (App. I).

Tests for purity: It is tested for mercurous chloride; carbonates and sulphated ash.

Mercurous chloride and carbonates are tested by trituration with acetic acid followed by heating to 70° with occasional shaking. A clear solution is obtained with no effervescence.

Assay: An accurately weighed amount (0.25 g) of NH_2HgCl is transferred to a stoppered flask containing water (50 ml) and potassium iodide (3 g). The mixture is shaken until solution is complete. The liberated alkalis, NH_3 and KOH are titrated with N/10 HCl, using solution of methyl orange as indicator:

$$NH_2HgCl + 2KI + H_2O = HgI_2 + NH_3 + KOH + KCl$$

1.0 ml of N/10 HCl is equivalent to 0.01261 g of NH_2HgCl.

Uses: It is used as an anti-infective substance.

Preparation: Ammoniated Mercury Ointment is also official in I.P. It is called White Precipitate Ointment and contains 2.5% of NH_2HgCl.

Ingredients:

Ammoniated Mercury, finely powdered .... 25 g
Simple Ointment .... 975 g

Preparation: Ammoniated mercury is triturated with a portion of the simple ointment to a smooth consistency and then the remainder of the simple ointment is added gradually and the preparation mixed thoroughly.

Tests for identity: The tests (1 to 3) listed above under Ammoniated Mercury are carried out with the residue after completely removing the ointment base with the help of a mixture of equal volumes of solvent ether and light petroleum.

Assay: The ointment is assayed by the above acid base titration method, except that the ointment is first treated with solvent ether and light petroleum to remove the fatty and greasy materials. An accurately weighed amount of ointment representing about 0.20 g of ammoniated mercury in it (in about 5 g) is taken and assayed as above.

Each ml of 0.1 N HCl is equivalent to 0.01261 NH_2HgCl.

Uses: See under ammoniated mercury.

ASTRINGENTS

Astringents are substances that precipitate surface proteins when applied topically. They have low cell penetrability and action is limited to the cell surface and interstitial spaces. Astringents are normally applied in very dilute solutions, since many are irritants or caustics in moderate to high concentrations. Most astringents are also antiseptics.

The astringent action is accompanied by contraction of the tissue, and hardening and pathological transcapillary movement of plasma protein is inhibited. Local edema, inflammation and exudation are thereby reduced. Mucous or other secretions may also be reduced and the affected area becomes drier.

Astringents are used therapeutically to reduce the volume of exudates from wounds and skin eruptions, to arrest hemorrhage by coagulating the blood, to check diarrhoea, reduce inflammation of mucous membranes, promote healing, toughen skin or decrease sweating due to their ability to constrict pores. They also possess deodorant properties due to their ability to destroy microorganisms that produced body odours.

Substances that possess astringent action include aluminium acetate, aluminium chloride, aluminium chlorohydrates, aluminium sulphate, calamine, zinc oxide, zinc sulphate, salts of manganese, bismuth, permanganates, tannins or related polyphenolic compounds.

ALUMINIUM SULPHATE

Chem. formula: $Al_2(SO_4)_3.xH_2O$ Mol. weight: 342.14 (anhyd.)

Aluminium sulphate contains not less than 51% and not more than 59% of $Al_2(SO_4)_3$. It contains varying amount of water of crystallization.

Preparation:

(1) It can be prepared by dissolving aluminium hydroxide in sulphuric acid.

$$2Al(OH)_3 + 3H_2SO_4 \longrightarrow Al_2(SO_4)_3 + 6H_2O$$

The solution is concentrated by removing water and left for crystallization.

(2) From **pyrites shale**, Al_2O_3, X SiO_2 + FeS_2

$$2FeS_2 + 2H_2O + 7O_2 \longrightarrow 2FeSO_4 + 2H_2SO_4$$

$$Al_2O_3 \ X \ SiO_2 + 3H_2SO_4 \longrightarrow Al_2(SO_4)_3 + X \ SiO_2 + 3H_2O$$

Description: It is a white, crystalline powder, shining plates or crystalline fragments, odourless, with sweet taste at first and then mildly astringent.

Solubility: It is very soluble in water, giving an acid solution, due to hydrolysis.

$$Al_2(SO_4)_3 + 6H_2O \longrightarrow 2Al(OH)_3 + 3H_2SO_4 \text{ insoluble in alcohol.}$$

Tests for identity: A solution (1 : 20) gives the reactions of aluminium and sulphates (App. I).

Reaction: It shows pH 3 to 4 when determined in a 2% w/v solution in CO_2-free water.

Tests for purity: It is tested for clarity and colour of solution; alkalis and alkaline earths; ammonium salts; arsenic; heavy metals and iron.

Test for clarity and colour of solution: A 5% w/v solution is clear and colourless.

Test for alkalis and alkaline earths: 1 g of sample is dissolved in 100 ml of water, to which methyl red solution as an indicator and enough dil. NH_3 solution to get a distinct yellow colour (pH 6.5) are added. The solution is diluted to 150 ml with water, boiled and filtered while hot. 75 ml of the filtrate is evoporated to dryness and ignited to constant weight. The wt. of the residue does not exceed 2 mg.

Test for ammonium salts: 1 g of sample is heated with 10 ml solution of NaOH on water bath for 1 minute. The colour of ammonium is not perceptible.

Test for arsenic: Does not exceed 3 ppm.

Test for heavy metals: Not more than 40 ppm, determined by dissolving 0.5 g of the sample in 1 ml of dil. CH_3COOH and sufficient water to produce 25 ml.

Test for iron: It is determined by adding potassium ferrocyanide solution to the sample solution (25 ml of a 1 in 150 solution) when no blue colour is produced immediately.

Assay: It is based upon the complexometric titrations. Disodium edetate is used as a sequestering agent. Xylenol orange is used as an indicator for metallic ions in acidic solution. It yields intensely red complexes with metals and is itself lemon yellow in acidic pH.

An accurately weighed quantity of the sample (0.6 g) is dissolved in 1 N HCl (2 ml) and water (50 ml) to which is added 0.05 M disodium edetate (50 ml) and neutralised to methyl red solution with 1 N NaOH. The solution is heated to boiling, left on a water bath for 10 minutes and cooled rapidly. Xylenol orange mixture (50 mg) and hexamine (5 g) are added and the solution is titrated with 0.05 M lead nitrite. A blank determination is also carried out.

Each ml of 0.05 M disodium edetate $\equiv$ 0.008554 g of $Al_2(SO_4)_3$.

Storage: It is stored in a well-closed container.

Uses: It is used as a pharmaceutical aid (for mineral carrier for adsorbed vaccines). It is a powerful astringent. It is widely used as a local anti-perspirant. It is used for water purification.

ALUM

Chem. formula: $KAl(SO_4)_2.12H_2O$ Mol. weight: 474.4

                    $K_2SO_4Al_2(SO_4)_3.24H_2O$

Alum is a potash alum, i.e. it is the potassium aluminium sulphate. Alums are double sulphates of a univalent metal and a trivalent metal. I.P requires it to contain aluminium equivalent to not less than 99.5% of $KAl(SO_4)_2.12H_2O$.

Preparation: Alum is prepared by adding a hot conc. solution of potassium sulphate to a hot solution of aluminium sulphate.

$$Al_2(SO_4)_3 + K_2SO_4 + 24H_2O \longrightarrow 2KAl(SO_4)_2.12H_2O$$

The alum crystallises out on cooling. By slow crystallization large characteristic, regular octahedral crystals are obtained. On being heated on water bath temperature alum melts in its water of crystallization. It loses the whole of its water below 20°C. leaving a white residue of anhydrous aluminium and potassium sulphate.

Description: It is available as a colourless, white powder or transparent crystalline mass. It is sweetish or astringent in taste and is freely soluble in water and insoluble in alcohol.

Tests for identity: It gives reactions characteristic of aluminium, potassium and sulphates.

$$Al_2O_3.3H_2O + 2NaOH \longrightarrow 2NaAlO_2 + 4H_2O$$

Bauxite $\quad\quad\quad\quad\quad\quad\quad\quad$ Sodium
$\quad\quad\quad\quad\quad\quad\quad\quad\quad\quad\quad$ metaluminate

$$NaAlO_2 + CO_2 + H_2O \longrightarrow NaHCO_3 + Al(OH)_3$$

$$2Al(OH)_3 + 3H_2SO_4 \longrightarrow Al_2(SO_4)_3 + 3H_2O$$

Tests for purity: It is tested for As; Cu; Zn; Fe and heavy metals. Potash alum is also required to comply with a test for ammonium salts.

Zinc is tested by comparison with a control and by dissolving 1 g of alum in 20 ml of water, adding 0.5 ml of dilute H_2SO_4 and 2 g of NH_4Cl and diluting the mixture to 20 ml of water. 1 ml of sol. of potassium ferricyanide is added and the solution is set aside for five minutes. Any opalescence which is produced is not greater than that produced in a control test made by adding 0.5 ml dilute HCl, 2 g of ammonium chloride and 1 ml of solution of potassium ferricyanide to 4 ml of 0.11% v/w $ZnSO_4$ and diluting the volume to 50 ml and setting aside for five minutes as in the case of test solution.

Ammonium salts are tested by comparison with a control test by dissolving 1 g of alum in 1000 ml of ammonia-free water. To the 10 ml of solution is added 40 ml of ammonia-free water and 2 ml of alkaline solution of potassium mercuric iodide. A colour, if produced, is not deeper than in a control made by adding 2 ml of alkaline solution of potassium mercuric iodide to 1 ml of dilute solution of ammonium chloride in 50 ml of ammonia-free water.

Assay: An accurately weighed amount (2 g) is dissolved in water (300 ml) and to the solution is added solution of ammonium chloride (20 ml) and 5 drops of methyl red and sufficient dil. ammonia solution to produce a distinct yellow colour in the mixture. The mixture is boiled and filtered. The precipitate is washed with 2.5 per cent w/v of solution of ammonium nitrate until it is free from chloride. The precipitate is dried to constant weight at a temperature above 120°C and the residue (Al_2O_3) is weighed.

1.0 g of residue is equivalent to 9.307 g of the alum.

Uses: It is used as a pharmaceutical aid and as an astringent. It is also considered as an antiseptic and used as local styptic. Barbers usually employ alum by wetting it and rubbing it on skin after shave, perhaps for its astringent and antiseptic action.

ZINC

Symbol: Zn   At. wt.: 65.38

Zinc widely and quite regularly occurs in animal tissues and it amounts on an average 20–30 microgram per 1 g of fresh tissue. Some organs, like genital organs, are especially rich in zinc. Its presence in insulin is of interest. Most of the dietary materials contain zinc (e.g. 1 litre of milk contains 4 mg) and hence an adult receives 10–15 mg of zinc daily and this amount far exceeds the requirement. Zinc is excreted in faeces.

Biochemically, zinc is found in association with some metalloenzymes like carbonic anhydrase, aldolase carboxy-peptidase etc. It is also found bound to RNA.

Earlier, zinc was supposed to be an essential dietary mineral and was regularly supplemented, but recently this view has changed and so far no one knows whether it is daily required and in how much quantity it is required. Food materials rich in zinc are milk, meat, fish, nuts, etc.

Zinc itself has no therapeutic value, but its compounds have astringent, anti-infective, antiseptic and protective properties.

Zinc compounds show very mild toxicity. Acute toxicity in some cases is seen with an intake of 1 g of zinc salts; 3–4 g of zinc sulphate or chloride is fatal. An immediately available antidote is sodium bicarbonate. Dimercaprol is an effective antidote for zinc toxicity, whose symptoms include periodic chills and fevers, malaise, coughing, headache and salivation.

The most important sources of zinc are zinc ores, Zinc blende (also known as sphalerite) (ZnS) and Calamine ($ZnCO_3$).

Zinc granulated and zinc powder are included under Appendix 7 in I.P. and are employed in tests. Also included in Appendix 7 are zinc acetate and zinc chloride.

ZINC SULPHATE

Chem. formula: $ZnSO_4.7H_2O$ Mol. wt.: 287.5

Zinc sulphate contains not less than 55.6 per cent and not more than 61% of $ZnSO_4$, corresponding to not less than 99.0 per cent and not more than the equivalent of 104.0 per cent of the hydrated salt, $ZnSO_4 \cdot 7H_2O$.

Preparation: Zinc sulphate is prepared by boiling an excess of metallic zinc with dilute sulphuric acid. The action is allowed to continue till evolution of hydrogen gas ceases.

$$Zn + H_2SO_4 \longrightarrow ZnSO_4 + H_2\uparrow$$

The solution is filtered to separate the undissolved zinc and evaporated to crystallisation.

In order to obtain purer product conforming to pharmacopoeial requirement, the solution after filteration is reacted with chlorine water to oxidise ferrous sulphate impurity, if any, to ferric state. The ferric salt is then precipitated as ferric hydroxide on agitating zinc carbonate or zinc oxide.

Description: Zinc sulphate occurs as colourless transparent crystals, prisms or needles or as a granular, crystalline powder. It is odourless and has an astringent and metallic taste. It effloresces in dry air.

It is very soluble in water (0.6 parts) and glycerin (2.5 parts) but insoluble in alcohol.

An aqueous solution of zinc sulphate is acidic to litmus, due to hydrolysis of the salt and has pH of about 5. The solution is acid to solution of phenol red and not acid to solution of methyl orange.

Tests for identity: It yields reactions characteristics of zinc and sulphates (App. I).

Tests for purity: It is tested for reaction (see above); aluminium; copper; manganese and nickel; As; Fe; chloride and alkalis and alkaline earths.

Tests for Al, Cu, Mg, Mn and Ni: It is performed by adding in excess dilute solution of ammonia to the solution (1 g in 20 ml of water) of the substance. The solution should remain colourless and produce no precipitate within thirty minutes.

The test for alkalis and alkaline earths: It is done by dissolving 2 g of the substance in about 150 ml of water contained in a 200 ml volumetric flask and precipitating the zinc completely by solution of ammonium sulphide and adding water to make 200 ml. The solution in the flask is mixed well and filtered through a dry filter rejecting the first portion of the filtrate. The subsequent 100 ml of the filtrate, after the addition of a few drops of sulphuric acid, is evaporated to dryness in a tared dish and then ignited to constant weight. The residue does not exceed 5 mg.

Assay: Zinc sulphate is also estimated by using complexometric titration. The titrant is disodium EDTA and the indicator is eriochrome black T solution .

Method: An accurately weighed amount of sample of about 0.3 g is dissolved in 100 ml of water to which 5 ml of ammonia-ammonium chloride solution and 0.1 ml of eriochrome black T solution are added. It is titrated with 0.05 M disodium EDTA until the solution is deep blue in colour.

Each ml of 0.05 M disodium EDTA $\equiv$ 0.01438 g of $ZnSO_4 \cdot 7H_2O$.

I.P. 2007 has modified the assay method which is given below.

An accurately weighed substance (about 0.5 g) is dissolved in 5 ml of 2 M acetic acid and diluted to 50 ml with water. To the resulting solution is added about 50 mg of xylenol orange triturate and sufficient hexamine to produce a violet-pink colour. After adding a further 2 g of hexamine, the solution is titrated with 0.1 M disodium edetate until the colour changes to yellow.

Each ml of 0.1 M disodium edetate $\equiv$ 0.02875 g of $ZnSO_4.7H_2O$.

Storage: Zinc sulphate is preserved in a well-closed container.

Uses: Zinc sulphate is used as an emetic and astringent. As emetic it is used as a reflex emetic. Its action is very rapid and does not cause local irritation to gastric mucosa. As an astringent it is usually found a component in some of the astringent solutions. Externally it is used as an ophthalmic astringent and its aqueous eye solutions have been used in 0.25 per cent concentration. But the eye solutions, if prepared without a borate buffer, are acidic (pH 5).

Usually Gifferd's borate buffer (pH 5.8 to 6.2) is used. If an alkaline solution is required, sodium citrate may be used as a sequestering agent (to keep the zinc ion from precipitating as the hydroxide).

Dose: 0.6 to 2 g.

Dental Products

Dental hygiene and dental therapeutics has acquired during the last thirty-forty years as much importance as general medical care. Different inorganic compounds are used as polishing, cleaning and anticaries agents in dentistry. Some of these agents are described in this chapter.

ANTICARIES AGENTS

Anticaries agents are substances used to prevent the tooth decay (caries). Caries is formed due to the action of acids, mostly lactic, obtained from oral bacterial metabolism of carbohydrate in the diet. The build up of plaque on the tooth surface aids the decay process by forming areas in which food particles can lodge. One of the objectives of brushing the teeth is to dislodge food particles and material from the teeth and leave a smooth surface on which it is difficult for food to adhere.

The most commonly used anticaries agent is fluoride. Ammoniated toothpastes are supposed to act by neutralizing lactic acid, although their use requires further study. Dentifrices containing antibiotics and antienzymes have also been tried.

Official anticaries products include sodium fluoride, stannous fluoride, sodium metaphosphate and dicalcium phosphate.

Fluorides: Tooth decay or dental caries prevention is the first and foremost problem widely prevalent throughout the world. The exact cause of dental caries is not clearly known. However, the use of fluorides in various forms e.g. drops, pastes, dentifrices etc. is quite common. The internal fluoride intake has been found to provide a better resistance to dental carries than its topical applications. Sodium fluoride supplements in the form of tablets and drops are dissolved in water or fruit juices for this purpose. A solution containing 2.2 mg of sodium fluoride (equivalent to 1.0 mg of fluoride anion) per day is recommended for children over three years of age and half this amount for children between two and three years of age.

SODIUM FLUORIDE

Chem. Form: NaF   Mol. wt.: 41.99

Description: It is a white powder or colourless crystalline material.

Solubility: It is soluble in water and practically insoluble in ethanol (95%).

Tests for identity:

(1) Dissolve 2.5 g in sufficient carbon dioxide-free water without heating to produce 100 ml (solution A). To 2 ml of solution A add 0.5 ml of calcium chloride solution; a gelatinous white precipitate is produced which dissolves on adding 5 ml of ferric chloride solution.

(2) Add about 4 mg to a mixture of 0.1 ml of alizarin red S solution and 0.1 ml of zirconyl nitrate solution and mix; the colour changes to yellow.

Tests for purity: It is tested for acidity and alkalinity; clarity and colour of solution; limits of chlorides; sulphate and fluorosilicate and loss on drying.

Assay: It is assayed by non-aqueous titration, using crystal violet solution as indicator. Each ml of 0.1 M perchloric acid is equivalent to 0.004199 g of NaF.

Uses: It is used as a preventive for dental caries, 1.5 to 3 ppm (equivalent to 0.7 to 1.3 ppm of fluoride ion) in drinking water and topically as a 2% solution to the teeth.

Usual dose: 2.2 mg (equivalent of 1 mg of fluoride ion) daily.

STANNOUS FLUORIDE

Chem. formula: SnF_2 Mol. wt.: 156.69

Description: It occurs as a white crystalline powder with bitter salty taste. It has a melting point about 213°C.

Solubility: It is freely soluble in water, practically insoluble in alcohol, ether and chloroform.

Uses: Stannous fluoride is used topically. It is not official in I.P.

DENTIFRICES

A dentifrice is a material used to clean the accessible surface of the teeth using preferably a tooth brush. Dentifrices are available as gels, pastes, powders, slurries, etc. They contain abrasives, such as phosphate salts, calcium carbonate, magnesium carbonate, hydrated aluminium oxide, silicates or dehydrated silica gels, along with binders, foaming agents, flavouring agents and humectants each comprising a few organic compounds resulting in different formulations. Some of the inorganic ingredients of commonly used tooth pastes include calcium carbonate, calcium monohydrogen phosphate, calcium pyrophosphate, sodium polyphosphate, stannous fluoride, stannous pyrophosphate, sodium monofluorophosphate, insoluble sodium metaphosphate, anhydrous dicalcium phosphate and pumice.

Dentifrices may be classified as:

- Dentifrices containing fluorides.
- Dentifrices containing polishing agents – an official product is pumice.
- Dentifrices containing desensitizing agents - that will desensitize the teeth to heat and cold. Official products include zinc chloride and zinc-eugenol cement. Ammoniacal silver nitrate solution was once used but is no longer in use.

PUMICE

It consists chiefly of complex silicates of aluminium, potassium and sodium. Pumice is a very light, hard, rough, porous, grayish mass or a gritty, grayish powder, odourless, tasteless and stable in the air. The powder is available in three grades of fineness of mesh size No. 200 (superfine), No. 150 (fine) and No. 60 (coarse).

It is insoluble in water and is not attacked by acids or alkali hydroxide solutions. It is used in the powdered form as a dental abrasive in tooth powders and tooth pastes. It does not find any place in any official literature now.

ZINC CHLORIDE

Chem. formula: $ZnCl_2$ Mol. wt.: 136.29

Description: It is a white crystalline powder or granules, without any odour. It is very deliquescent.

Solubility: It is very soluble in water and soluble in other polar solvents such as alcohol and glycerin. It should contain 95 to 100.5% of $ZnCl_2$.

Tests for identity:

   (1) To 2.0 g of $ZnCl_2$ in 38 ml of freshly boiled and cooled water is added 2 N HCl dropwise until the sol. is complete. The resulting sol. gives the reaction of zinc salts (App. I).

   (2) A 5% w/v sol. in 2 N HNO_3 gives the reaction of chlorides (App. I).

pH: 4.6 to 6.0 determined by using specified amount of drug (1 g) in freshly boiled and cooled water (9 ml).

Tests for purity: It is tested for ammonium salts; alkalis and alkaline earths; lead; SO_4 and oxychloride.

Ammonium salts: They are determined by adding 1 N NaOH to a dilute solution of drug and warming the solution, which should not give odour of NH_3.

Alkalis and alkaline earths: Not more than 1% (I.P., p. 548)

Lead: It should comply with limit test by comparing sample with standard preparation (I.P. 85, p. 548).

Sulphate: A specified amount of sample (2 g) should comply with the limit test for sulphates.

Oxychloride: A specified amount of sample of drug (1.5 g) is dissolved in freshly boiled and cooled water (1.5 ml). To the solution, which should be clear, is added alcohol (7.5 ml). The solution changes to cloudy appearance but becomes clear by adding 2 N HCl (0.2 ml).

Assay: It is done by following the complexometric titration method.

Method: An accurately weighed amount of sample of about 3 g is dissolved in about 125 ml of water to which is added 3 g of ammonium chloride and sufficient water to produce 250 ml. To 25 ml of the resulting solution is added 100 ml of water, 10 ml of strong ammonia-ammonium chloride solution and 1 ml of eriochrome black T solution. The solution is titrated with 0.05 M disodium EDTA to a deep blue end point.

Each ml of 0.05 M disodium EDTA $\equiv$ 0.006815 g of $ZnCl_2$.

Uses: It is used as an astringent and dentin desensitizer externally, as a 10% topical solution. It is also used as a pharmaceutical aid for insulin preparations.

Most of the other inorganic compounds used in formulations of dental products mentioned above have been described elsewhere in the book. Those mentioned in the diploma course in Pharmacy syllabus also include calcium carbonate and strontium chloride. But apart from calcium carbonate which is described under pharmaceutical aids, others are no more official in I.P. 2007.

10

Complexing and Chelating Agents Used in Therapy

Many toxic effects of excessive metal-ion concentrations can be treated by agents that are capable of forming strong co-ordination complexes through chelation, thus facilitating the excretion of the metal. These agents are used in the treatment of heavy metal poisoning from such elements as iron, lead, copper, cobalt, nickel, mercury and zinc and to treat certain metabolic disorders resulting from the accumulation of abnormal amounts of metals such as iron and copper in various tissues, by chelation therapy. The standard chelating agents used for this purpose are calcium disodium edetate, disodium edetate, dimercaprol and D-penicillamine.

The association of two or more interacting molecules or ions forms *complexes*. Co-ordination complexes are formed by co-ordinate bonds in which a pair of electrons is to some degree transferred from one interactant to another. Molecular complexes are formed by noncovalent forces (electrostatic, charge-transfer, hydrogen bonding and hydrophobic effects) between substrate and ligand.

Chelates are compounds with a partial ring of atoms that close up by holding an atom, usually a metal, in a molecular claw. Such molecules, which can form a ring structure with a metal, are called *ligands*. Chelating agents may be used for sequestration of metals, stabilization of drugs vulnerable to oxidation in presence of trace metals, treatment of heavy metal poisoning, certain metabolic disorders where metals such as iron and copper are accumulated in abnormal amounts in various tissues.

The formation of a complex can result in the alteration of various properties of the drug like solubility, light absorption, conductance, partitioning behaviour and chemical reactivity.

Complexation is also used to stabilize drugs. Boric acid chelation of the catechol function of epinephrine stabilizes epinephrine against attack by bisulphate and sulphate.

Dimercaprol (British antilewisite; BAL) chelates a number of heavy metals, and is used as an antidote in heavy metal poisoning. Edetate sodium chelates calcium (and magnesium) in addition to various heavy metals. It is used widely in therapy to lower plasma calcium levels. Other chelating agents include calcium disodium edetate (EDTA), penicillamine and deferoxamine.

CALCIUM DISODIUM EDETATE (USP)

Calcium disodium ethylenediaminetetraacetate hydrate

Chem. formula: $C_{10}H_{12}CaN_2Na_2O_8.xH_2O$ Mol. Wt.: 374.28

Preparation: It is prepared by boiling an aqueous solution of disodium edetate with a slight excess of an equimolar quantity of calcium carbonate until carbon dioxide ceases to evolve. The hot solution is filtered and the salt crystallized.

Description: It is a mixture of the dihydrate and trihydrate (predominantly the dihydrate) and occurs as white crystalline granules or a white crystalline powder and is stable in air. It is odourless, slightly hygroscopic with a faint saline taste. The salt is freely soluble in water, giving a weakly alkaline solution.

Assay: It is assayed by titration with M/20 lead nitrate.

1000 ml of M/20 lead nitrate are equivalent to $1/20 \ C_{10}H_{12}CaN_2Na_2O_8$.

Uses: It is mainly used in the treatment of lead poisoning. It may also be used to remove some other heavy metals from the body. The usual route of administration is by intravenous injection.

Dose: Intravenous infusion for adults: 1 g in 250–500 ml of isotonic solution over a period of one hour two times a day for five days; for children: up to 35 mg/kg as 0.2 to 0.4% isotonic solution twice a day. Intramuscular for adults: 75 mg/kg administered as a 20% solution in 0.5% procaine hydrochloride twice a day; for children: up to 35 mg/kg of a 20% solution in 0.5% procaine hydrochloride solution twice a day in divided doses at 8–12 hours interval.

DISODIUM EDETATE (I.P.)

Disodium ethylenediaminetetraacetate dihydrate

Chem. formula: $C_{10}H_{14}N_2Na_2O_8 \cdot 2H_2O$ Mol. Wt.: 372.24

Preparation: (Ethylenedinitrilo) tetraacetic acid (editic acid) is dissolved in a hot solution containing two equivalents of sodium hydroxide and the disodium salt is crystallized.

Description: It is a white, crystalline powder and is odourless.

Solubility: It is soluble in water and is sparingly soluble in ethanol (95%), practically insoluble in chloroform and ether.

Tests for identity:

(a) The infra-red absorption spectrum 4 is concordant with the reference spectrum of disodium edetate or with spectrum obtained from disodium edetate RS.

(b) Dissolve 2 g in 25 ml of water, add 6 ml of lead nitrate solution, shake and add 3 ml of potassium iodide solution; no yellow precipitate is produced. Make alkaline to red litmus paper with 2 M ammonia and add 5 ml of ammonium oxalate solution; no precipitate is produced.

(c) Dissolve 0.5 g in 10 ml of water, add 0.5 ml of a 10% w/v solution of calcium chloride, make alkaline to red litmus paper with 2 M ammonia and add 3 ml of ammonium oxalate solution; no precipitate is produced.

(d) Gives the reactions of sodium salts (I.P.).

Tests for purity: It is tested for pH; clarity and colour of solution and heavy metals and iron.

Assay: It is assayed by titration with 0.1 M lead nitrate using xylenol orange triturate as indicator.

Each ml of 0.1 M lead nitrate $\equiv$ 0.03722 g of $C_{10}H_{14}N_2Na_2O_8 \cdot 2H_2$.

Uses: It is used as a chelating agent in metal poisoning.

Dose: Intravenous injection, 50 mg per kg of body weight up to a maximum of 3 g per day.

DISODIUM EDETATE INJECTION (I.P.)

Disodium Edetate Injection is a sterile solution of Disodium Edetate in water for injection, containing varying amounts of disodium and trisodium salts as a result of pH adjustment. The pH is between 6.5 and 7.5.

Usual strengths: 3 g per 15 ml and 3 g per 20 ml.

Tests of identity: To volume equivalent to about 1 g of disodium edetate add 3 M hydrochloric acid to adjust the pH to 5.0 and evaporate to dryness on a steam-bath. The residue so obtained complies with tests a, b and c described under Disodium Edetate.

pH: Between 6.5 and 7.5.

Assay: Same as that for disodium edetate above.

An accurate volume containing about 0.6 g of disodium edetate is diluted with water to make upto 100 ml. To the mixed solution 2 g of hexamine and 2 M hydrochloric acid are added and the solution is titrated with 0.1 M lead nitrate using about 50 mg of xylenol orange triturate as an indicator.

Each ml of 0.1 M lead nitrate $\equiv$ 0.03722 g of $C_{10}H_{14}N_2Na_2O_8 \cdot 2H_2O$.

Storage: It is stored in single dose containers.

11

Gases and Vapours

Official gases include oxygen, carbon dioxide, helium, nitrogen and nitrous oxide. Some inorganic gases used in therapy are discussed in this chapter. These include oxygen and nitrous oxide. Some volatile vapours used as respiratory stimulants are also discussed.

OXYGEN

A common sentence in primary school textbooks is "All living things breathe" and "all living things need oxygen." Indeed atmospheric oxygen is essential for the survival of life on Earth. Oxygen is necessary in normal oxidative metabolism for the production of useful energy. Severe oxygen deprivation causes anatomic and physiologic disorders that can lead to permanent local damage.

The mitochondria of each cell have a tightly integrated enzyme system which catalyses a series of oxidative reductive reactions ending with the reduction of atomic oxygen and forming the oxide anion. This quickly combines with protons forming water, which along with CO_2 is the end point of combustion. Energy released during each oxidation reduction step in the mitochondrial enzyme system is used by the cell to synthesise adenosine triphosphate (ATP) by the process of oxidative phosphorylation. This may be considered the 'energy storehouse' for all normal oxidative metabolic reactions.

Atmospheric oxygen reaches the cells through its diffusion from the alveoli of the lungs to the blood where they are held by the haemoglobin (present in red blood cells), and transported through the circulatory system to various parts of the body. Blood contains 15 g of haemoglobin per 100 ml, and 100 ml of blood can hold 20 ml of oxygen.

Insufficiency of normal oxygen requirements in the body may be classified under the following classes:

1. *Anoxic*: Where the oxygen tension in the blood is lowered. Hence oxygen supply in the tissues is inadequate. The reasons may be lowered oxygen tension in the atmospheric air (due to high altitude or increase in inert gases normally present), disturbed pulmonary function or defect in the cardiac septum allowing mixture of arterial and venous blood. Oxygen therapy has thus found use is such conditions as asthma, massive collapse of the lungs, atelectasis of the newborn (incomplete expansion of the lungs at birth), bronchopneumonia, congestive heart failure, coronary thrombosis, cerebral thrombosis, etc.

2. *Anemic*: This is the condition where oxygen tension is normal, but haemoglobin content is inadequate to supply enough oxygen to the tissues. This condition may result from hemorrhage, defective red blood cell formation, or carbon monoxide poisoning. Oxygen therapy in such conditions aims at increasing the amount of oxygen dissolved in the plasma for the patient to survive until normal conditions are restored.

3. *Stagnant*: This occurs when general circulation is retarded or inadequate. Therapy for oxygen is not usually indicated and can be treated with cardiotonic drugs that increase the circulation.

4. *Histotoxic*: Here tissue cell oxidation may be interfered resulting in released energy that cannot be utilizd by the cell to form ATP. Certain toxic substances, such as cyanide, block electron transport thereby stopping the cell from carrying out metabolism requiring oxidation and reduction. Here traditional oxygen therapy is directed towards neutralization of toxic materials, and counteracting some of the lethal effects of cyanide.

ANAESTHETICS

Nitrous oxide, also called "laughing gas" (because it causes delirium), is the only inorganic gas used as an anaesthetic. Nitrous oxide is to be administered concomitantly with oxygen (20–25%). Failure to do so can result in death by suffocation and brain damage from hypoxia.

Nitrous oxide is usually administered with suitable sedatives like barbiturate to obtain a deep enough anaesthesia for surgery. It does not have muscle relaxant properties, and has a quick recovery time.

RESPIRATORY STIMULANTS

Respiratory stimulants being dealt in this chapter are agents/vapours used to revive an unconscious person who may have fainted.

Official inorganic agents include ammonium carbonate and aromatic ammonia spirit. Concentrated solutions should not be used as respiratory stimulants.

OXYGEN

Chem. formula: O_2 Mol. weight : 32.00

Oxygen is the major constituent of air and water, besides making up nearly one-half of the solid crust of earth. Oxygen constitutes about one-fifth by weight of air in the free state, seven-eight by weight of water and quite appreciable fractional part by weight of minerals, such as calcium carbonate ($CaCO_3$), manganese dioxide (MnO_2), ferric oxide (Fe_2O_3), etc.

Oxygen of I.P. contains not less than 99.0% v/v of O_2. The residue consists either of argon with a trace of nitrogen or hydrogen. It is made available in compressed form in metallic cylinders.

Preparation:
   (1) Oxygen is usually prepared by electrolysis of water.
   (2) Industrially oxygen is obtained by physically separating it from the air. This is done by fractionation of liquid air.

Description: It is an odourless, tasteless gas which is highly reactive chemically. It combines directly under suitable conditions with all elements except a few including mercury, silver, gold, etc. One volume dissolves in 32 volumes of water and in 3.6 volumes of alcohol at one atmospheric pressure and at 20°C. Its specific gravity at 0°C and at 760 mm of mercury is 1.429 g.

Tests for identity:

(1) A glowing splinter of wood bursts into flame on being plunged into the gas.

(2) When mixed with an equal volume of nitric oxide, red fumes are produced (distinction from nitrous oxide).

(3) It is absorbed when shaken with alkaline pyrogallol solution, the solution being dark brown.

Tests for purity: It is tested for alkalinity and acidity; carbon monoxide; carbon dioxide; halogens and oxidising substances.

Assay: Assay is carried out using 100 ml of the gas. The apparatus comprises essentially of a gas burette with two bulbs of suitable size. 100 ml of the gas being examined is used by placing spirals of freshly cleaned copper wire and 125 ml of ammonia buffer, pH 10.9, in the pipette. The volume of the residual gas in the burette should not be more than 1.0 ml.

Labelling and storage: Oxygen is preserved in metallic cylinders, which should not have been treated with any toxic, sleep inducing compound that will be irritating to respiratory tract. The shoulder of the cylinder is painted white and the remainder is painted black. The cylinder carries the name and symbol of oxygen which are stencilled in paint on the shoulder.

Uses: Oxygen gas is essential for proper respiratory functions and in normal course it is inhaled from the air, but it is employed as a therapeutic and medicinal gas in the treatment of a variety of hypoxia conditions and a condition where artificial respiration is to be given and the patient is put on oxygen in an unconscious and other serious conditions.

CARBON DIOXIDE

Chem. formula: CO_2 Mol. weight: 44.01

Carbon dioxide is one of the medicinal gases and contains not less than 99% v/v of CO_2. It is usually compressed in metal cylinders. It is not official in I.P. now.

Preparation: Carbon dioxide is prepared by the action of acids on any mineral carbonate.

$$CaCO_3 + 2HCl \longrightarrow CaCl_2 + H_2O + CO_2\uparrow$$

Carbon dioxide so produced is not pure and hence it is passed through potassium carbonate solution at room temperature, when potassium carbonate gets saturated and is converted into potassium bicarbonate. On boiling the solution of potassium bicarbonate at 100°C, pure carbon dioxide is liberated as follows:

$$2KHCO_3 \xrightarrow{\;100°\;} CO_2\uparrow + K_2CO_3 + H_2O$$

Pure carbon dioxide so obtained is then liquefied under pressure in steel cylinders and marketed.

Carbon dioxide is also obtained as a by-product in the fermentation of sugar molasses.

Description: It is a heavy colourless gas. Its aqueous solution is faintly acidic in taste. It can be liquefied under pressure. It is soluble in water in equal parts. One litre of carbon dioxide at 0°C and at one atmospheric pressure weighs 1.977 g.

Tests for identity:

(1) It can extinguish fire.

(2) On being passed through a solution of barium hydroxide a white precipitate is produced, which dissolves in acetic acid with effervescence.

Tests for purity: It is tested for the presence of acid and sulphur dioxide and phosphine; hydrogen sulphide and organic reducing substances and carbon monoxide.

For acid and sulphur dioxide: It is tested by comparing the colour of a carbon dioxide-free water containing methyl orange through which is passed a measured volume of carbon dioxide with that of a sample of carbon dioxide-free water containing 1 ml of 0.01 HCl and same amount of methyl orange. The colour produced in the sample should not show deeper shade of red colour than that of the blank.

Phosphine, hydrogen sulphide and organic reducing substances are detected when the gas is passed through an ammonical silver ammonium nitrate solution. The experiment is repeated by omitting carbon dioxide for purpose of comparison. No turbidity of dark colour due to the formation of silver phosphide of silver sulphide is produced (I.P., p. 153).

Carbon monoxide is tested by treating a sample of dilute oxalated blood with pyrogallol and tannic acid and shaking the contents and setting aside the mixture for forty minutes. The precipitate assumes a greyish brown colour and no red colour is seen. (In case carbon monoxide is present the contents will show red colour.)

Assay: It is assayed by gasometric method on the basis of the following principle:

The decrease in the volume of gas, when a suitable agent is used to absorb the gas, is measured and reduced to standard conditions of temperature and pressure. The absorbing agent used is 50% KOH solution.

The I.P. 1985 method* uses a nitrometer, consisting of a measuring tube and a balancing tube, connected by means of rubber tubing (Fig. 11.1). They are called Hempel burette and Hempel absorption pipette, respectively.

Uses: It is used as a respiratory stimulant. On being inhaled it raises the carbon dioxide content of the blood. Only in low concentration of up to 10% in the air or gas mixture, it is used to stimulate the

---

* The I.P. 85 method is mentioned below.

Place sufficient quantity of mercury in 100 ml nitrometer or a gas burette provided with a two-way stopcock and a two-way outlet and properly connected with a balancing tube. Connect one of the outlet tubes of the nitrometer with a gas pipette of suitable capacity. Place in the pipette about 125 ml of a 50 per cent w/v solution of potassium hydroxide. Draw the liquid (free from air bubbles) through the capillary opening, connection and stopcock opening in the nitrometer by reducing the pressure in the nitrometer tube and opening the stopcock controlling the connection with the gas pipette. Close the stopcock. Having completely filled the nitrometer, the other stopcock opening and the other intake tube with mercury, draw into the nitrometer rube, by reducing the pressure in the tube, exactly 100 ml of carbon dioxide at N.T.P. Close the stopcock. Increase the pressure on the gas in the nitrometer tube and open the stopcock controlling the connection with the gas pipette. Force the entire volume of gas into the pipette. Close the stopcock and rock the pipette gently providing frequent contact of the liquid and the gas. At the end of five minutes when most of the gas has been absorbed by the liquid, facilitate the absorption of the remainder by drawing some of the liquid into nitrometer rube, and forcing the residual gas back upon the surface of the liquid in the gas pipette. Again rock the pipette until no further dimunition in the volume of gas occurs. Draw the residual gas, if any, into the nitrometer tube and measure its volume, not more than 1 ml of gas remains.*

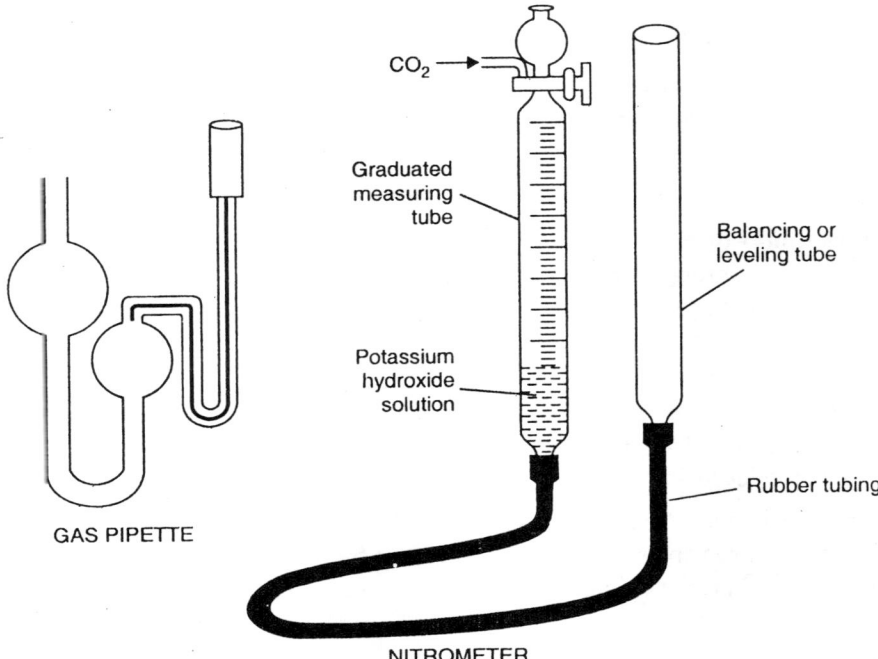

$CO_2 \rightarrow$

Graduated
measuring
tube

Balancing or
leveling tube

Potassium
hydroxide
solution

Rubber tubing

GAS PIPETTE

NITROMETER

Fig. 11.1. Hempel pipette and Hempel burette (Hempel apparatus).

respiratory and cardioaccelerator centres. In concentrations of 20% or more it is very fatal and in very high concentrat ons, it produces convulsions and respiratory depression.

Carbon dioxide is usually administered by inhalation in concentrations of 5% to 7.5% mixed with oxygen.

Labelling: The gas is usually marketed in metal cylinders, painted grey with the name of the gas clearly stated on the cylinders. The symbol CO_2 is also stencilled in paint.

Nitrogen in the free state is available upto 75% in atmospheric air. It is available in the form of nitrites and nitrates in the soil of the earth. In the combined form, protein is one of the essential constituents of plants and animals.

The main source for synthesizing nitrogen compounds is atmospheric nitrogen, sodium nitrate and coal.

---

* Gasometric methods of analysis: These methods, which are meant for assaying gases, involve measurement of gases and they are of two kinds: (1) Production of gas, which is produced or liberated in a chemical reaction in the given assay procedure. The gas that is produced or liberated is corrected to standard conditions of temperature (0°C) and atmospheric pressure (760 m). (2) Decrease in gas volume, which results when the gas gets absorbed in an appropriate or suitable agent (chemical/solution). The decrease in the volume of one or one of the absorbed gases present is measured and reduced to standard conditions of temperature and pressure.

In the pharmacopoeia mostly the second type of method is prescribed for assaying the gases. Gases assayed in I.P. are: nitrous oxide and oxygen. Carbon dioxide has been official in I.P., B.P. and U.S.P.

Nitrogen compounds are used mainly in synthesizing explosives, chemicals, medicines, dyes and for preserving food.

NITROUS OXIDE

Chem. formula: N_2O Mol. wt.: 44.01

It is official in B.P., U.S.P. and I.P. Nitrous oxide contains not less than 95% v/v of N_2O in the gaseous phase.

Preparation: It can be easily prepared on laboratory scale by the action of heat on ammonium nitrate.

$$NH_4CO_3 \xrightarrow{\Delta} N_2O + 2H_2O$$

The temp. must be a little above the m.p. of NH_4NO_3, otherwise at high temp. it may become dangerously explosive. It may also give by-products at high temp. (Nitrogen, higher oxides of nitrogen and ammonia).

Description: It is a colourless gas but under 50 atm./15°C pressure it goes into liquid state. It is odourless and tasteless.

Solubility: It is soluble in water (1 : 1.4), alcohol, solvent ether and oils.

Tests for identity:

(1) A glowing splinter of wood bursts into flame on contact with the gas.

(2) It is not absorbed by alkaline-pyrogallol solution.

Tests for purity: It is tested for acidity; alkalinity; arsenic and phosphine; carbon dioxide; carbon monoxide; halogen and hydrogen sulphide; nitric oxide and nitrogen dioxide; reducing substances; oxidising substances and water.

Acidity/alkalinity: It is done by comparing colour of standard solution with sample. In this experiment effects of acidity or alkalinity of the gas sample are seen on a solution of methyl orange-bromocresol green solution, which has been adjusted to about the middle of its transition interval by addition of 0.01 N HCl. It is better to use methyl red solution in determination of alkalinity (I.P. 85, p. 338).

Arsenic and phosphine: It is tested through a mercuric chloride paper attached to a glass tube, as in the limit test for arsenic. No visible stain should be produced.

CO_2: Not more than 300 ppm v/v. It is done by comparison of colour of the standard with the sample using 0.3 N $Ba(OH)_2$. Any turbidity produced is not more intense than that produced by adding 1 ml of 0.11% w/v sol. of $NaHCO_3$ in CO_2-free water to 50 ml of 0.3 N $Ba(OH)_2$.

CO: Not more than 10 ppm v/v.

Halogens and hydrogen sulphide: The test consists in passing the gas into a solution of $AgNO_3$, neither opalescence nor darkening should be produced.

Nitric oxide and nitrogen dioxide: Not more than 2 ppm v/v. They are determined by a spectro-photometric method, comparison being made with a control mixture prepared from sodium nitrite (I.P., p. 1457).

Reducing substances: Using $KMnO_4$ as oxidizing agent by passing solution of gas through water containing $KMnO_4$. The colour is not completely discharged.

Oxidising substances: The test is performed by using soluble starch and potassium iodide in water along with 1 drop of glacial acetic acid for preparing solution. No colour is produced by passing gas through this solution.

Water: It is tested by using magnesium perchlorate as absorptive media. The increase in weight of media by passing one litre of gas does not exceed 2 mg.

Assay: The assay of nitrous oxide is carried out using 100 ml of gas as per I.P.

Storage: It is stored in safe metal cylinders under compression at a temp not exceeding 37°.

Labelling:

(1) The colour of cylinder should be blue.

(2) The name of the gas must be written on it.

(3) The shoulder of the cylinder is labelled with the name of the gas or the symbol "N_2O" stencilled in paint.

Uses: It is used as a general anaesthetic by inhalation and as an analgesic.

Dose: 60–80% with oxygen 20–40% as required.

AROMATIC SPIRIT AMMONIA

Synonym: Spirit of Sal. Volatile.

Aromatic spirit of ammonia is one of the important pharmaceutical preparations, which is treated in detail in pharmaceutics. However, its inclusion here is found relevant, since it contains ammonium carbonate and strong solution of ammonia as the major components, to which the therapeutic value is attributed.

The spirit contains about 2% w/v of free ammonia (limit 1, 12–1–1.25) calculated as NH_3 and 3% w/v ammonium carbonate (limit 2.76–3.24), calculated as ammonium carbonate. It contains 64–70% w/v of alcohol, besides lemon oil and nutmeg oil, which are used mainly as flavouring agents.

Ingredients:

Ammonium Bicarbonate	25 g
Ammonia Solution Strong	70 ml
Lemon oil	5 ml
Nutmeg oil	3 ml
Alcohol (90 per cent)	150 ml
Purified water, sufficient to produce	1000 ml

Assay: The spirit is assayed both for ammonium carbonate and for free ammonia.

Ammonium carbonate: The spirit (20 ml) contained in a stoppered flask is mixed with 1 N sodium hydroxide (25 ml) and to the mixture is added sodium or barium chloride (40 ml). The flask is heated on a water bath for 15 minutes with the stopper inserted loosly and cooled. Solution of formaldehyde (40 ml), after it is neutralised to solution of thymol blue, is added to the cooled flask contents and the excess of alkali is titrated with 1 N hydrochloric acid, using solution of thymol blue as indicator till grey colour is obtained.

Each ml of 1 N sodium hydroxide is equivalent to 0.04805 g of $(NH_4)_2CO_3$.

Free ammonia: To the spirit (20 ml) is added 1 N hydrochloric acid (50 ml) and after the mixture has been boiled and cooled, it is titrated with 1 N hydrochloric acid, using solution of methyl red as an indicator. For purpose of calculation one has to substract from the volume of HCl used in this titration the volume of sodium hydroxide consumed in first titration (i.e. assay for ammonium carbonate). The amount of NH_3 is then calculated from the remainder Sodium Carbonate.

Each ml of 1 N HCl is equivalent to 0.01703 of NH_3.

Storage: It is stored in small, well-closed container. Rubber stoppers are not used as they absorb ammonia.

Uses: Aromatic spirit of ammonia is used as a respiratory stimulant by inhalation. It is also used as a flavouring agent. It is said to accelerate heart and cause vaso-constriction.

12

Miscellaneous Agents

This chapter will deal with the Sclerosing Agents, Expectorants, Emetics, Poisons and Antidotes and Sedatives.

SCLEROSING AGENTS

Sclerosing agents are irritant drugs that are of sufficient activity to damage cells, but they are not so potent as to destroy a large number of cells at the site of application. Such agents promote fibrosis and thereby strengthen supporting structures. Their use can result in the intimal surface of blood vessels breaking down, thereby initiating thrombosis. This action is used in the reduction of varicose veins and hemorrhoids.

Sclerotherapy is the most important initial treatment undertaken in variceal bleeding (bleeding from an abnormally dilated and lengthened vein), artery, or lymph vessel (varix) and is undertaken, if possible, at the time of diagnostic endoscopy. It is also the most widely used method for preventing recurrent esophageal variceal bleeding.

Sclerosing agents can be harmful when improperly used and even when used sometimes need to be used with caution. Examples of sclerosing agents are morrhuate sodium injection and sodium tetradecyl sulphate.

MORHUATE SODIUM INJECTION
(Scleromate)

It is a sterile solution of the sodium salts of the fatty acids of cod liver oil and contains 50 mg of sodium morhuate per ml. An antimicrobial agent (not more than 0.5%) and ethy/benzyl alcohol (not more than 3%) is normally added.

Preparation: It is prepared by heating cod liver oil with alcoholic sodium hydroxide until completely saponified. The solution is diluted with water and the alcohol is removed by distillation. Dilute sulphuric acid is then added to the aqueous solution and the liberated organic acids are extracted with a suitable solvent such as ether. The acids are neutralized with aqueous sodium hydroxide solution and used for the preparation of injection.

Uses: It has been used as a sclerosing and fibrosing agent for obliterating varicose veins. It has been official in USP.

SODIUM TETRADECYL SULPHATE
(STS; Sotradecol)

$$CH_3(CH_2)_3 \underset{\underset{C_2H_5}{|}}{CH}(CH_2)_2 \underset{\underset{}{|}}{\overset{\overset{CH_2CH(CH_3)_2}{|}}{CH}}OSONa$$

Chem. formula: $C_{14}H_{29}NaO_4$ Mol. weight: 316.43

Preparation: It is prepared by reacting tetradecyl alcohol (meristyl alcohol) with chlorosulphonic acid and neutralizing the resulting hydrogen sulphate ester with sodium carbonate.

Description: It is a white, waxy, odourless solid and is soluble in water, alcohol or ether.

Uses: It has been used as a buffered solution in the obliteration of varicose veins and internal haemorrhoids. For this purpose the solution is injected directly into the vein. Since it is an anionic surface-active agent, it is also used as a wetting agent for spreading tropical antiseptics.

EXPECTORANTS

Expectorants are used orally to loosen and liquefy mucus, soothe irritated bronchial mucosa and make coughs more productive. They act by decreasing the viscosity of the bronchial secretions, thereby facilitating their elimination and by increasing the amount of respiratory tract fluid. Expectorants are used in the treatment of respiratory disorders in which secretions are purulent, viscid or excessive, and as an adjunct in bronchopulmonary disorders.

Expectorants that are generally recognized as safe and effective are antimony potassium tartrate, iodides, ipecac fluid extract, guaifenesin and squill. Ammonium chloride and carbonate and ammonium and potassium iodides are commonly used as expectorants. If the iodides are used in solution, they must be protected by an antioxidant, e.g. sodium thiosulphate.

Water vapour is an excellent expectorant and humidification of room air and adequate fluid intake are also important therapeutically.

The following two expectorants have been described in the chapters shown against each one of them.

(i) Ammonium Chloride (See Chapter 5).
(ii) Potassium Iodide (See Chapter 8).

EMETICS

An emetic is a drug that induces vomiting. The final result is to evacuate the stomach. The clinical value of emetics is diminished with the use of the stomach tube, which is a safer and more efficient method for emptying the stomach. Emetics should not be used in unconscious or comatose patients, or those with central nervous system depression or shock. They are also contraindicated in poisoning caused by corrosive or petroleum products. Emetics are sometimes used in low doses in cough preparations to stimulate flow of respiratory tract secretions. Example of an inorganic emetic is antimony potassium tartrate (official as an antischistosomal agent) and it has been described in Chapter 8.

(i) Antimony Sodium Tartrate (see Chapter 8).

(ii) Antimony Potassium Tartrate.

These compounds and their injections have been official in B.P., U.S.P. and I.P., but slowly have not been finding favour for their continuous inclusion in them.

POISONS AND ANTIDOTES

Acute poisoning is an urgent medical problem and calls for emergency. It may be accidental (particularly in children below five), a true attempted suicidal, parasuicidal (intentional and self-inflicted but not suicidal) or homicidal.

Poisoning may occur as a result of food, industrial and agricultural poisons. Commonly used drugs that are abused for poisoning are benzodiazepines, barbiturates, tricyclic antidepressants, salicylates, paracetamol and dextropropoxyphene. Specific antidotes are available in only a small percentage of acute poisonings. Treatment is, therefore, dependent on a sound knowledge of the poison involved, clinical assessment and minimizing the absorption of the poison.

Aside from use of antidotes and inactivation of poison, the treatment of poisoning is symptomatic and supportive. Problems requiring supportive care include coma, respiratory insufficiency, convulsions, shock, vomiting, diarrhea, fluid and electrolyte disturbances, cerebral edema, kidney failure and damage to other organs.

Antidotes may belong to any of the following classes:

- Physiological antidote (counteracts the physiological effects of the poison).
- Chemical antidote (acts by changing the chemical nature of the poison).
- Mechanical antidote (prevents the absorption of the poison into the body).

Examples of inorganic agents used as antidotes are given in the Table below.

Antidote (inorganic agent)	Antidote type
Sodium nitrite	Physiological – converts haemoglobin to methemoglobin in order to bind cyanide.
Sodium thiosulphate	Chemical – causes conversion of systemic toxic cyanide to nontoxic thiocyanate.
Activated charcoal	Mechanical – adsorbs the poison prior to absorption.
Cupric sulphate/magnesium sulphate, Na_2HPO_4	Mechanical – inactivates and precipitates the toxic material as insoluble salts, thereby preventing their absorption.

SODIUM NITRITE

Chem. formula: $NaNO_2$ Mol. weight: 69.00

Sodium nitrite contains not less than 97% of $NaNO_2$ calculated with reference to the substance dried over silica gel for four hours. It is official in USP.

Preparation:

(1) It can be prepared by passing nitric oxide (NO) and oxygen (O_2) through a solution of sodium carbonate (Na_2CO_3) or by passing NO_2 and NO in a solution of sodium hydroxide (NaOH).

$$4NO + O_2 + 2Na_2CO_3 \longrightarrow 4NaNO_2 + 2CO_2$$

or
$$NO_2 + NO + 2NaOH \longrightarrow 2NaNO_2 + H_2O$$

(2) Sodium nitrite can be prepared by fusing sodium nitrate and adding sufficient metallic lead to completely reduce sodium nitrate to sodium nitrite; heating is continued till the reaction is complete. The mass is lixiviated with water, filtered (to remove insoluble lead oxide) and the filtrate is crystallised.

$$NaNO_3 + Pb \longrightarrow NaNO_2 + PbO$$

Description: Sodium nitrite occurs as a white to slightly yellowish white granular powder or white, opaque, fused mass or stick, which is deliquescent, odourless and saline in taste. It is soluble in water (1.5 parts) and only sparingly soluble in alcohol. A solution is alkaline to litmus paper.

Tests for identity: The substance yields reactions characteristic of sodium and nitrites (App. I).

On being treated with dilute H_2SO_4 at about 15°C nitrous acid is liberated which is not stable at room temperature and so it gets immediately decomposed to H_2O, NO and HNO_3 (at room temperature). NO is oxidised to give NO_2.

$$2NaNO_2 + H_2SO_4 \longrightarrow Na_2SO_4 + 2HNO_2$$

$$3HNO_2 \rightleftharpoons H_2O + 2NO\uparrow + HNO_3$$

$$2NO + O_2 \longrightarrow 2NO_2$$

Tests for purity: It is tested for heavy metals, Cl, SO_4 and loss on drying.

Limit of heavy metals is 20 parts per million.

Assay: It depends on the oxidation of nitrite to nitrate, i.e. $NaNO_2$ solution is prepared and it is added slowly to N/10 potassium permanganate solution acidified with sulphuric acid. The nitrite solution is run into permanganate solution and not vice-versa. It is because of the fact that acidification of solution of sodium nitrite results in the formation of nitrous acid (HNO_2) which gets decomposed readily, losing oxides of nitrogen. In this procedure, however, nitrous acid is formed in the presence of excess of permanganate solution and hence nitrous acid is oxidised before any loss takes place. (In order to avoid decomposition of HNO_2, the tip of the pipette should be kept below the level of solution.) A known excess of standard oxalic acid is added and the mixture, after it is heated, is back titrated with standard potassium permanganate solution.

Procedure: An accurately weighed amount (about 1 g) is dissolved in water and the volume is made up to 100 ml. 10 ml of this solution is added with the help of a pipette to a mixture of 50 ml of 0.1 N potassium permanganate, 100 ml of water and 5 ml of sulphuric acid, immersing the tip of the pipette beneath the surface of the mixture at 40°C, allowed to stand for 5 minutes and after the addition of 25 ml of 0.1 N oxalic acid the mixture is heated to about 80°C and titrated with 0.1 N potassium permanganate.

$$10NaNO_2 + 4KMnO_4 + 11H_2SO_4 \longrightarrow 10HNO_3 + 2K_2SO_4 + 5Na_2SO_4 + 6H_2O + 4MnSO_4$$

$$NaNO_2 + H_2SO_4 \longrightarrow HNO_2 + NaHSO_4$$

$$HNO_2 + O \longrightarrow HNO_3$$

1000 ml of N/10 $KMnO_4$ are equivalent to 1/20 $NaNO_2$.

Or Each ml of N/10 $KMnO_4$ is equivalent to 0.00345 g of $NaNO_2$.

Storage: Sodium nitrite is preserved in a well-closed container.

Uses: It is used as an antidote for cyanide poisoning and is administered intravenously in large doses to cause methemoglobinaemia.

Dose: 30 to 120 mg.

SODIUM THIOSULPHATE

Sodium thiosulphate has been described in Chapter 4.

SEDATIVES

Sedatives are agents that produce a quieting effect along with relaxation and rest, though not necessarily sleep. Hypnotic refers to the production of sleep. A drug may be sedative in small doses, whereas a large dose of the same drug may act as a hypnotic.

Sedative drugs are used to calm excitement and reduce motor activity without inducing sleep in the management of neurosis and to dispel anxiety and apprehension accompanying disease states like hypertension, cardiac failure and coronary artery disease. Anxiety can display as fatigue, dizziness, palpitations, indigestion, bowel disturbances, headaches, muscle aches, insomnia, excessive perspiration, tremors of hand or voice and other signs of nervous tension.

Agents used as sedatives and hypnotics include potassium bromide, sodium bromide, chloral hydrate, ethchlorvynol, paraldehyde, ethinamate, meprobamate, barbiturates, benzodiazepines, etc.

POTASSIUM BROMIDE

Formula: KBr   Mol. weight: 119.0

Potassium bromide contains not less than 98.5% of KBr calculated with reference to the substance dried at 105°.

Preparation:

(1) Potassium bromide is prepared by adding bromine in slight excess to a concentrated solution of potassium hydroxide. Potassium bromide and potassium bromate are formed. The pale yellow solution is evaporated to dryness and the residue is heated with charcoal to reduce potassium bromate to potassium bromide, which is extracted with water. The solution after filtration is evaporated to crystallization.

$$6KOH + 3 Br_2 \longrightarrow KBrO_3 + 5KBr + 3H_2O$$

$$KBrO_3 + 3C \longrightarrow KBr + 3CO$$

(2) Potassium bromide is also prepared by first obtaining a bromide of iron by treating moist iron foils with bromine as follows:

$$3Fe + 4Br_2 \longrightarrow Fe_3Br_8$$
Ferroso
ferric
bromide

$$Fe_3Br_8 + 4K_2CO_3 + 4H_2O \longrightarrow 8KBr + Fe_3(OH)_3 + 3CO_2$$
Ferroso ferric
hydroxide

The bromide of iron, i.e. Ferroso-Ferric Bromide is then boiled with potassium carbonate solution and filtered. The filtrate is then evaporated to dryness. The dried residue is again extracted with water and recrystallized.

Description: It consists of colourless, transparent or opaque crystals or white granular powder which, though colourless, has saline and salty bitter taste. It is soluble in 1.5 parts of water, in 250 parts of alcohol and in 5 parts of glycerin.

Tests for identity: It gives reactions characteristic of potassium and bromide (see App. I).

Tests for purity: It is tested for acidity and alkalinity; As; Ba; heavy metals; Na; Cl; bromate; alkali and loss on drying; calcium and magnesium; iron and iodides.

Test for chloride: Test for chloride is performed by dissolving one g of the substance in 75 ml of water and 25 ml of nitric acid in a distillation flask fitted with bung carrying a thermometer and a tapered air inlet tube which is adjusted in such a way that it is above the surface of the liquid. A gentle steam of air is passed and the flask is heated to 105°. The inlet tube is lowered into the liquid and the heating is continued for few minutes at the same temperature at 105°. Heating is discontinued and a brisk steam of air is passed for 10 minutes. To the solution is now added 0.1 N silver nitrate and 5 drops of nitrobenzene and the solution is shaken. The excess of silver nitrate is titrated with 0.1 N ammonium thiocyanate, using solution of Ferric Ammonium Sulphate as indicator and shaking vigorously near the end-point. Not less than 3.7 ml of 0.1 N ammonium thiocyanate is required.

$$Cl^- + AgNO_3 \longrightarrow AgCl\downarrow + NO_3$$
$$AgNO_3 + NH_4SCN \longrightarrow NH_4NO_3 + AgSCN$$

Test for bromate: It is represented by taking 1 g of the powdered substance and adding 1 ml of dilute sulphuric acid. No yellow colour is produced immediately.

Assay: It is based upon volumetric titration. Hot concentrated H_2SO_4 decomposes KBr to give a mixture of bromine and hydrobromic acid.

$$2KBr + Conc. \; H_2SO_4 \longrightarrow K_2SO_4 + 2HBr$$
$$2HBr + H_2SO_4 \longrightarrow 2H_2O + Br_2 + SO_2\uparrow$$
$$2KMnO_4 + 3H_2SO_4 \longrightarrow K_2SO_4 + 2MnSO_4 + 3H_2O + 5[O]$$

Potassium permanganate acts as a powerful oxidising agent in neutral, alkaline or acidic solution.

$$MnO_4 + 8H^+ + 5e \longrightarrow Mn^{2+} + 4H_2O$$

$KMnO_4$ itself acts as an indicator. The solution remains pink so long as it contains the permanganate ion.

In this estimation as H_2SO_4 is used in dilute solution, it does not react with $KMnO_4$.

An accurately weighed substance about 1.2 g is dissolved in water and diluted to 100 ml with water. To 10 ml of the solution is added 100 ml of water, 10 ml of H_2SO_4 and a few glass beads. The contents are heated to boiling and titrated with 0.1 N $KMnO_4$ added dropwise until pink colour just persists.

1 ml of 0.1 N $KMnO_4 \equiv 0.01190$ g of KBr.

Storage: It is preserved in a well-closed container.

Uses: It is used as a sedative similar to sodium bromide (see sodium bromide).

SODIUM BROMIDE

Chem. formula: NaBr   Mol. weight: 102.9

Sodium bromide contains not less than 98.5% of NaBr calculated with reference to the substance dried to constant weight at 105°.

Preparation:

(1) When bromine, in slight excess, is added to a concentrated solution of sodium hydroxide, sodium bromate and sodium bromide are formed. The pale yellow solution is evaporated to dryness and the residue is heated with charcoal to convert sodium bromate into sodium bromide.

$$6NaOH + 3Br_2 \longrightarrow NaBrO_3 + 5NaBr + 3H_2O$$

$$NaBrO_3 + 3C \longrightarrow NaBr + 3CO$$

The product is then extracted with water and filtered. The filtrate is evaporated to dryness.

(2) Sodium bromide can also be manufactured from a bromide of iron which is prepared by treating moist iron foils with bromine.

$$3Fe + 4Br_2 \longrightarrow Fe_3Br_8$$
Ferrosoferric bromide

The above compound is then boiled with sodium carbonate solution and filtered. The filtrate is then evaporated to dryness to crystallize the products.

$$Fe_3Br_8 + 4Na_2CO_3 + 4H_2O \longrightarrow 8NaBr + Fe_3(OH)_8 + 4CO_2$$
Ferrosoferric hydroxide

Description: It consists of white odourless cubic crystals or white granular powder, which has saline and bitter taste. It absorbs moisture when exposed to air. It is soluble in water (1 g in 1.2 ml) and forms a dihydrate. In alcohol 1 g is dissolved in 30 ml.

Tests for identity: It gives reaction for Na and bromides (App. I).

Tests for purity: It is tested for As; Ba; Fe; bromide; SO_4; alkali; lead; Cl and loss on drying. The type and nature of impurities can be imagined if one takes into consideration the above methods of preparation.

Tests for bromate depend on the interaction of bromate and bromide in the presence of dilute sulphuric acid with liberation of bromine.

$$HBrO_3 + 5HBr \longrightarrow 3Br_2 + 3H_2O$$

Test for Chloride: The test depends on the fact that bromides are more readily oxidised than chlorides. The substance (dissolved in water – 1 g in 75 ml of H_2O) is heated with HNO_3 at a temp. of about 105°C which oxidises bromide to bromine; heating is continued for one or two more minutes. The heat source is removed and a stream of air is passed for 10 minutes to expel bromine. A few drops of silver nitrate and 5 ml of nitrobenzene are added. The excess of N/10 $AgNO_3$ is titrated against ammonium thiocyanate.

$$AgNO_3 + Cl^- \longrightarrow AgCl\downarrow + NO_3$$
$$AgNO_3 + NH_4SCN \longrightarrow AgSCN + NH_4NO_3$$

Ammonium thiocyanate reacts with ferric alum:

$$3NH_4SCN + FeNH_2(SO_4)_2 \longrightarrow Fe(SCN)_3 + 2(NH_4)_2SO_4$$
$$\text{Ferric ammonium}$$
$$\text{sulphate}$$

Limit for 1 gm. NaBr should not be less than 3.7% ml of N/10 NH_4SCN. This method is a modified Volhard's method.

Assay: The substance is dissolved in water and acidified with HNO_3 and titrated with a known excess of N/10 $AgNO_3$ and 5 ml of nitrobenzene. It is shaken well and titrated with N/10 NH_4SCN using ferric alum as indicator.

$$AgNO_3 + NaBr \longrightarrow AgBr + NaNO_3$$
$$AgNO_3 + NH_4SCN \longrightarrow AgSCN + NH_4NO_3$$

1000 ml of 0.1 N $AgNO_3$ is equivalent to 1/10 NaBr.

Or each ml of 0.1 N silver nitrate is equivalent to 0.01029 g of NaBr.

Storage: Sodium bromide is preserved in a well-closed container.

Uses: It is used as a sedative, which induces sleep.

(See also Potassium Bromide.)

VITAMINS

Vitamins are a group of organic substances, present in minute amounts in natural foodstuffs, that are essential to normal metabolism; insufficient amounts in the diet may cause deficiency diseases.

CALCIUM PANTOTHENATE
(Synonym: Calcium D Pantothenate)

$$\left[HOCH_2 - \underset{\underset{CH_3}{|}}{\overset{\overset{CH_3}{|}}{C}} - \underset{\underset{H}{|}}{\overset{\overset{OH}{|}}{C}} - CONHCH_2CH_2COO^- \right]_2 Ca^{2+}$$

Chem. formula: $C_{18}H_{32}CaN_2O_{10}$ Mol. weight: 476.54

It is the calcium salt of the D-isomer of (R)–3–(2,4–dihydroxy–3,3–dimethylbutyramido) propionic acid (pantothenic acid). It contains 90.0% to 110.0% of $C_{18}H_{32}CaN_2O_{10}$, calculated with reference to the dried substance.

Because of its wide distribution in nature it was named "Pantothenic" from the Greek word Pantothen, meaning from all sides.

Description: It is a white powder without odour and with bitter taste. It is slightly hygroscopic.

Solubility: It is freely soluble in water, soluble in glycerin and practically insoluble in alcohol, chloroform and solvent ether.

Tests for identity:

(1) A solution (1 in 20) gives reaction of calcium (I.P. App. 3.1).

(2) When a specified amount of sample (50 mg) in 1 N NaOH (5 ml) is boiled for one minute, cooled and to it is added two drops of $FeCl_3$ test-solution, a strong yellow colour is produced.

(3) On addition of copper sulphate solution to the substance (50 mg) in 1 N NaOH (2 ml) a blue colour is obtained.

Tests for purity: It is tested for specific optical rotation; pH; heavy metals and calcium.

Specific optical rotation: Between +25.0° and +27.5°, determined in a 5% w/v solution.

pH: Between 7.0 and 9.0, determined in 5% w/v solution.

Heavy metals: Not more than 40 ppm, determined by dissolving the substance (0.5 g) in water (25 ml).

Calcium: Between 8.2% and 8.6%.

Assay: It is determined as per assay of Calcium Gluconate, using substance (0.8 g) in water (50 ml). Each ml of the remainder $\equiv 0.002004$ g of Ca.

Nitrogen: Between 5.7% to 6.0% calculated with reference to the dried substance. The estimation is carried out by general method for determination of nitrogen, using 0.5 g of the substance.

Each ml of 0.1 N $H_2SO_4 \equiv 0.001401$ g of N.

Loss on drying: Not more than 5.0% of substance (1 g) by drying in oven at 105°.

Assay: The assay is carried out as per assay of Calcium Pantothenate.

An accurately weighed substance (1.8 g) is dissolved in 50 ml of anhydrous glacial acetic acid. Non-aqueous titration is carried out and the end point is determined potentiometrically. A blank titration is also carried out

Each ml of 0.1 M perchloric acid $\equiv 0.02383$ g of $C_{18}H_{32}CaN_2O_{10}$.

Uses: It is a member of vitamin B complex (constituent of coenzyme A).

Dose: 10 to 100 mg daily.

Storage: It is stored in a well-closed container.

SODIUM ASCORBATE

Chem. formula: $C_6H_7NaO_6$ Mol. weight: 198.1

Sodium ascorbate is monosodium L-ascorbate (vitamin C).

It contains not less than 99.0 per cent and not more than 101.0 per cent of $C_6H_7NaO_6$ calculated with reference to the dried substance.

Description: It occurs as white or faintly yellow crystals or crystalline powder, odourless or almost odourless. It darkens gradually on exposure to light.

Solubility: It is freely soluble in water, very slightly soluble in ethanol (95%), practically insoluble in chloroform and in ether.

Tests for identity:

(1) The infra-red absorption spectrum of a mineral oil dispersion is concordant with the spectrum obtained from sodium ascorbate R.

(2) To 4 ml of a 2% w/v solution add 1 ml of 0.1 M hydrochloric acid; add a few ml of 2,6–dichlorophenol-indophenol solution, which gets decolourised.

(3) A 2% w/v solution gives the reactions of sodium salts (App. I).

pH: Between 7.0 and 8.0, determined in a 10% w/v solution.

Clarity and colour of solution: A 5.0% w/v solution in carbon dioxide-free water is clear and not more intensely coloured than reference solution BYS7 (App. 2.4.1).

Specific optical rotation: Between $+103°$ and $+108°$, determined in a 10% w/v solution.

Assay: An accurately weighed amount of sodium ascorbate (0.2 g) is dissolved in a mixture of carbon dioxide-free water and 25 ml of 1 M sulphuric acid. The solution is titrated immediately with 0.05 M iodine, using 1 ml of starch solution as indicator, until a persistent, violet blue colour is obtained.

1 ml of 0.05 M iodine is equivalent to 0.009905 g of $C_6H_7NaO_6$.

HYPOGLYCEMIC AGENTS

Hypoglycemic agents are compounds from several different chemical classes that are capable of lowering blood sugar.

INSULIN ZINC SUSPENSION (AMORPHOUS)

Amorph. I.Z.S., Prompt Insulin Zinc Suspension.

It contains not less than 90.0 per cent and not more that 110.0 per cent of the stated number of units of insulin.

Insulin Zinc Suspension (Amorphous) is a sterile, buffered suspension of insulin in the form of a complex obtained by the addition of zinc chloride to insulin in a manner such that the solid phase of the suspension is amorphous. It may be prepared by adding aseptically to crystalline insulin having a potency not less than 23 units per mg, calculated with reference to the dried substance, a suitable quantity of zinc chloride, an appropriate amount of a suitable substance to render the preparation isotonic with blood and a sufficient quantity of a suitable bactericide. It is distributed aseptically into sterile containers which are then sealed so as to exclude microorganisms.

Description: White suspension which on standing deposits a white sediment and leaves an almost colourless supernatant liquid. The sediment is readily resuspended on gentle shaking. When examined under a microscope, the particles in the suspension are seen to have no uniform shape and rarely exceed 2 μm in maximum dimension.

Tests for identity: In the high performance liquid chromatographic assay, the principal peak due to insulin in the chromatogram obtained with solution (1) has a retention time similar to that of the principal peak in the chromatogram obtained with solution (2), (3) or (4), as appropriate (I.P., p. 399).

pH: Between 6.9 and 7.5.

Total Zinc: Not more than 0.00095% w/v (for preparations containing 40 units per ml) and not more than 0.014% w/v (for preparations containing 80 units per ml).

Zinc in solution: Not more than 70% of the total zinc (for preparations containing 40 units per ml) and not more than 55% of the total zinc (for preparations containing 80 units per ml).

Insulin in solution: Complies with the test described under Isophane Insulin Injection (I.P. 2.4.14).

Other requirements: Complies with the requirements of tests stated under injectable preparations (injections).

Assay: Carry out the method for high performance liquid chromatography using (a) a stainless steel column (25 cm × 4.6 mm) packed with a stationary phase Ultrasphere ODS (5 μm) and maintained at 45°, (b) as the mobile phase with a flow rate of 1 ml per minute and maintained at a temperature of not less than 20° a mixture of 72.5 volumes of 0.1 M sodium dihydrogen phosphate adjusted to pH 2.0 with phosphoric acid and 27.5 volumes of acetonitrile, the mixture being adjusted so that the retention time of the principal peak of bovine insulin is about 20 minutes and (c) a detection wavelength of about 214 nm and as per I.P. specifications.

Storage: Store in multiple dose containers at a temperature between 2° and 8°. It should not be allowed to freeze.

Labelling: The label states (1) the strength in terms of the number of units per ml; (2) the animal source or sources of the insulin; (3) that the preparation should not be allowed to freeze; (4) that the container should be gently shaken before a dose is withdrawn; (5) the storage conditions.

Uses: It is used as a hypoglycaemic agent for insulin-dependent patients.

Dose: By subcutaneous injection, in accordance with the needs of the patient.

Usual strengths: 40 units per ml, 80 units per ml.

INSULIN ZINC SUSPENSION (CRYSTALLINE)

Cryst. I.Z.S.; Extended Insulin Zinc Suspension.

It contains not less than 90.0 per cent and not more than 110.0 per cent of the stated number of units of insulin.

It is a sterile, buffered suspension of insulin in the form of a complex obtained by the addition of zinc chloride to insulin in a manner such that the insulin is in the form of crystals insoluble in water. It may be prepared by adding aseptically to crystalline insulin having a potency not less than 23 units per mg, calculated with reference to the dried substance, a suitable quantity of zinc chloride, an appropriate amount of a suitable substance to render the preparation isotonic with blood and a sufficient quantity of a suitable bactericide. The solution is partially neutralized to allow crystallization to occur and the pH of the crystalline suspension is distributed aseptically into sterile containers which are then sealed so as to exclude microorganisms.

Description: White suspension which on standing deposits a white sediment and leaves an almost colourless supernatant liquid. The sediment is readily resuspended on gentle shaking. When examined under a microscope, the particles in the suspension are seen to be rhombohedral crystals, the majority having a maximum dimension greater than 10 μm but rarely exceedings 40 μm.

Identification, pH, total zinc, zinc in solution: Complies with the requirements stated under insulin zinc suspension.

Insulin extractable with buffered acetone solution: Note more than 15%.

Insulin in solution: Complies with the test described above in I.Z.S. (I.P. 2.4.14).

Other requirements: Complies with the requirements of tests stated under injectable preparations (injections).

Assay: Same as described under Insulin Zinc Suspension (Amorphous) above.

Storage: Store in multiple dose containers at a temperature between 20 and 80. It should not be allowed to freeze.

Labelling: The label states (1) the strength in terms of the number of units per ml; (2) the animal source or sources of the insulin; (3) that the preparation should not be allowed to freeze; (4) that the container should be gently shaken before a dose is withdrawn; (5) the storage conditions.

Uses: It is used as a hypoglycemic agent for insulin-dependent patients.

Dose: By subcutaneous injection, in accordance with the needs of the patient.

Usual strengths: 40 units per ml, 80 units per ml.

PROTAMINE ZINC INSULIN INJECTION

Protamine Zinc Insulin.

It contains not less than 90.0 per cent and not more than 110.0 per cent of the stated number of units of Insulin.

Preparation: Protamine Zinc Insulin Injection is a sterile buffered suspension of insulin in the form of a complex obtained by the addition of a suitable protamine and zinc chloride. It may be prepared by assaying a sterile solution of crystalline insulin having a potency not less than 23 unit per mg, calculated with reference to the dried substance, adjusting its potency so that when diluted with the other constituents in sterile form, it contains 'the requisite number of units per ml, and adding aseptically to it a sulphate protamine in the proportion of 1.0 to 1.7 mg of protamine sulphate for each 100 units of insulin. It contains Sodium Phosphate as buffering agent, sufficient amount of a suitable substance to render the preparation isotonic with blood and a sufficient amount of a suitable bactericide. It is distributed aseptically into sterile containers which are then sealed so as to exclude microorganisms.

Description: White suspension which on standing deposits a white sediment and leaves an almost colourless supernatant liquid. The sediment is readily resuspended on gentle shaking.

Tests for identity: In the HPLC assay, the principal peak due to insulin in the chromatogram obtained with solution (1) has a retention time similar to that of the principal peak in the chromatogram obtained with solutions (2), (3) or (4), as appropriate.

pH: Between 6.9 and 7.5.

Glycerin (if present): Between 1.4 and 1.75% w/v.

Total zinc: Not less than 20 μg per 100 units of insulin.

Insulin in solution: Complies with the test described under Isophane Insulin Injection in I.P.

Other requirements: Complies with the requirements of tests stated under Injectable Preparations (Injections).

Assay: Same as described under Insulin Zinc Suspension (Amorphous) above.

Storage: Store in multiple dose container at a temperature between 2° and 8°. It should not be allowed to freeze.

Labelling: The label states (1) the strength in terms of the number of units per ml; (2) the animal source or sources of the insulin; (3) that the preparation should not be allowed to freeze; (4) that the container should be gently shaken before a dose is withdrawn; (5) the storage conditions.

Uses: It is used as a hypoglycemic agent for insulin-dependent patients.

Dose: By subcutaneous injection, in accordance with the needs of the patient.

Usual strengths: 40 units per ml.

ANALGESICS

Analgesics are agents which relieve pain by acting centrally to alleviate pain threshold without disturbing consciousness and altering other sensory modalities.

SODIUM SALICYLATE

Chem. formula: $C_7H_5O_3Na$ or $C_6H_4(OH).CO_2Na$ 　　　　　　　　　　　　**Mol. weight:** 160.1

Sodium salicylate contains not less than 99.5% of $C_7H_5O_7Na$ calculated with reference to substance dried at 105°.

Preparation: A weighed quantity of salicylic acid is suspended in water and to this $NaHCO_3$ is added. The solution is heated till it becomes clear.

The solution is then filtered and evaporated to dryness at a temperature below 100°. It can be recrystallised from alcohol.

Description: It is a white colourless, pearly crystalline powder or flakes. It has a faint characteristic odour and sweetish saline taste. It is soluble in water (1 part), alcohol (10 parts) but insoluble in chloroform and solvent ether. If a concentrated solution is made crystals of hexahydrate ($C_6H_4OH \cdot COONa \cdot 6H_2O$) are deposited.

Tests for identity:

(1) The salt gives reactions characteristic of sodium (App. I).

(2) It gives a violet colour with a solution of ferric chloride. The test is indicative of salicylates and is performed by taking 5 ml of a 0.1 per cent w/v solution and adding a drop of test solution of ferric chloride and noting the violet colour.

(3) A concentrated solution of sodium salicylate on being acidified with dilute sulphuric acid gives white crystalline precipitate of salicylic acid, which on being washed and dried melts at 158–161°C. The test is performed by taking 5 ml of 0.5 per cent w/v solution, adding 1 ml of dilute sulphuric acid and collecting the precipitate.

Tests for purity: It is tested for As; heavy metals; Cl; SO_4 and loss on drying.

For reaction: A 10 per cent w/v solution is tested which should be neutral or acidic to litmus.

For heavy metals: 2 g is dissolved in 46 ml of water to which is added with constant stirring 4 ml of dilute HCl. The solution is filtered and 25 ml of filtrate is used for the test; limit of heavy metal is 20 parts per million.

Assay: Sodium salicylate is a salt of strong base and a weak acid.

It will react and neutralise hydrochloric acid/sulphuric acid as follows:

$$C_6H_4(OH).COONa + HCl \longrightarrow C_6H_4(OH).CO_2H + NaCl$$

$$2C_6H_4(OH).COONa + H_2SO_4 \longrightarrow 2C_6H_4(OH).COOH + Na_2SO_4$$

An accurately weighed amount, 3 g, is dissolved in 50 ml of water and to the solution is added 50 ml of solvent ether and a few drops of solution of bromophenol blue and the solution is titrated with 0.5 N sulphuric acid with constant shaking, until the colour of the indicator begins to change.

The lower layer is separated and the upper ethereal layer is washed with 10 ml of water and this washing is added to the separated lower aqueous layer. A further quantity of 20 ml of solvent ether is added to the aqueous layer and the titration is completed with 0.5 N sulphuric acid with constant shaking.

(The solvent ether is added to dissolve the liberated salicylic acid which is liberated when the sodium salicylate is titrated with 0.5 N sulphuric acid.)

1000 ml of 0.5 N H_2SO_4 is equivalent to 1/2 $C_6H_4(OH)COONa$.

Or 1 ml of 0.5 N sulphuric acid is equivalent to 0.08005 g of $C_7H_5O_3Na$.

I.P. 2007 gives a new assay method, in which an accurately weighed amount (0.15 g) is dissolved in anhydrous glacial acetic acid (30 ml) and the solution is titrated with 0.1 M perchloric acid. The end point is determined potentiometrically. A blank titration is carried out.

1 ml of 0.1 M perchloric acid is equivalent to 0.01601 g of $C_7H_5NaO_3$.

Storage: Sodium salicylate is preserved in a well-closed container and protected from light.

Uses: It is used as an antipyretic and analgesic and is thus widely employed for the relief of pain and lowering of fever. It also causes relief in acute gout (accumulation of uric acid) and rheumatic fever.

Dose: 500 mg to 4 g daily in divided doses.

ANTIDEPRESSANTS

Antidepressants are agents used in the treatment of depression or to relieve depression symptoms without inducing mental excitement or delirium or fits. Some agents, like lithium carbonate, are used prophylactically as a mood stabilizer in manic-depressive illness.

LITHIUM CARBONATE

Chem. formula: Li_2CO_3 Mol. weight: 73.9

Preparation: It is prepared by adding ammonium carbonate to a solution of a lithium salt.

$$Li_2SO_4 + (NH_4)_2CO_3 \longrightarrow Li_2CO_3 + (NH_4)_2SO_4$$

Description: Li_2CO_3 is a white, crystaline powder, odourless but with a slight alkaline taste.

Solubility: It is sparingly soluble in water and insoluble in alcohol.

Tests for identity:

(A) Dissolve 0.2 g in 5 ml of hydrochloric acid, boil, add 2 ml of sodium hydroxide solution and 5 ml of disodium hydrogen phosphate solution and boil; a white precipitate is produced.

(B) Moisten a small quantity with hydrochloric acid and introduce on a platinum wire into the flame of a Bunsen burner; a red colour is imparted to the flame.

(C) It gives reactions of carbonates (App. I).

Tests for purity: It is tested for As; calcium and magnesium; chlorides; heavy metals; aluminium and iron; potassium; sodium; sulphate and loss on drying.

Calcium and magnesium: 1.0 g of the substance is dissolved in 30 ml of N hydrochloric acid and neutralised with dil. NH_3 sol. This is filtered if necessary and divided into two equal portions. To one portion is added 1 ml of ammonium oxalate sol. when no turbidity or ppt. is produced on standing for five minutes. To the second portion is added 1 ml of $NaHPO_4$ sol. when no turbidity or ppt. is produced on standing for five minutes.

Chlorides: 1 g dissolved in water with the addition of HNO_3 (5 ml) complies with the limit test for chlorides (App. I).

Heavy metals: Not more than 20 ppm (I.P. 2.3.13).

Aluminium and iron: Determined as per method described in I.P.

Potassium: Not more than 0.1 of K, determined as per method described in I.P.

Sodium: Not more than 0.2% of Na, determined as per method described in I.P.

Sulphate: 1 g dissolved in water with addition of dil. HCl complies with the limit test for sulphates.

Loss on drying: Not more than 0.5% at 105°C (App. IV).

Assay: It is based on simple acid-base volumetric titration:

$$Li_2CO_3 + 2HCl \longrightarrow 2LiCl + H_2CO_3$$
$$H_2CO_3 \longrightarrow H_2O + CO_2\uparrow$$
$$HCl + NaOH \longrightarrow NaCl + H_2O$$

An accurately weighed amount of about 0.5 g is dissolved in 25 ml of 1 M HCl, titrated with 1 M NaOH using methyl orange solution as indicator.

Each ml of 1 M HCl ≡ 0.03695 g of Li_2CO_3.

Storage: It is stored in well-closed containers.

Use: It is used as an antidepressant in doses of 0.25 - 1.6 g daily.

LITHIUM CARBONATE TABLETS

According to I.P. standards, Lithium Carbonate tablets contain not less than 95% and not more than 105% of the stated amount of Li_2CO_3.

Dissolution: Dissolution test is carried out as per the method described in I.P. Not less than 60% of the stated amount of Li_2CO_3 in the tablets dissolves in 30 minutes.

Other requirements: Complies with the requirements stated under tablets.

Assay: 20 tablets are weighed and powdered. An accurately weighed quantity of the powder equivalent to 1.0 g of Lithium Carbonate is assayed as described under Lithium Carbonate.

13

Inorganic Radiopharmaceuticals

A radiopharmaceutical or radioactive medicine may be defined as a preparation containing a radionuclide in the form of an element, a salt or a complex. It exists as a solid, liquid or gas and is intended for *in vivo* use.

Some of the important terms used in connection with radiopharmaceutical preparations are as follows:

Specific Activity

The specific activity of a preparation of a radioactive material is the radioactivity of the radionuclide involved per unit weight of the element or of the compound concerned.

Radioactive Concentration

The radioactive concentration is the radioactivity of the radionuclide involved per unit volume of the solution in which it is present (it is necessary to state the date and, for radionuclides of short half-life, the hour at which the statement of radioactive concentration is valid).

Carrier

It is a stable isotope of the radionuclide involved, that is added to the radioactive preparation in the same chemical form as that in which the radionuclide is present.

Radionuclide Purity/Radioactive Purity/Radioisotope Purity

It is the ratio, expressed as a percentage of the radioactivity of the radionuclide concerned, to the local activity of the source.

Radiochemical Purity

It is the ratio, expressed as a percentage of the radioactivity of the radionuclide involved, that is present in the source in the chemical form declared to the total radioactivity of that radionuclide present in the source.

The determination of radiochemical purity consists of separating the different chemical substances containing the radionuclide and estimating the radioactivity associated with the declared chemical substance.

Chemical Purity

The ratio, expressed as a percentage of the weight of substance present in the declared chemical form to the total weight contained in the source, irrespective of any excipients or solvents.

Half-Life of Radiopharmaceuticals

It is defined as the time required for a radionuclide to decay to one half of its initial value. It is denoted by $t_{1/2}$. Each radioactive element has its own characteristic $t_{1/2}$.

The half-life values are a measure of the stability of radionuclides, the larger the value the more stable the nuclide.

The half-life of a radionuclide is measured using a suitable detection apparatus such as a Geiger-Muller counter or a scintillation counter.

Half-life values of radionuclides in a preparation are of crucial importance for selecting and calculating the quantity of a radionuclide required for medical work. Too long a half-life can lead to a high level of residual radioactivity in the patient which would constitute a serious health risk.

Curie: The activity of radioactive isotopes is expressed in terms of the curie (c) and is equivalent to the amount of radioactive material providing 3.7×10^{10} atomic disintegrations per second (dps). The actual quantities of material corresponding to one curie varies with the particular isotope involved.

Specifications of Radiopharmaceuticals

All radiopharmaceutical preparations should comply with the general requirements stated in the pharmacopoeias and with the requirements for the individual preparation used for clinical and other purposes.

Radiopharmaceuticals constitute a special class of drugs according to the Drugs and Cosmetic Act. They exhibit spontaneous disintegration of unstable nuclei with the emission of nuclear particles or photons for external detection in medical care.

The specifications of radiopharmaceuticals are given in monographs in pharmacopoeias and similar publications. These monographs usually include:

   (i) A method of identifying the radioisotope by means of its half-life, the type and energy of its emissions.
  (ii) The physical characteristics of the preparation.
 (iii) The radionuclide and radiochemical purity with respect to specific isotopes.
  (iv) Limit tests for non-radioactive chemical impurities.
   (v) The limits of alkalinity and acidity allowed for the preparation.
  (vi) The stability of the preparation and any storage condition.
 (vii) Storage conditions and the time limit for its use.
(viii) A radioactivity assay procedure.
  (ix) Contraindications to use.

Application of Radiopharmaceuticals

Radiopharmaceuticals have two main applications in medicine and may be described as:

(i) **Therapeutic radiopharmaceuticals:** These are used in the treatment of diseases and contain enough radioactivity to produce the intended specific effects in tissues.

(ii) **Diagnostic pharmaceuticals:** These are used as an aid to the diagnosis of diseases. These may be divided into two types:

   (a) Radiopharmaceutical used for measuring physiological parameters in tracer techniques, such as ^{51}Cr-EDTA for measuring glomerular filtration rate.

   (b) Radiopharmaceutical used for diagnostic imaging such as ^{99m}TC-methylene diphosphonate (MDP) used in bone scanning. These contain γ-emitting radionuclides since their interaction with tissue is much less than that of particulate emitters (α and β particles) and will cause significantly less damage to tissues.

Radiopharmaceuticals are usually administered to the patients by the i.v. route and get distributed into a particualr organ. The radiation emitted may be detected externally by a γ-camera used as a scintillation detector to monitor the distribution of image of radiopharmaceutical within the patient's body. A γ-camera used in conjunction with a computer system can produce static images of an organ as well as the movement of radiopharmaceutical through the organ. The dynamic images reflect the functioning of the organ. The images may be created in all three planes by a process known as single photon emission computerised tomography (SPECT).

The radionuclides commonly used for the preparation of radiopharmaceuticals employed in diagnosis have short physical half-lives. The shorter the half-life, the fewer total number of atoms necessary for the production of a given unit of activity. Therefore, the atoms for a short half-life radionuclide do not exist very long before emitting radiation. This allows a patient to receive fewer total atoms and increases the degree of safety for the patient during diagnostic procedures.

The discipline of nuclear pharmacy (radiopharmacy) is concerned with the manufacture of radiopharmaceuticals. The safe production of radiopharmaceuticals involves compliance with good manufacturing practice and good radiation protection practice. The radiopharmaceuticals used in medicine should provide high quality clinical information and also be safe for both patient and user alike.

A *Qualified Nuclear Pharmacist* is a pharmacist who holds a current license issued by the board, and who is either certified as a Nuclear Pharmacist by the Board of Pharmaceutical Specialities (USA) or have satisfied the prescribed requirements.

Preparation of Radiopharmaceuticals

The majority of radiopharmaceuticals are intended for intravenous (i.v.) administration. It is, therefore, understood that these preparations have to be sterile. However, in preparations like these a terminal sterilization by autoclaving is not possible due to their short half-lives, hence these injections must be prepared using aseptic techniques.

All the radiopharmaceuticals do not use metal atoms as the radionuclide. But when a molecule is radiolabelled with a metal atom, sometimes the metal atom does not change the biological properties of the molecule into which it is incorporated. However, sometimes it changes the biological properties of the molecule considerably. The former molecule is classified as *metal-tagged* radiopharmaceutical and the latter as *metal-essential* radiopharmaceutical. In *metal-essential* radiopharmaceuticals, the presence of radioactive metal atom is absolutely essential in determining the site where that molecule will distribute in the body. Therefore, in the design of a radiopharmaceutical it should be kept in mind as to how the addition of a metal atom will affect a particular molecule. It is, therefore, important to select the compounds that are likely to distribute to the organs or tissues of interest.

The consideration of structure-distribution relationship (SDR) is necessary in the design of radiopharmaceuticals to be used as radiodiagnostic agents. The object of SDR is to optimize target sites of the radiopharmaceutical in question. This may involve investigation of changes in the pharmacokinetic behaviour of the proposed radiopharmaceutical as a result of small variations in its structure, such as the addition of specific functional groups to the compound. Consequently the most effective compound is selected for both animal and human testing.

Quality Assurance of Radiopharmaceuticals

It involves the appropriate chemical, physical and biological tests on radiopharmaceuticals to ensure the suitability of the preparations for human use. These activities also include proper interpretation of the results, evaluation of analytical methods, calibration of the equipment and instrument used, and appropriate record-keeping. Radiopharmaceuticals must meet all pharmacopoeial specifications ihcluding radionuclide purity, radiochemical purity, chemical purity, pH, particle size, sterility, bacterial endotoxin and specific activity.

Storage

Radiopharmaceutical preparations should be kept in an air-tight container in a place sufficiently covered to avoid irradiation of personnel by primary or secondary emissions and complying with national and international regulations concerning the storage of radioactive substances.

It should be kept in mind that the radiopharmaceutical preparations are intended for use within a short time.

During the storage of radiopharmaceutical preparations, containers and solutions tend to darken due to radiation emitted by the radionuclide. Such darkening does not, however, indicate the deterioration of the preparations.

Lebelling

The lebel on the container states the following:
(1) The preparation is radioactive.
(2) The name of the preparation.
(3) The name of the manufacturer.
(4) An identification number
(5) The preparation is intended for medical use.
(6) In case of :
  (i) Liquid preparations: The total radioactivity in the container and/or the radioactive concentration per ml at a stated date and, if necessary, hour and the volume of liquid in the container;
  (ii) Solid preparations: Freeze-dried preparations – the total radioactivity at a stated date and, if necessary, hour. For capsules – the radioactivity of each capsule at a stated date and, if necessary, hour and the number of capsules in the container.

(7) The route of administration.

(8) For any preparations to be administered parenterally, the name and concentration of any anti-microbial preservatives.

(9) The date after which the preparation is not intended to be used.

(10) Any special storage conditions.

Handling of Radiopharmaceutical Preparations

Radioactive preparations should be handled with care as it involves a degree of risk. It should be undertaken only with the use of appropriate protective clothing, shielding, tools and procedures, and carried out in a laboratory classified as being suitable for the type of radioactive work under investigation. The International Commission on Radiation Protection (ICRP) has recommended limits of radiation to which a worker can be exposed. All work should be undertaken under proper surveillance and within the current limits set by the ICRP. Laboratories and personnel should be monitored with appropriately positioned equipment (like film badge detector on the chest/back; finger detector if handling syringes; etc.) suitable for detecting the sources being handled. A procedure for dealing with spillages must be established before work with a radionuclide commences. A general protocol used by some laboratories using short half-life radionuclides is to seal the laboratory and allow five half-lives to pass before entering and cleaning up. This is not practical if the radionuclide has a long half-life.

The Biological Effects of Radiation

Various changes/alterations in the normal metabolic processes can occur as a result of the passage of radiation through the cells of living tissue, resulting in the formation of ions and free radicals. These changes can result in :

1. The death of the organism or animal.
2. A reduction of the ability of cells to divide.
3. Abnorma cell division leading to cancers.
4. Change in genetic material
5. Increase in the rate of ageing.

The disruption of normal cell metabolism is mainly due to the interaction of the radiation with the large amounts of water that occur in all living tissue.

$$H_2O + radiation \longrightarrow H^+ + OH + e^-$$

The hydroxyl free radicals formed in this process are very reactive and immediately react with any neighbouring molecules such as proteins and DNA to produce substances that are foreign to the tissue. These reactions and the compounds they produce change and/or disrupt the normal course of the metabolic processes occurring in the tissue. Hydroxyl free radicals also react to form hydrogen and hydrogen peroxide that are toxic to cells. It is interesting to note that the symptoms of radiation sickness are similar to those of hydrogen peroxide poisoning. Disruption and alteration of biological processes may also occur by the direct interaction of the radiation with the organic molecules in the process.

The disruption and alterations to metabolism often results in a cascade effect, the substances formed by the initial effect of the radiation causing further disruptions and alterations to other metabolic processes. This in turn leads to further metabolic interference and so on. The initial radiation effect is magnified by the succession of secondary processes it initiates as shown in figure below.

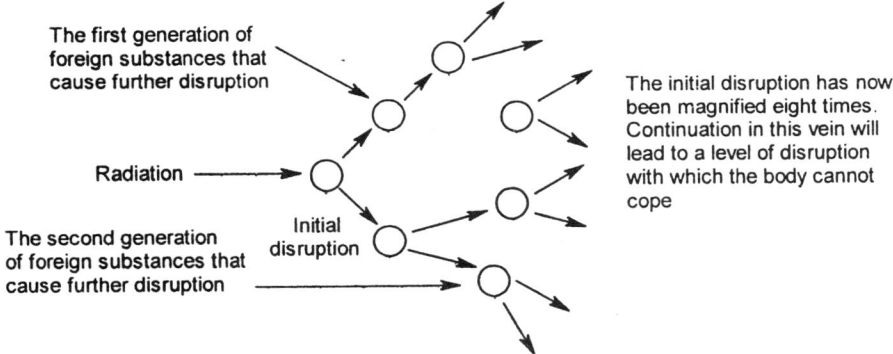

The first generation of foreign substances that cause further disruption

Radiation

The second generation of foreign substances that cause further disruption

Initial disruption

The initial disruption has now been magnified eight times. Continuation in this vein will lead to a level of disruption with which the body cannot cope

Fig. 13.1. A schematic representation of the cascade effect of radiation.

Exposure to low doses of low energy radiation over a long period of time is more likely to result in genetic mutations and cancers than low exposure to high energy radiation. Exposure to high energy radiation and high doses of low energy radiation over long periods of time will usually kill a cell or stop it reproducing. This is why high doses of low energy radiation are used to treat cancer. It is also the reason for carefully monitoring the amount of low energy radiation to which a patient is exposed in diagnostic investigations.

The biological effects of radiation depend on the type of radiation as well as its energy. Heavy particles, such as α particles and neutrons, produce dense clusters of ions and radicals along a short radiation path length whilst γ and X-rays leave ions and radicals at scattered intervals along much longer path lengths. These differences in behaviour make it difficult to compare quantitatively the biological effect of the different types of radiation on the same type of tissue. However, it has been compared in terms of the linear energy transfer (LET) value for the radiation. This is the average energy deposited per unit path length by the radiation. Cells are more likely to be able to repair the damage caused by non-lethal doses of radiation with a low LET value than radiation with a high LET value.

General Requirements for Radiopharmaceutical Preparations

All radiopharmaceutical preparations should comply with the general requirements stated in the pharmacopoeias and with the specific requirements for the individual preparation used for clinical and other purposes.

SODIUM CHROMATE [^{51}CR] STERILE SOLUTION

Preparation: It is a sterile solution of sodium chromate [^{51}Cr] made isotonic with blood by the addition ol sodium chloride.

Chromium-51 is a radioactive isotope of chromium and may be prepared by the neutron irradiatior of chromium, either of natural isotope composition or enriched in chromium-50,

Content of chromium-51 activity at the date and hour stated on the label: 90.0 to.110.0%.

Half-life of chromium-51: 27.7 days; emission: γ-radiation.

Characteristics: A clear, colourless or slightly yellow solution.

Identification:

A. The X-ray spectrum does not differ significantly from that of a standardized chromium-51 solution.

B. In the radiochemical purity test (see below) the distribution of radioactivity in the chromatogram is an indication of the identification of the preparation.

Acidity or alkalinity: pH 6.0 to 8.5.

Radiochemical purity: It is carried out by ascending paper chromatography using a solvent system water–ethanol (96%) – 10 M ammonia (125 : 50 : 25). The distribution of radioactivity in the chromatogram is determined using a suitable instrument. Not less than 90% of the total radioactivity is found in the spot with an Rf-value of about 0.9 due to sodium chromate.

Assay: The actiyity of the preparation may be determined using a suitable counting equipment by comparison with a standardized chromium-51 solution or by measurement in an instrument calibrated with the aid of such a solution.

Storage: Sodium chromate $[^{51}Cr]$ sterile solution should be used not later than three months stated on the label.

Uses: Sodium chromate $[^{51}Cr]$ solution is used diagnostically to determine red blood cell mass, volume and survival time and for scanning the spleen. The use of sodium chromate $[^{51}Cr]$ in scanning the spleen involves damaging the red blood cells with heat after incubation with the isotope. The damaged cells are then reinjected by i.v. where they are rapidly taken up by the spleen. The amount of radioactivity in this organ is taken as an indication of its ability to function properly.

Doses: I.V. doses for red blood cell volume range from 25 to 100 µc. Doses for red blood cell survival range from 150 - 250 µc.

IODINATED [^{125}I] ALBUMIN INJECTION

Preparation: It is a sterile solution of albumin that has been iodinated with iodine-125 and subsequently freed from iodide $[^{125}I]$ ion, made isotonic with blood by the addition of sodium chloride and containing a suitable antimicrobial preservative such as benzyl alcohol. It is prepared from albumin solution and contains not less than 1% of protein.

Content of iodine-125 activity stated on the label at the date stated on the label: 85.0 to 115.0%.

Half-life of iodine-125 : 60.1 days, emission: γ-radiation and X-rays

Characteristics: It is a clear, colourless or faintly yellow solution.

Identification:

A. The γ-ray and X-ray spectrum does not differ significantly from that of a standarized Iodine-125 solution.

B. On examination in an ultracentrifuge it has the sedimentation coefficient of normal human albumin.

Acidity or alkalinity: pH, 6.5 to 8.5.

Radiochemical purity: It is determined by paper electrophoresis using a volume containing not less than 0.5 mg of albumin applied to a strip of filter paper and a solution containing 5 g of barbitone sodium, 3.25 g of sodium acetate, 4 g of sodium octanoate and 34.2 ml of 0.1 M HCl in sufficient water to produce 100 ml. Not less than 95% of radioactivity on the paper occurs in a position corresponding to that which would be occupied by treating normal human albumin at the same time and in the same manner.

Assay: The activity is determined by comparison with a standardized iodine-125 solution or by measurement in an instrument calibrated with such a solution.

Storage: Iodinated [^{125}I] Albumin injection should be stored at a temperature of 2° to 8°C.

All the tests described under Iodinated [^{125}I] Albumin are applied to iodinated [^{131}I] albumin.

Uses: Radioiodinated serum albumin preparations are used to determine the plasma volume, and simultaneously with sodium chromate Cr-51 and ferric citrate Fe–59 to determine total blood volume. These preparations are also used to study circulation time and cardiac output. They are useful diagnostic aids for localizing neoplasms of the brain. They have also been used to evaluate the circulation of cerebrospinal fluid.

These preparations have the advantages of emitting low energy radiation with no β particles. Therefore radiation exposure to the patient is minimized.

Doses: The i.v. doses for blood and plasma volume studies range from 3 to 20 μc for both ^{125}I and ^{131}I and for brain, lung and liver scanning range from 200 to 500 μc.

CYANOCOBALAMIN [^{57}CO] SOLUTION

Preparation: Cyanocobalamin [^{57}Co] may be prepared by the growth of appropriate microorganisms on a medium containing cobalt(II) [^{57}Co] ion.

Content of Cobalt-57 activity at the date stated on the label: 90.0 to 110.0%.

Half-life of Cobalt-57 : 271 days, emission: γ radiation.

Characteristics: It is a clear, colourless or slightly pink solution.

Identification:

    A. The γ-ray spectrum does not differ significantly from that of a standarized cobalt-57 solution.

    B. In the radiochemical purity test (see below), the principal peak in the radiochromogram obtained with the test solution has a retention time similar to that of the peak in the chromatogram obtained with a reference solution.

Acidity: pH, 4.0 to 6.0.

Radiochemical purity: This is determined by liquid chromatography using a stationary phase of silica modified by chemically-bonded octylsilyl groups, and a mobile phase of 1% of w/v disodium hydrogen orthophosphate - methanol (73.5 : 26.5 v/v) adjusted to pH 3.5 with orthophosphoric acid at a detection wavelength of 351. The percentage of cobalt-57 present as cyanocobalamin is determined by normalization.

Assay: The activity is determined by comparison with a standardized cobalt-57 solution.

Storage: Cyanocobalamin [^{57}Co] solution should be stored at a temperature of 2° to 8°C and protected from light.

Uses: Cyanocobalamin [^{57}Co] solution is used in diagnostic procedures for pernicious anaemia. It is also used to study the effect of the liver on the intestinal absorption of vitamin B$_{12}$.

The radioactivity from an oral dose of the solution is detectable in the urine of the normal patient and absent or at a very low level in the urine of patients with pernicious anaemia, since the patients lack intrinsic factor, which is necessary for the proper intestinal absorption of vitamin B$_{12}$.

Doses: For oral and i.m. injection the range is 0.5 to 1.0 µc corresponding to 0.5 to 2.0 µg of cyanocobalamin.

CYANOCOBALAMIN [^{57}Co] CAPSULES

Preparation: Cyanocobalamin [^{57}Co] may be prepared by the growth of appropriate microorganisms on a medium containing cobalt(II) [^{57}Co] ion.

Content of Cobalt-57 activity at the date stated on the label: 90.0 to 110.0%

Half-life of Cobalt-57: 271 days; emission: γ radiation.

Characteristics: Hard gelatin capsules.

Identification:

A. The γ-ray spectrum does not differ significantly from that of a standarized cobalt–57 solution.

B. In radiochemical purity test (see below) the retention time of the principal peak in the radiochromatogram obtained with the test solution is similar to the peak in the chromatogram obtained with the reference solution.

Radiochemical purity: This is determined by liquid chromatography using the centrifuged supernatant solution of the dissolved contents of a capsule in one ml of water, a stationary phase of silica modified by chemically-bonded octylsilyl groups, and the mobile phase comprising 1% w/v disodium hydrogen orthophosphate - methanol (73.5 : 26.5 v/v), adjusted to pH 3.5 with orthophosphoric acid and a detection wavelength of 361 mm. The percentage of cobalt–57 present as cyanocobalamin is determined by normalization.

Disintegration: Complies with the requirement of hard capsules, using only one capsule.

Uniformity of content: The radioactivity of one capsule is measured, the procedure is repeated with further nine capsules and the average radioactivity for capsule is determined. The radioactivity of no capsule differs by more than 10% from the average radioactivity (RSD < 3.5%).

Assay: The average of 10 or more individual results obtained in the tests for uniformity of content is used to determine average radioactivity per capsule.

Storage: Cyanocobalamin [^{57}Co] capsules should be kept in an airtight container protected from light and stored at a temperature of 2° to 8°C.

Use: Same as for Cyanocobalamin [^{57}Co] solution.

Dose: Same as for Cyanocobalamin [^{57}Co] solution.

FERRIC CITRATE [^{59}Fe] INJECTION

Ferric Citrate [^{39}Fe] injection is a sterile solution containing iron [^{59}Fe] in the iron (III) state, 1.0% w/v of sodium citrate and sufficient sodium chloride to make it isotonic with blood.

Content of iron-59 activity at the date stated on the label: 90.0 to 110.0%.

Half-life of iron-59: 44.6 days; emission: γ-radiation.

Characteristics: It is a clear colourless or faintly orange brown solution.

Identification:

    A. The γ-ray spectrum does not differ significantly from of a standarized iron-59 solution.

    B. A suitable quantity is boiled with an excess of mercury (II) sulphate solution, filtered, the filtrate boiled and 0.15 ml of dilute potassium permanganate solution added. The colour is discharged and a white precipitate is produced.

Acidity or alkalinity: pH 6.0 to 8.0.

Total iron: Complies with the limit tests for iron.

Assay: The activity is determined by comparison with a standardized iron-59 solution or by measurement in an instrument calibrated with such a solution.

Labelling: The label states the content of total iron.

Uses: The preparation is used for determining the mechanism or estimating the status of erythropoiesis and of iron metabolism in normal and diseased persons. The parameters of iron metabolism, which can be measured, include clearance of iron from the plasma, appearance of iron in the red cells, appearance of iron in various sites and absorption of iron from the intestine. Suitable tests for these parameters and the inferences drawn from them are based on the fact that blood plasma is a medium in which iron is in continuous flux. Iron-59 has sufficient γ-radiation energy for scintillation counting of the radioactivity in various tissues associated with erythrocyte formation and destruction, such as in spleen, sacrum and liver from outside the body.

Doses: The usual oral and i.v. dose for ferrous citrate Fe-59 is 2 to 5 µc and may increase to 10 µc. Ferric chloride Fe-59 is also used for the same purposes and at the same dosage as the above compound in sterile solution.

COLLOIDAL GOLD [^{198}Au] INJECTION

It is a sterile, apyrogenic, colloidal dispersion of gold-198 stabilised with gelatin and contains reducing agents such as glucose or ascorbic acid.

Content of gold-198 activity at the date and hour mentioned on the label: 90.0 to 110.0%.

Half-life of gold-l98: 2.70 days; emission : β and γ radiations.

Characteristics: A dark red liquid, which does not deposit metal on the surface of the container.

Identification:

    A. The γ-ray spectrum does not differ significantly from that of a standarized gold-198 solution.

    B. In the test for radiochemical purity (see below), the distribution of radioactivity in the chromatogram is an indication of the identification of the preparation.

Acidity or alkalinity: pH 4.0 to 8.0

Radiochemical purity: It is determined by using ascending paper chromatography using a mobile phase consisting of acetone - water - hydrochloric acid (70 : 20 : 10). The distribution of radioactivity is determined using a suitable instrument. The spot corresponding to colloidal gold contains not less than 98% of the total radioactivity of the chromatogram.

Assay: The activity is determined by comparison with a standardized gold-198 solution or by measurement in an instrument calibrated with such a solution.

Labelling: The particle size range of the gold is stated on the label.

Uses: Gold-198 solutions are most frequently used for therapeutic purposes. They are administered by intracavitary injection into the pleural and peritoneal cavities as an aid in the management of pleural effusion (accumulation of serous fluid in pleural cavity) and ascites (accumulation of serous fluid in the peritoneal cavity). These fluid accumulations when secondary to neoplastic disease in the area can be inhibited by the effect of β-radiation on the cancerous tissue cells. Another use of this preparation is made as a prophylactic benefit against the growth of more tumors after surgical removal of tumors from a major cavity.

The colloidal gold Au-198 solutions are also used for diagnostic scanning of liver. Liver scanning with Au-198 is used in determining the position, shape and size of the organ as well as to obtain information on the distribution of the isotope concerning the functioning of the Kupffer's cells. The isotope does not enter the tumor tissue, abscesses or cysts; therefore, these appear as light areas in the liver scans.

Doses: The usual dose of gold Au-198 injection for pleural effusion is 35 to 75 mc and for ascites is 100 to 125 mc. The i.v. dose is around 300 μc with a range of 100 to 500 μc.

SODIUM IODIDE [^{131}I] SOLUTION

Sodium Iodide [^{131}I] solution is a solution suitable for oral administration containing iodine-131 in the form of sodium iodide and containing sodium thiosulphate or other suitable reducing agent. It is suitable for oral administration.

Content of iodine-131 activity at the date and hour stated on the label: 90.0 to 110.0%.

Half-life of iodine-131: 8.04 days; emission: γ-radiation.

Characteristics: It is a clear colourless solution.

Identification:

    A. The γ-ray spectrum does not differ significantly from that of a standarized iodine-131 solution.

    B. In the test for purity (see below), the distribution of radioactivity in the chromatogram is an indication of the identification of the preparation.

Radiochemical purity: Ascending paper chromatography is used to determine the radiochemical purity of iodine-131 using a mobile phase consisting of methanol - water (75 : 25 v/v). The distribution of radioactivity is determined using a suitable instrument. The spot corresponding to the iodide contains not less than 95% of the total radioactivity of the chromatogram.

Assay: The activity is determined by comparison with a standardized iodine-131 solution or by measurement in an instrument calibrated with such a solution.

SODIUM IODIDE [^{125}I] SOLUTION

All the tests described under sodium iodide [^{131}I] solution are applied to sodium iodide [^{125}I] solution.

Uses: It is the most common isotope and chemical form used as a diagnostic aid to study the function of thyroid gland and in scanning the thyroid to determine size, position and possible tumor location. The study of thyroid function involves the measurement of uptake of radioactive iodine in a 24-hour period after oral administration or i.v. injection. The normal patient will take up from 15 to 45% of the administered dose in 24 hours. If the uptake is less than 10%, the patient is hypothyroid and an uptake of over 50% indicates hyperthyroidism.

In thyroid scanning the radioactive dose is about 2–3 times than that used in uptake studies. Scanning of the gland in the neck area provides a picture of its size, shape and location as well as areas of high and low iodine concentrating ability. Most of the tissue effect of iodine-131 is due to β-radiation, which will penetrate 2–3 mm into tissue.

Sodium iodide [^{131}I] is also employed to destroy thyroid tissue or to alter the function of its tissue size. The particular use of the isotope is in disease states, such as hyperthyroidism, thyroid carcinoma and severe cardiac disease. Severe cardiac diseases like angina pectoris, and congestive heart disease may be eased by the use of the isotope required to induce hypothyroid state in order to reduce the work load of the heart.

Scanning can be done with iodine-125 which has lower energy and hence an advantage of lower radiation exposure to the patient. I-125 does not emit β radiation and, therefore, has minimum damage potential. The shelf life of iodine-125 preparations is longer than that of iodine-131 preparations giving them a longer shelf life in the laboratory.

Sodium iodide [^{125}I] is used in the treatment of hyperthyroidism to impair the hormone-synthesizing capability of the apex of the thyroid cells. It has been demonstrated that the properties of iodine-125 are more desirable than iodine-131 in this therapy. The lower energy and shorter path length radiation from iodine-125 are advantageous in limiting its deleterious effect on cell muscles without impairing its effect on areas of hormone synthesis. The concept behind this therapy is to avoid overtreatment of hyperthyroidism.

Doses: Diagnostic preparations of sodium iodide [^{131}I] or [^{125}I] are available in capsule or solution form. Oral or i.v. doses for uptake or general thyroid scanning range from 5 to 50 μc. Metastatic thyroid cancer scanning requires doses around 300 μc. Oral or i.v. doses for therapeutic purposes may vary. In hyperthyroidism doses range from 80 to 120 μc/g of gland tissue. Thyroid cancer is treated with doses ranging from 100 to 200 mc. Cardiac diseases need 10 to 25 mc, which may be repeated in 2 to 6 weeks.

SODIUM PHOSPHATE [^{32}P] INJECTION

Sodium Phosphate [^{32}P] injection is a sterile solution of disodium and monosodium orthophosphate [^{32}P] that is made isotonic with blood by the addition of sodium chloride.

Content of phosphorus-32 at the date and hour stated on the label: 90.0 to 110.0%.

Half-life of phosphorus-32 : 14.3 days; emission: β-radiation.

Characteristics: It is a clear colourless solution.

Identification:

A. The β-ray spectrum or the β-ray absorption curve does not differ significantly from that of a standardized phosphorus-30 solution measured under the same conditions.

B. In the test for radiochemical purity (see below), the distribution of the radioactivity in the chromatogram is an indication of the identification of the preparation.

Acidity or alkalinity: pH 6.0 to 8.0.

Radiochemical purity: It is determined by ascending paper chromatography using a mobile phase consisting of propan-2-ol – water – 10 M ammonia (75 : 25 : 0.3 v/v) with 5 g trichloroacetic acid dissolved in it The radioactive spot is located by autoradiography or by measuring the radioactivity of the whole chromatogram. Not less than 95% of the total radioactivity corresponds to the spot of orthophosphoric acid.

Assay: The activity is determined by comparison with a standardized phosphorus-32 solution or by measurement in an instrument calibrated with such a solution.

Uses: Sodium phosphate [^{32}P] is used for both diagnosis and treatment of neoplastic diseases. Since phosphate is utilised in cell metabolism, the rapidly proliferating cells as in the case of cancer show up the highest turnover of phosphate, compared with those of the non-cancerou cells. The primary diagnostic use of this preparation is in the localization of intraocular and cerebral tumors. The β-radiation from phosphorus–32 has sufficient energy to penetrate in tissues of about 8 mm. It is particularly helpful in the location of eye tumors which are relatively near the surface.

Sodium phosphate [^{32}P] is therapeutically used in diseases associated with both red and white blood cells. It is used in the treatment of polycythemia vera, which involves increase in the number and absolute mass of red blood cells. The effect of radioactivity in this disease is primarily through the reduction in erythrocytes formation.

It is also used in the palliative treatment of chronic granulocytic or myelocytic leukemia that results in an increase in the number of white blood cells.

Dose: For diagnostic purposes doses range from 250 to 500 μc with counts being taken at one hour, 24 hours and 48 hours over both eyes.

Therapeutic doses in polycythemia vera range from 2-10 mc with an average of 6 mc i.e. the dose is 75% of this dose.

TECHNETIUM [^{99M}Tc] ALBUMIN INJECTION

It is a sterile, apyrogenic solution of albumin labelled with technetium-99m.

Content of technetium-99m at the date and hour stated on the label: 90.0 to 110.0%.

Half-life of technetium-99m: 6.02 hours; emission: γ-radiation.

Identification:

A The γ-ray spectrum does not differ significantly from that of a standardized technetium-99m solution, either by direct comparison or by using an instrument calibrated with such a solution.

B. Using antiserum to normal human serum, compare normal human serum and the injection being examined by immunoelectrophoresis. The main component of the injection corresponds to the main component of the normal human serum.

Acidity: pH 2.0 to 6.5.

Radiochemical purity: It is determined by thin-layer chromatography using silica gel as an adsorbent and butan-2-one as the mobile phase. The distribution of radioactivity on the chromatogram is determined using a suitable instrument. Not more than 5.0% of the radioactivity due to technetium-99m corresponds to technetium in the form of pertechnetate ion.

Assay: The activity is determined by comparison with a standardized technetium-99m solution or by measurement in an instrument calibrated with such a solution.

Lebelling The amount of albumin and the quantity of tin per ml, if any, are stated on the label.

Uses: Technetium-99m is used in several chemical forms for a number of diagnostic purposes. It has the advantages of short half-life, emission of single γ-photon, absence of β-radiation and its damaging effects on tissues, lack of chemical toxicity and administration of large doses of radioactivity to the patient.

The common chemical forms of Tc-99m are sodium pertechnetate salt and a colloidal preparation of technetium sulphide. Other frequently used forms include technetium serum albumin, technetium colloidal sulphur, technetium colloidal tin, technetium etifenin, technetium macrosalb, technetium medronate, technetium microspheres, technetium pentetate, technetium succimer and technetium tin pyrophosphate in the form of injections.

Sodium pertechnetate Tc-99m is used as a diagnostic agent for brain scan in determining the presence and location of neoplastic and non-neoplastic agents. The uptake of this salt by thyroid gland renders this isotope useful for thyroid function studies.

Technetium sulphide Tc-99m colloidal solution which, when injected intravenously, is taken up by reticuloendothelial cells in liver, spleen and bone marrow, enables the scintillation scans of all the three organs to be obtained. The quantity of the scan is better than that obtainable with gold-198, with less radiation exposure to the patient.

Doses: For brain scanning sodium pertechnetate Tc-99m may be administered orally or by i.v. injection in doses of 200 μc/kg of body weight. The average dose of adult is 10 mc. For thyroid function tests doses of around 500 μc are required. Liver and spleen scanning can be done with doses of 1 to 3 mc. For bone marrow tests 4 to 10 mc is required. In all instances colloidal solutions are injected by i.v. route.

PART III

Appendices

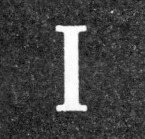
Qualitative Reactions of Some Common Substances and Radicals

A large number of inorganic compounds are tested for their identity on the basis of qualitative reactions and tests given by their radicals and by substances, obtained through some special treatment. These reactions and tests are given under this appendix hereunder.

Acetates

Acetates, when warmed with sulphuric acid, yield acetic acid, which has a characteristic odour when warmed with sulphuric acid and a small quantity of alcohol, they yield ethyl acetate which has a characteristic odour.

Neutral acetates are decomposed by heating, yielding a characteristic acetous odour.

With neutral or slightly acid solution of acetates, solution of ferric chloride gives a deep-red colour, and the resulting liquid on boiling yields a reddish-brown precipitate. On adding hydrochloric acid the red solution turns yellow.

Acetates when heated with calcium oxide, yield acetone, detected by the indigo-blue colour obtained when the vapours impinge on filter-paper, which has been moistened with a 2 per cent w/v solution of o-nitrobenzaldehyde in alcohol, dried and then moistened with solution of sodium hydroxide.

Aluminium

Solutions of aluminium salts yield with dilute ammonia solution or with solution of ammonium sulphide a white gelatinous precipitate soluble in hydrochloric acid, in acetic acid, and in solution of sodium hydroxide but nearly insoluble in dilute solution of ammonia and in solutions of ammonium salts and quite insoluble in these solutions when the mixture is boiled.

Solutions of aluminium salts to which have been added five drops of a freshly prepared 0.05 per cent w/v solution of quinalizarin in a 1 per cent w/v solution of sodium hydroxide heated to boiling, cooled and acidified with excess of acetic acid, yield a reddish-violet colour.

Amines, Primary, Aromatic

When solution of primary aromatic amines, prepared by dissolving 0.1 g in 2 ml of dilute hydrochloric acid with the aid of heat, if necessary, are cooled in ice, treated with 4 ml of a 1 per cent w/v solution of sodium nitrite and the mixture poured into 2 ml solution of B-naphthol containing 1 g of sodium acetate a heavy precipitate is produced, the colour of which varies from orange yellow to scarlet depending on the substance under test.

Ammonium Salt

Many ammonium salts volatilise, when strongly heated, leaving no residue. When they are heated with solution of sodium hydroxide, ammonia is evolved, recognised by its odour, by its reaction on moist red litmus paper and by its ability to produce black stain on filter-paper impregnated with solution of mercurous nitrate.

Antimony

Slightly acid solutions of antimony compounds yield, with hydrogen sulphide, an orange-coloured precipitate soluble in solution of sodium hydroxide, in solution of ammonium sulphide, and in warm hydrochloric acid with evolution of hydrogen sulphide but almost insoluble in solution of ammonium carbonate.

Solutions of antimony compounds react with nascent hydrogen, generated by the interaction of granulated zinc and dilute sulphuric acid, to yield stibine. A cold porcelain tile held in the flame of this gas acquires dark metallic deposit, which is not appreciably dissolved by solutions of chlorinated soda.

Solutions of antimony compounds acidified with dilute nitric acid, and filtered, if necessary, yield a white microcrystalline precipitate with a 5.0 per cent w/v solution of pyrogallol in water.

Arsenic

Solutions of arsenic compounds, containing hydrochloric acid, yield with hydrogen sulphide a yellow precipitate, soluble in solution of sodium hydroxide, in solution of ammonium sulphide and in solution of ammonium carbonate, but reprecipitated on the addition of hydrochloric acid.

Solutions of arsenic compounds treated with nascent hydrogen generated by the interaction of granulated zinc and dilute sulphuric acid, yield arsine. A cold porcelain tile held in the flame of this gas acquires a dark metallic deposit, which is readily dissolved by solution of chlorinated soda.

Solution of arsenic compounds yield with solution of stannous chloride brown precipitate.

Solution of arsenious compounds, treated with nascent hydrogen generated by the interaction of granulated zinc and solution of sodium hydroxide, slowly yield hydrogen arsenide; this gas gives a black stain to a filter paper moistened with solution of silver nitrate and placed as a cap over the tube in which the test is being performed.

Arsenates

Solutions of arsenates in the presence of hydrochloric acid liberate iodine from solution of potassium iodide.

Solutions of arsenates yield a reddish-chocolate precipitate with solution of silver ammonio-nitrate and a white, crystalline precipitate with solution of magnesium ammonio-sulphate.

Arsenites

Solutions of arsenites to which sodium bicarbonate has been added decolourise solution of iodine.

Solutions of arsenites yield a yellow precipitate with solution of silver ammonio-nitrate.

Barium

Solutions of barium salt yield a white precipitate with dilute sulphuric acid. This precipitate is insoluble in hydrochloric acid and in nitric acid.

Barium salts impart a yellowish-green colour to a non-luminous flame, appearing blue when viewed through green glass.

Benzoates

Benzoates do not char when heated with sulphuric acid but yield a white sublimate on the sides of the tube.

Solutions of benzoates yield a white crystalline precipitate with dilute hydrochloric acid readily soluble on shaking, in solvent ether or chloroform.

Neutral solutions of benzoates yield with test-solution of ferric chloride a buff-coloured precipitate which is soluble in hydrochloric acid with the simultaneous separation of a white crystalline precipitate of benzoic acid.

Neutral solutions of benzoates do not decolourise a few drops of solution of bromine.

Bismuth

Solutions of bismuth salts yield with hydrogen sulphide a brownish-black precipitate insoluble in solution of sodium hydroxide, in dilute hydrochloric acid and in solution of ammonium sulphide, but soluble in warm nitric acid.

Solutions of bismuth salts, which are not too acidic yield with a dilute solution of sodium chloride in water in large excess, a white precipitate in solutions of tartaric acid.

Solutions of bismuth salts yield with solution of potassium iodide a dark-brown precipitate, soluble in excess of the reagent, giving a yellowish-green solution which, on diluting well with water, yields an orange precipitate.

Solutions of bismuth salts acidified with dilute nitric acid give with a 10 per cent w/v solution of thiourea in water, a deep-yellow colour.

Bromides

When a bromide is heated with sulphuric acid and manganese dioxide or potassium dichromate, bromine is liberated, the vapour gives an orange-yellow colour to filter-paper moistened with solution of starch.

Solutions of bromides give, with solution of silver nitrate, a yellowish-curdy precipitate somewhat soluble in ammonia solution but almost insoluble in dilute ammonia solution and dilute nitric acid.

From solutions of bromides, bromine is liberated by solution of chlorine. The bromine is soluble in two or three drops of carbon disulphide or chloroform forming a reddish solution. Addition of a saturated solution of phenol to the aqueous solution containing liberated bromine yields a white precipitate.

In testing for bromides in the presence of iodides, all iodine must be first removed by boiling the aqueous solution with excess of lead dioxide.

Calcium

Solutions of calcium salts yield, with solution of ammonium carbonate, a white precipitate which after boiling and cooling the mixture, is insoluble in solution of ammonium chloride.

Solutions of calcium salts yield, with solution of ammonium oxalate, a white precipitate soluble in hydrochloric acid but insoluble in acetic acid.

With solution of potassium chromate, strong solutions of calcium salts yield a yellow, crystalline precipitate on shaking, the precipitate being soluble on diluting well with water or on adding acetic acid.

Solutions of calcium salts yield no immediate precipitate with solution of potassium ferrocyanide, but on the addition of an excess of the reagent in the presence of an excess of ammonium chloride, yield a white precipitate.

Carbonates and Bicarbonates

Carbonates and bicarbonates effervesce with dilute acids, liberating carbon dioxide; the gas is colourless and produces a white precipitate in solution of calcium hydroxide.

Solutions of carbonates produce a brownish-red precipitate with solution of mercuric chloride; solutions of bicarbonates produce a white precipitate.

Solutions of carbonates yield, with solution of silver nitrate, white precipitate which becomes yellow on the addition of excess of the reagent and brown on boiling the mixture. The precipitate is soluble in dilute ammonia solution and in dilute nitric acid.

Solutions of carbonates produce, at room temperature, a white precipitate with solution of magnesium sulphate. Solutions of bicarbonates yield no precipitate with the reagent at room temperature, but on boiling the mixture a white precipitate is formed.

Solutions of bicarbonates, on boiling, liberate carbon dioxide which produces a white precipitate in solution of calcium hydroxide.

Chlorides

Chlorides, heated with manganese dioxide-sulphuric acid, yield chlorine, recognisable by its colour and by giving a blue colour with potassium iodide and solution of starch.

Solutions of chlorides yield, with solution of silver nitrate, a white, curdy precipitate soluble in dilute ammonia solution but insoluble in nitric acid.

Citrates

Citrates, on heating with sulphuric acid in a tube placed in a boiling water-bath, give only pale-yellow colour and evolve carbon dioxide and carbon monoxide.

Neutral solutions of citrates boiled, with an excess of solution of calcium chloride, yield a white granular precipitate soluble in acetic acid.

Neutral solutions of citrates yield, with an excess of solution of silver nitrate, a white precipitate soluble in nitric acid and dilute ammonia solution. No mirror is formed on the test tube when this ammoniacal solution is warmed.

Solutions of citrate boiled with an excess of solution of mercuric sulphate, and filtered, if necessary, yield a solution which after boiling and addition of a few drops of solution of potassium permanganate decolorise the reagent and yield a white precipitate.

Copper

Solutions of copper salts yield a brownish-black precipitate with hydrogen sulphide insoluble in dilute hydrochloric acid and solution of sodium hydroxide, almost insoluble in solution of ammonium sulphide but decomposed and dissolved by boiling nitric acid.

Solutions of copper salts yield with solution of sodium hydroxide a light blue precipitate which becomes brownish-black on boiling.

Solutions of copper salts yield with solution of potassium iodide a brownish precipitate and a brown aqueous liquid giving a deep blue colour with solution of starch.

Strong solutions of copper salts yield with solution of ammonium thiocyanate a black precipitate becoming white on the addition of sulphurous acid.

Solutions of copper salts yield with dilute ammonia solution a greenish blue precipitate which readily dissolves in excess of the precipitant forming a deep blue solution.

Cupric salts in solution produce with solution of potassium ferrocyanide a reddish brown precipitate or, in very dilute solution, a reddish-brown colour.

Cyanides

Solutions of cyanides produce, with solution of silver nitrate, a white curdy precipitate, soluble in solution of potassium cyanide and in dilute ammonia solution and slowly soluble in boiling nitric acid.

When to a solution of cyanide are added a few small crystals of ferrous sulphate and just sufficient solution of sodium hydroxide to precipitate the iron and the mixture is boiled and just acidified with dilute hydrochloric acid, a blue colour of precipitate is produced.

Solutions of cyanides evaporated to dryness with solution of ammonium polysulphide yield residue which, after being acidified with a few drops of hydrochloric acid, give a blood-red colour with solution of ferric chloride.

Solutions of cyanides yield a grey precipitate of metallic mercury with solution of mercurous nitrate.

Gold

Metallic gold is soluble in a mixture of 3 volumes of hydrochloric acid and one volume of nitric acid, yielding a solution of chloroauric acid, and is insoluble in concentrated mineral acids.

Solutions of gold compounds yield, with hydrogen sulphide, a black precipitate insoluble in dilute hydrochloric acid, but soluble in solution of ammonium polysulphide, from which it is reprecipitated on the addition of dilute hydrochloric acid.

Auric compounds in neutral or weaker acid solution yield, with solution of stannous chloride; a purple colour and, with solution of hydrogen peroxide and solution of sodium hydroxide, a precipitate which appears brownish-black by reflected light and bluish-green by transmitted light.

Iodides

Iodides heated with sulphuric acid and manganese dioxide or potassium dichromate evolve violet vapours of iodine. Solutions of iodides yield with solution of silver nitrate, a yellow, curdy precipitate in dilute ammonia solution and in dilute nitric acid.

Solution of iodides with solution of potassium iodate and dilute acetic acid liberate iodine, which colours chloroform reddish-violet and solution of starch blue.

Solutions of iodides produce, with solution of mercuric chloride, a scarlet precipitate slightly soluble in excess of this reagent and very soluble in excess of solution of potassium iodide.

A small quantity of solution of chlorine added to solutions of iodides liberates iodine which colours chloroform reddish-violet and solution of starch deep blue.

Iron

Reactions common to ferrous and ferric salts.

Solutions of iron salts in dilute hydrochloric acid after the addition of a sufficient quantity of solution of potassium permanganate to produce a faint pink colour, give with solution of ammonium thiocyanate a blood-red colour, which is extracted by solvent ether, or amyl alcohol and which is discharged on the addition of solution of mercuric chloride or of phosphoric acid.

(a) Ferric salts

Solution of ammonium nitrosophenylhydroxyl amine in the presence of hydrochloric acid gives reddish-brown precipitate soluble in solvent ether.

Solution of potassium ferricyanide produces a reddish-brown colour but no precipitate.

Solution of sodium hydroxide produces, in the absence of citrates and tartrates, a reddish-brown precipitate soluble in solution of citric acid in water, or of tartaric acid in water.

Solutions of ferric salts, strongly acidified with acetic acid, give with a 0.2 per cent w/v solution of 7-iodo-8-hydroxyquinoline-5-sulphonic acid in water, a stable green colour.

(b) Ferrous salts

Solution of potassium ferrocyanide produces a white precipitate rapidly turning blue, and insoluble in dilute hydrochloric acid.

Solution of potassium ferricyanide produces a dark-blue precipitate insoluble in dilute hydrochloric acid and decomposed by solution of sodium hydroxide.

Solution of sodium hydroxide produces a dull green precipitate which on filtering and exposing to the atmosphere changes to a brownish colour.

Lead

Strong solutions of lead salts yield with hydrochloric acid a white precipitate soluble in boiling water and redeposited as crystals when the solution is cooled.

Solutions of lead salts which are not very strongly acid yield with hydrogen sulphide a black precipitate insoluble in dilute hydrochloric acid and in solution of ammonium sulphide but soluble in hot dilute nitric acid.

Solutions of lead salts yield with dilute sulphuric acid a white precipitate almost insoluble in water, more nearly insoluble in dilute sulphuric acid and in alcohol (90 per cent), but soluble in dilute solution of ammonium acetate.

Solutions of lead salts yield with solution of potassium iodide a yellow precipitate which dissolves on boiling and reprecipitates as glistening plates on cooling.

Solutions of lead salts yield with solution of potassium chromate a yellow precipitate readily soluble in solution of sodium hydroxide and in hot nitric acid, sparingly soluble in dilute nitric acid and insoluble in acetic acid.

Solutions of lead salts to which has been added solution of potassium cyanide and made alkaline with ammonia solution produce a brick-red coloured lower layer on shaking with lead free-solution of diphenylthiocarbazone.

Lignin

Lignified cell walls are coloured bright red when soaked in solution of phloroglucinol and adding a drop or two of hydrochloric acid.

Solution of aniline hydrochloride colours lignified tissues yellow.

Magnesium

Solutions of magnesium salts yield a white precipitate with solution of ammonium carbonate, especially on boiling, but yield no precipitate in the presence of solution of ammonium chloride.

Solutions of magnesium salts yield a white crystalline precipitate with solution of sodium phosphate in the presence of ammonium salts and dilute ammonia solution.

Solutions of magnesium salts yield with solution of sodium hydroxide a white precipitate insoluble in excess of the reagent, but soluble in solution of ammonium chloride.

Solutions of magnesium salts yield with solution of sodium hydroxide and solution of diphenylcarbazide a pink precipitate.

Mercury

Reactions common to mercurous and mercuric salts.

Hydrogen sulphide produces a black precipitate, insoluble in solution of ammonium sulphide and in boiling dilute nitric acid.

Bright copper foil immersed in a solution free from excess of nitric acid becomes coated with a deposit of mercury, which on rubbing becomes bright, the mercury may be volatilised from the foil by heat and obtained in globules.

Solution of stannous chloride added in excess gives a white precipitate rapidly turning grey with excess of the reagent.

Mercuric salts

Solution of sodium hydroxide yields a yellow precipitate.

Solution of potassium iodide, added to a neutral solution, produces a scarlet precipitate, soluble in excess of the precipitant and in a considerable excess of the solution of the mercuric salt.

Mercurous salt

Solution of sodium hydroxide yields a black precipitate.

Hydrochloric acid yields a white precipitate insoluble in water and blackened by dilute ammonia solution.

Solution of potassium iodide yields a greenish, yellow precipitate decomposed on addition of an excess reagent, giving dark-grey, finely-divided mercury.

Nitrates

Nitrates liberate red fumes when warmed with sulphuric acid and copper.

Solutions of nitrates do not yield a brown colour with solution of ferrous sulphate, but when to a mixture of the reagent and the solution being tested sulphuric acid is cautiously added to form a lower layer, a brown colour is produced, at the junction of the two liquids.

When solutions of nitrates are mixed cautiously with sulphuric acid and a crystal of brucine is added a red colour is produced.

Solutions of nitrates previously boiled with solution of sodium hydroxide to free them from traces of ammonium compounds, on boiling with zinc powder and solution of sodium hydroxide liberate ammonia, detected by its odour, by its action on moistened red litmus paper and by the darkening produced on a filter-paper previously impregnated with solution of mercurous nitrate.

Nitrites

Nitrites when heated with dilute sulphuric acid evolve red fumes.

On adding to a solution of a nitrite a few drops of dilute sulphuric acid and solution of potassium iodide and solution of starch, a blue colour is produced.

Solutions of nitrites produce with solution of ferrous sulphate a deep brown colour.

Solutions of nitrites with urea and dilute sulphuric acid yield carbon dioxide, the gas producing a white precipitate in solution of calcium hydroxide.

Phosphates

Solutions of ortho-phosphates give the following reactions:

Solution of silver ammonio-nitrate yields a light yellow precipitate, readily soluble in dilute of ammonia solution and in cold dilute nitric acid.

Solution of magnesium ammonio-sulphate yields a white, crystalline precipitate.

Solution of ammonium molybdate with an equal volume of nitric acid yields, on warming, a yellow precipitate.

On adding, to a dilute solution of a phosphate, one-fifth of its volume of solution of ammonium molybdate with sulphuric acid, followed by one-fifth of its volume of methylaminophenol with sulphite, and heating for 30 minutes in a water-bath, a blue colour is produced.

Potassium

Potassium compounds moistened with hydrochloric acid and introduced on platinum wire into the flame of a Bunsen burner, give violet colour to the flame.

Moderately strong solutions of potassium salts, which have been previously ignited to remove ammonium salts, give a white, crystalline precipitate with perchloric acid.

Solutions of potassium salts, which have been previously ignited to free them from ammonium salts and from which iodine has been removed, give a yellow precipitate with solution of sodium cobaltinitrite and acetic acid.

Protein

Solutions of proteins yield, when heated with solution of mercury nitrate, a brick red precipitate.

Solutions of proteins yield, when heated with nitric acid, a yellow colour which becomes more yellow or brownish, on the addition of solution of sodium hydroxide.

Solutions of proteins yield, on the addition of solution of sodium hydroxide and a few drops of solution of copper sulphate, a pinkish-violet colour.

Salicylates

Salicylates char slowly on warming with sulphuric acid, evolving carbon monoxide and sulphur dioxide.

Salicylates heated with excess of soda lime evolve phenol recognised by its characteristic odour and its inflammability.

Solutions of salicylates, with dilute hydrochloric acid, yield a crystalline precipitate of salicylic acid, soluble in solution of ammonium acetate, in solvent ether and in chloroform.

Neutral solutions of salicylates give, with solution of ferric chloride, an intense reddish-violet colour which remain on addition of a little acetic acid, but disappears on addition of dilute hydrochloric acid, a white crystalline precipitate of salicylic acid separating.

Silver

Solutions of silver salts yield a white, curdy precipitate with solutions of chlorides or with hydrochloric acid. The precipitate is soluble in dilute ammonia solution and insoluble in nitric acid.

Solutions of silver salts yield, with solution of potassium chromate, a red precipitate soluble in nitric acid.

Solutions of silver salts yield a cream-coloured precipitate with solution of potassium iodide. The precipitate is insoluble in dilute ammonia solution and in nitric acid.

Sodium

Sodium compounds, moistened with hydrochloric acid and introduced on a platinum wire into the flame of a Bunsen burner, give a yellow colour to the flame.

Solutions of sodium salts yield, with solution of uranyl zinc acetate, a yellow crystalline precipitate.

Sulphates

Solutions of sulphates yield, with solution of barium chloride, a white precipitate insoluble in hydrochloric acid.

Solutions of sulphates yield, with solution of lead acetate, a white precipitate soluble in solution of ammonium acetate and in solution of sodium hydroxide.

Sulphites and bisulphites

Sulphites and bisulphites heated with hydrochloric acid evolve sulphur dioxide, a colourless gas with a pungent smell of burning sulphur.

Solutions of sulphites and bisulphites decolourise solution of iodine, the resulting solution gives the reactions for sulphates.

Solutions of sulphites and bisulphites decolourise solution of potassium permanganate in the presence of dilute sulphuric acid.

Solutions of sulphites and bisulphites yield with solution of lead acetate a white precipitate, soluble in cold dilute nitric acid and giving a white precipitate on boiling the mixture.

Tartrates

Tartrates heated with sulphuric acid in boiling water-bath char rapidly evolving carbon dioxide and carbon monoxide.

Neutral solutions of tartrates produce with excess of solution of calcium chloride in the cold, a white, granular precipitate soluble in acetic acid.

Neutral solutions of tartrates yields, with excess of solution of silver nitrate, a white precipitate soluble in nitric acid and in dilute ammonia solution, the ammoniacal solution containing just enough ammonium hydroxide to dissolve the silver precipitate, on heating deposits metallic silver as a mirror on the sides of the test tube.

On adding to a solution of tartaric acid in water or of a tartrate acidified with acetic acid, a drop of solution of ferrous sulphate, a few drops of solution of hydrogen peroxide and an excess of solution of sodium hydroxide a purple or violet colour is produced.

Solutions of tartrates mixed with a few drops of a 10 per cent w/v solution of potassium bromide, a few drops of a 2 per cent w/v solution of resorcinol and sulphuric acid, give an intense colouration on warming, and on cautiously pouring the cooled solution into water a red colouration is obtained.

Thiosulphates

Solutions of thiosulphates give with hydrochloric acid a white precipitate of sulphur which soon turns to yellow and evolves sulphur dioxide, colourless gas with a pungent smell of burning sulphur.

Strong solutions of thiosulphates give with solution of barium chloride a white precipitate which is soluble in hydrochloric acid with separation of sulphur and evolution of sulphur dioxide.

Solutions of thiosulphates decolourise solution of iodine, the decolourised solutions do not give the reaction for sulphates.

Solutions of thiosulphates decolourise solution of bromine, the decolorised solution gives the reactions for sulphates.

Solutions of thiosulphates give with solution of lead acetate a white precipitate soluble in excess of the reagents; on boiling the suspension a black precipitate is obtained.

Zinc

Neutral solutions of zinc salts yield with solution of ammonium sulphide, or with hydrogen sulphide and solution of sodium hydroxide, a white precipitate soluble in hydrochloric acid but insoluble in acetic acid.

Solution of zinc salts yield with solution of potassium ferrocyanide a white precipitate insoluble in dilute hydrochloric acid.

Solutions of zinc salts acidified with phosphoric acid and mixed with 0.05 ml of 0.1 per cent w/v solution of copper sulphate and 2 ml of solution of mercuric ammonium thiocyanate yield a violet precipitate.

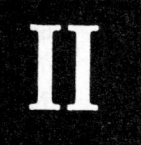

Determination of Weight Per Millilitre and Specific Gravity

Weight per Millilitre

Weight per millilitre of a liquid is determined by dividing the weight in air, expressed in grammes, of the quantity of the liquid which fills a pycnometer at 20° or 25° by the capacity of the pycnometer at 20° or 25° respectively, expressed in millilitres. The capacity of the pycnometer at these temperatures is ascertained from the weight in g of quantity of water required to fill the pycnometer. The following data are assumed:

Weight of 1 ml of water in air at:

20°	0.99719 g
25°	0.99602 g

Ordinary deviations in the density of air do not affect the result of a determination significantly for pharmacopoeial purposes.

Specific Gravity

The specific gravity of a substance is the weight of a given volume of that substance at a stated temperature as compared with the weight of an equal volume of water at the same temperature, all weighings being taken in air. A suitable pycnometer may be used for the determination.

Specific gravity at 15° and the percentage of glycerin of w/w in aqueous solutions

Sp. gr.	Percentage	Sp. gr.	Percentage	Sp. gr.	Percentage
1.0000	0	1.0858	34	1.1799	68
1.0024	1	1.0885	35	1.1827	69
1.0048	2	1.0912	36	1.1855	70
1.0072	3	1.0939	37	1.1882	71
1.0096	4	1.0966	38	1.1909	72
1.0120	5	1.0993	39	1.1936	73
1.0144	6	1.1020	40	1.1963	74
1.0168	7	1.1047	41	1.1990	75
1.0192	8	1.1074	42	1.2017	76
1.0216	9	1.1101	43	1.2044	77
1.0240	10	1.1128	44	1.2071	78
1.0265	11	1.1155	45	1.2089	79
1.0290	12	1.1182	46	1.2125	80
1.0315	13	1.1209	47	1.2152	81
1.0340	14	1.1236	48	1.2179	82
1.0365	15	1.1263	49	1.2206	83
1.0390	16	1.1290	50	1.2233	84
0.0415	17	1.1318	51	1.2260	85
1.0440	18	1.1346	52	1.2287	86
1.0465	19	1.1374	53	1.2314	87
1.0490	20	1.1402	54	1.2341	88
1.0516	21	1.1430	55	1.2368	89
1.0542	22	1.1458	56	1.2395	90
1.0568	23	1.1486	57	1.2421	91
1.0594	24	1.1514	58	1.2447	92
1.0620	25	1.1542	59	1.2473	93
1.0646	26	1.1570	60	1.2499	94
1.0672	27	1.1599	61	1.2525	95
1.0698	28	1.1628	62	1.2550	96
1.0724	29	1.1657	63	1.2575	97
1.0750	30	1.1686	64	1.2600	98
1.0777	31	1.1715	65	1.2615	99
1.0804	32	1.1743	66	1.2650	100
1.0831	33	1.1771	—		

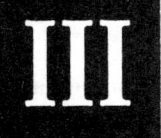
Determination of Water

Drugs and pharmaceutical aids contain varying amount of water, which may be present in the form of water of dehydration (as part and parcel of the compound) or as water absorbed superficially by the substance. Since the amount of water in one and the same drug/pharmaceutical aid may vary depending upon the condition of storage and preservation and handling of the materials, the pharmacopoeias all over the world prescribe limit for the content of water to achieve uniformity in the quality of drugs, which are invariably used for finished pharmaceutical products and formulations. Big manufacturing houses have to mostly purchase huge raw materials on the moisture-free basis and their finished products have to similarly conform to specified uniform qualities.

Even in day to day work scientists have to know the water-content of drugs and other chemicals to be able to achieve uniformity in their results.

Although there are a few methods, which have to be used keeping in view the nature of material to be handled for determination of water, I.P. describes only one method, namely Karl Fischer Method. This method depends upon the reaction of water, which is to be determined with iodine and sulphur dioxide in pyridine-methanol solution. The pyridine prevents loss of sulphur dioxide from the reagent by forming an additive compound and it also helps in the completion of reaction with water by combining with the products of reaction, which take place as follows:

$$I_2 + SO_2 + H_2O \rightleftharpoons 2HI + SO_3$$

$$\underset{\text{Pyridine}}{C_5H_5N} + \underset{\substack{\text{Sulphur} \\ \text{trioxide}}}{SO_3} \longrightarrow \underset{\substack{\text{Pyridine sulphur} \\ \text{trioxide additive}}}{C_6H_5N.SO_3}$$

The Karl Fischer reagent consists of iodine, sulphur dioxide and pyridine and methanol. Presence of methanol is necessary, as otherwise pyridine sulphur trioxide complex would react with water as follows:

$$C_5H_5N.SO_3 + HOH \longrightarrow C_5H_5NH + H_2SO_4$$

The reaction between water and the reagent is complex and the stoichiometrical relationships are uncertain and, therefore, it is desirable to standardise the reagent emperically against weighed amount of water. The reagent is required to be prepared with special precautions and stored and used carefully. It should be standardised periodically.

The Karl Fischer Method as given in I.P. appendix is reproduced here.

Trimetric (Karl Fischer) Method

The titrimetric determination of water depends upon the fact that a solution of sulphur dioxide and iodine in pyridine and methyl alcohol reacts with water stoichiometrically. Since reagents and solutions used in the test are sensitive to water, precautions should be taken to rigidly exclude the atmospheric moisture. The end-point of the titration may be determined electrometrically or visually in colourless solution by a change from a canary-yellow to an amber colour. The end-point in coloured solutions is likely to be obscured and is best determined electrometrically. The apparatus consists of a simple electrical circuit which serves to pass 5 to 10 microamperes of direct current between a pair of platinum electrodes immersed in the solution to be titrated. At the end-point of the titration a slight excess of the reagent increases the flow of current to between 50 and 150 microamperes for thirty seconds or longer, depending upon the solution being titrated. The time is shortest for substances which react with the reagent.

Apparatus: An apparatus which provides for efficient exclusion of atmospheric moisture and determination of the end-point may be used. The apparatus generally comprises of a closed system consisting of one or two automatic burettes and tightly covered titration vessel fitted with the necessary electrodes and a magnetic stirrer. The air in the system is kept dry with a suitable desiccant (phosphorous pentoxide, anhydrous granular calcium chloride, or silica gel).

Karl Fischer reagent: Dissolve 63 g of iodine in 100 ml of dehydrated pyridine, cool in ice and pass sulphur dioxide in solution until a gain of 32.3 g has occurred, taking care to avoid absorption of atmospheric moisture. Add sufficient dehydrated methyl alcohol to produce 500 ml and allow to stand for twenty-four hours. One ml of this solution when freshly prepared is equivalent to approximately 5 mg of water, but it deteriorates gradually, therefore, standardise it within one hour before use, or daily if in continuous use. The solution should be protected from light while in use. Store any bulk stock of the reagent in a suitably sealed, glass-stoppered container fully protected from light, and in the cold. Stabilised solution of Karl Fischer Reagent, if commercially available may be used.

Primary standardisation of the reagent: Place about 36 ml of methyl alcohol in the titration vessel, and add sufficient Karl Fischer reagent to give the characteristic end-point. Add quickly 150 to 350 mg accurately weighed, sodium tartrate by difference, and titrate to the end-point. The water equivalence factor F, in mg of water per ml of reagent, is given by the formula 0.1566 W/V, in which W is weight, in mg, of the sodium tartrate, and V is the volume, in ml, of the reagent required.

Secondary standardisation of the reagent: The reagent may alternatively be standardised for each day's use against a water-methyl alcohol solution standardised as follows:

Add 2 ml of water to 1000 ml of methyl alcohol. Retain a portion of the methanol for a blank determination. Place 25 ml, accurately measured, of the water-methanol solution in the titration vessel, and titrate with Karl Fischer Reagent. Similarly carry out a blank titration on 25 ml, accurately measured of the methanol used, and make any necessary correction. The water content in mg per ml, of the water-methanol solution is given by the formula VF/25, in which V is the volume of Karl Fischer Reagent corrected for the blank methyl alcohol titration, and F is the water equivalence factor of the reagent determined against sodium tartrate as directed under primary standardisation of the reagent.

Procedure: Unless otherwise specified, add about 25 ml of methyl alcohol to the titration flask and titrate to the end-point with Karl Fischer Reagent, disregarding the volume consumed, since it does not enter into the calculations. Weigh or measure sufficient sample to contain preferably 10 to 50 ml of water and quickly transfer it to the titration flask. Stir vigorously, and again titrate with Karl Fischer Reagent.

The water content of the sample, in mg, is the product, SF, in which S is the volume of reagent used to titrate the sample and F is the water equivalence factor defined above.

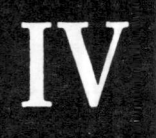

Determination of Loss on Drying

The following procedure determines the amount of volatile matter of any kind (including water) that can be driven off under the conditions specified.

Loss on drying is the loss in weight in per cent w/w determined by means of the procedure given below. Unless otherwise directed in the monograph, carry out the test on 1.0 g of the substance, previously mixed well. If the sample is in the form of large crystals, reduce the size by quickly crushing to a powder.

Method

Weigh a glass-stoppered, shallow weighing bottle that has been dried for 30 minutes under the same conditions to be employed in the determination. Put the sample in the bottle, cover it and accurately weigh the bottle and the contents. Distribute the sample as evenly as practicable by gentle sidewise shaking to a depth not exceeding 10 mm. Place the loaded bottle in the drying chamber (oven or desiccator), remove the stopper and leave it also in the chamber. Dry the sample for the time specified in the monograph or to constant weight, at the prescribed temperature under one of the following conditions. Shown in brackets are the words used in the individual monograph for the drying conditions:

(a) In a desiccator dry over phosphorous pentoxide at atmospheric pressure and at room temperature ("desiccator").

(b) Dry over phosphorous pentoxide, in vacuum at a pressure not exceeding 20 Torr at room temperature ("in vacuo").

(c) Dry over phosphorous pentoxide, in vacuum at a pressure not exceeding 20 Torr at a higher temperature ("in vacuo with indication of temperature and time").

(d) Dry in an oven at the temperature indicated in the monograph ("in oven with temperature range of monograph").

After drying is completed, open the drying chamber, close the bottle promptly and allow it to come to room temperature (where applicable) in a desiccator before weighing.

Note: Where drying in a desiccator is specified, care must be taken to keep the desiccant fully effective by frequent replacement.

---

* The term 'constant weight' means that two consecutive weighings do not differ by more than 0.5 mg, the second weighing being made after an additional one hour of drying under the specific conditions.

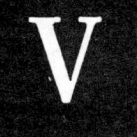

Classification of Pharmaceutical
and Medicinal Compounds
and Preparations

The inorganic compounds used as therapeutic and diagnostic agents and as pharmaceutical aids/ necessities are classified alphabetically under this appendix. Many a time some of the inorganic compounds, specially those used therapeutically, have two or more uses. However, they are categorized mostly by keeping their main uses in view. Hence quite a few of them may be found included in different categories. At places a more prominent and/or secondary use/action is shown within brackets against the compounds. In this revised edition, explanation under each of the therapeutics is given before the classification so that the students have ready information about the same without consulting any pharmacology book.

Acidifiers

There are two types of acidifiers. They are gastric acidifiers and acidifiers of urine.

Gastric acidifiers

These are drugs which help digestion of food in the alimentary tract. Hydrochloric acid is a normal secretion of the gastric juice which helps to activate proteolytic enzyme pepsinogen into pepsin and also in maintaining pH of the gastric contents for optimal activity of the enzyme. Dilute hydrochloric acid in doses of 2–8 ml is indicated in achlorhydria, pernicious anaemia, cancer of stomach and gastrogenous diarrhoea. Dilute acid is usually given with milk. Dilute phosphoric acid, 0.25–5 ml, is used as a stomachic to increase the gastric secretion.

Hydrochloric acid

. Phosphoric acid

Urine acidifiers

Urine acidifiers are those compounds which on being ingestion result in lowering the pH of urine. They are used to help excretion of certain drugs or drug metabolites through urine.

Sodium acid phosphate

Absorbents

Absorbents are agents which attract and suck up gases or secretions from a wound.

Soda lime (Carbon dioxide absorbent)

Adsorbents

Adsorbents are neutral and chemically inert drugs, which when administered orally or mechanically adhere on to the surfaces of unwanted substances like gases, toxins, bacteria, alkaloids etc. from the lumen of the alimentary tract and delay or inhibit their absorption. Activated wood charcoal is used to adsorb gases from stomach and intestines. Light kaolin is used to remove toxins and poisonous substances from intestinal lumen.

Active wood charcoal

Light kaolin

Anticoagulants

Anticoagulants and drugs which inhibit or retard the process of coagulation of blood. Sodium citrate acts by preventing the action of ionic calcium.

Sodium citrate

Antidepressants

Drugs which relieve depressive symptoms without inducing mental excitement or delirium or fits are called antidepressants. Lithium carbonate is used prophylactically as a mood-stabiliser in manic-depressive illness. Lithium carbonate is also used to calm manic patients.

Lithium carbonate

Antipyretics and analgesics

They are drugs which reduce body temperature and relieve body pain.

Sodium salicylate

Antifungal, antimicrobial, antiprotozoal and antiseptic agents

Antifungal agents are drugs which inhibit the growth of common mycotic organism or kill the infection-causing fungal organism.

Antimicrobial agents are drugs which prevent the growth of microorganisms, like gram-positive and gram-negative bacteria.

Antiprotozoal agents are drugs which are used to treat protozoal infections, like malaria, amoebiasis, trichomoniasis, giardiasis, trypanosomiasis, leishmaniasis and schistosomiasis. Each type of protozoal infection is treated with different types of drugs.

Antischistosomal drugs are specifically used in the treatment of schistosomiasis.

Antiseptics are substances which are non-toxic for superficial application to living tissues in order to kill pathogenic microbes or prevent their growth.

Ammoniated mercury (anti-infective)

Ammoniated mercury ointment

Borax (bacteriostatic)
Borax glycerine
Boric acid (local anti-infective)
Calcium mandalate (anti-bacterial)
Hydrogen peroxide
Iodine (local anti-infective, germicide, fungicide)
Yellow mercuric oxide (local anti-bacterial ophthalmic agent)
Oleated mercury (anti-infective)
Potassium permanganate (oxidant)
Silver nitrate (local anti-infective)
Mild silver protein (local anti-infective)
Strong silver protein (local anti-infective)
Sodium benzoate (fungistatic)
Sodium metabisulphite (preservative)
Sodium perborate (local anti-infective)
Precipitated sulphur (scabicide)
Sublimed sulphur (scabicide)
Zinc undecylenate (fungistatic)

Antischistosomal and leishmaniacidal agents

Antimony sodium tartrate
Sodium antimony gluconate

Astringents

Astringents are substances which precipitate proteins.

When they are applied locally or topically they behave as protein precipitants and show low cell penetrability. Their action is essentially limited to the cell surface and the interstitial spaces. The astringent action causes contraction and wrinkling of the tissue. On topical application of skin or mucous membrane they precipitate proteins of exudate or secretions, thus reducing them. They are also used therapeutically to arrest haemorrhage by coagulating the blood. They also control diarrhoea, reduce inflammation of mucous membrane and promote healing and toughen the skin and reduce sweating.

Alum
Bismuth subcarbonate
Bismuth subgallate
Calamine (protective)
Calamine lotion (protective)
Calcium hydroxide (protective)
Copper sulphate
Lead acetate

Zinc oxide

Zinc stearate

Zinc sulphate

Cathartics and purgatives

Cathartics and purgatives are drugs which cause evacuation of the bowels. Hence they are used in constipation and also to remove worms present in the large intestine.

Magnesium sulphate

Dried magnesium sulphate

Mercurous chloride (calomel)

Mercury with chalk (purgative)

Potassium acid tartrate (purgative)

Sodium phosphate

Dried sodium phosphate

Sodium potassium tartrate

Diagnostic agents

Diagnostic agents are drugs that help to detect functional activity or structural changes in the organ concerned. There are mainly two groups of diagnostic agents available (i) agents for determination of functional activity, (ii) contrast media for roentgenography. As barium sulphate is completely insoluble, it is not absorbed, and being opaque to x-ray, it is chiefly used as a contrast medium for radiological examinations of the alimentary canal.

Barium sulphate

Sodium benzoate

Diuretics

Diuretics are drugs which increase the flow of urine. Ammonium chloride is an acidifying diuretic. Potassium salts act as saline diuretic. Potassium salts make the reaction of urine alkaline and, therefore, have some special value in reducing the chances of crystalluria due to sulphonamides. Potassium salts also have diaphoretic effect.

Ammonia chloride (systemic acidifier)

Potassium acetate (diaphoretic)

Potassium citrate (osmotic)

Electrolytes replenisher

Electrolytes replenishers are agents which are administered to repair either acute or chronic states of depletion or deficiency of electrolytes. These inorganic elements are usually administered intravenously in the form of isotonic solution for the repair of dehydration.

Calcium chloride hydrated

Calcium gluconate

Calcium lactate
Calcium levulinate
Calcium pantothenate
Dibasic calcium phosphate
Potassium bicarbonate
Potassium chloride
Sodium chloride

Emetics are drugs which induce vomiting and may act either reflexly through the stomach or centrally on the chemoreceptor trigger zone. Zinc sulphate is a reflex emetic.

Zinc sulphate

Expectorants and antitussives

Expectorants are drugs which stimulate the secretory activity of the respiratory tract and thus reduce the viscosity of mucus and help its expulsion. Hence, they are useful in dry cough.

Antitussives are agents which suppress coughing.

Ammonium chloride
Potassium iodide (source of iodine)

Gastric antacids

Antacids are basic compounds which react with gastric acid to form neutral salts. They neutralize acid in the gastric contents. They are used in peptic ulcer.

Aluminium hydroxide gel
Dried hydroxide gel
Bismuth subcarbonate
Bismuth subgallate
Magnesium carbonate heavy (laxative)
Magnesium carbonate light
Magnesium oxide heavy
Magnesium oxide light
Magnesium trisilicate
Milk of magnesia (laxative)
Potassium bicarbonate
Sodium bicarbonate
Sodium carbonate
Sodium citrate

General anaesthetics

General anaesthetics are drugs which produce complete reversible loss of consciousness in which all the sensations of the body are lost and most of the reflexes are abolished.

Nitrous oxide.

Haematopoietics (haematinics)

Haematopoietics (haematinics) are agents which give rise to an increase of the haemoglobin content of the blood. These agents are used in anaemia.

Ferrous gluconate

Ferrous sulphate

Dried ferrous sulphate

Iron and ammonium citrate (ferric ammonium citrate)

Iron

Respiratory stimulants

Respiratory stimulants are drugs which stimulate the respiratory movements and are known as respiratory stimulants.

Aromatic spirit of ammonia

Carbon dioxide

Oxygen (essential for respiration)

Sedatives and hypnotics

Sedatives are drugs which produce merely a quietening effect on the central nervous system. Hypnotics are drugs employed to induce sleep resembling natural sleep.

Potassium bromide

Sodium bromide

Pharmaceutical aids/necessities

Pharmaceutical aids/necessities are agents used in pharmaceutical preparations and are mostly meant for external use.

Alum

Ammonia solution strong

Ammonia solution dilute

Ammonium bicarbonate

Bentonite

Borax

Boric acid

Calcium phosphate

Dried ferrous sulphate

Hydrochloric acid

Hypophosphorous acid

Heavy kaolin

Lead monoxide

Magnesium chloride

Magnesium stearate

Mercury

Phosphoric acid

Plaster of Paris (surgical aid)

Potassium hydroxide

Potassium hydroxide solution

Sodium carbonate

Sodium hydroxide

Sodium nitrite (antidote for cyanide poisoning)

Sodium perborate (oxidant)

Sodium thiosulphate (antidote for cyanide poisoning)

Sulphuric acid

Purified talc

Titanium dioxide (tropical protectant)

Zinc chloride

Zinc oxide

Zinc stearate

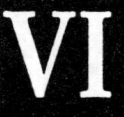
$^{12}C = 12$

Element	Symbol	Atomic weight	Element	Symbol	Atomic weight
Aluminium	Al	26.9815	Gold	Au	196.9665
Antimony	Sb	121.757	Hafnium	Hf	178.49
Argon	Ar	39.948	Helium	He	4.0026
Arsenic	As	74.9216	Holmium	Ho	163.9303
Barium	Ba	137.327	Hydrogen	H	1.0079
Beryllium	Be	9.0122	Indium	In	114.82
Bismuth	Bi	208.9804	Iodine	I	126.9045
Boron	B	10.811	Iridium	Ir	192.22
Bromine	Br	79.904	Iron	Fe	55.847
Cadmium	Cd	112.411	Krypton	Kr	83.80
Caesium	Cs	132.9054	Lanthanum	La	138.9055
Calcium	Ca	40.078	Lead	Pb	207.2
Carbon	C	12.011	Lithium	Li	6.941
Cerium	Ce	140.115	Lutetium	Lu	174.967
Chlorine	Cl	35.4527	Magnesium	Mg	24.3050
Chromium	Cr	51.9961	Manganese	Mn	54.9381
Cobalt	Co	58.9332	Mercury	Hg	200.59
Copper	Cu	63.546	Molybdenum	Mo	95.94
Dysprosium	Dy	162.50	Neodymium	Nd	144.24
Erbium	Er	167.26	Neon	Ne	20.1797
Europium	Eu	151.965	Nickel	Ni	58.6934
Fluorine	F	18.9984	Niobium	Nb	92.9064
Gadilinium	Gd	157.25	Nitrogen	N	14.0067
Gallium	Ga	69.723	Osmium	Os	190.2
Germanium	Ge	72.61	Oxygen	O	15.9994

Element	Symbol	Atomic weight	Element	Symbol	Atomic weight
Palladium	Pd	106.42	Tantalum	Ta	180.9479
Phosphorus	P	30.9738	Technetium	Tc	(97)
Platinum	Pt	195.08	Tellurium	Te	127.60
Potassium	K	39.0983	Terbium	Tb	158.9253
Praseodymium	Pr	140.9077	Thallium	Tl	204.3833
Rhenium	Re	186.207	Thorium	Th	232.0381
Rhodium	Rh	102.9055	Thulium	Tm	168.9342
Rubidium	Rb	85.4678	Tin	Sn	118.70
Ruthenium	Ru	101.07	Titanium	Ti	47.88
Samarium	Sm	150.36	Tungsten	W	183.85
Scandium	Sc	44.9559	Uranium	U	238.0289
Selenium	Se	78.96	Vanadium	V	50.9415
Silicon	Si	28.0855	Xenon	Xe	131.29
Silver	Ag	107.8682	Ytterbium	Yb	173.04
Sodium	Na	22.9898	Yttrium	Y	88.9059
Strontium	Sr	87.62	Zinc	Zn	65.39
Sulphur	S	32.066	Zirconium	Zr	91.224

The above-mentioned atomic weights are those published in 1989 by the International Union of Pure and Applied Chemistry (*Pure App. Chem.* 1991, 63, 978).

APPENDIX

VII

Modern Periodic Table of Elements

Metals

Metalloids

Non-metals

The zigzag line separates the metals from the non-metals.

1	2	3	4	5	6	7	8	9	10	11	12	13	14	15	16	17	18
1 **H** 1.0079																	2 **He** 4.0026
3 **Li** 6.941	4 **Be** 9.0122											5 **B** 10.811	6 **C** 12.011	7 **N** 14.007	8 **O** 15.999	9 **F** 18.998	10 **Ne** 20.180
11 **Na** 22.990	12 **Mg** 24.305											13 **Al** 26.982	14 **Si** 28.086	15 **P** 30.974	16 **S** 32.065	17 **Cl** 35.453	18 **Ar** 39.948
19 **K** 39.098	20 **Ca** 40.078	21 **Sc** 44.956	22 **Ti** 47.867	23 **V** 50.942	24 **Cr** 51.996	25 **Mn** 54.938	26 **Fe** 55.845	27 **Co** 58.933	28 **Ni** 58.693	29 **Cu** 63.546	30 **Zn** 65.409	31 **Ga** 69.723	32 **Ge** 72.64	33 **As** 74.922	34 **Se** 78.96	35 **Br** 79.904	36 **Kr** 83.798
37 **Rb** 85.468	38 **Sr** 87.62	39 **Y** 88.906	40 **Zr** 91.224	41 **Nb** 92.906	42 **Mo** 95.94	43 **Tc** (98)	44 **Ru** 101.07	45 **Rh** 102.91	46 **Pd** 106.42	47 **Ag** 107.87	48 **Cd** 112.41	49 **In** 114.82	50 **Sn** 118.71	51 **Sb** 121.76	52 **Te** 127.60	53 **I** 126.90	54 **Xe** 131.29
55 **Cs** 132.91	56 **Ba** 137.33	57-71 *	72 **Hf** 178.49	73 **Ta** 180.95	74 **W** 183.84	75 **Re** 186.21	76 **Os** 190.23	77 **Ir** 192.22	78 **Pt** 195.08	79 **Au** 196.97	80 **Hg** 200.59	81 **Tl** 204.38	82 **Pb** 207.2	83 **Bi** 208.98	84 **Po** (209)	85 **At** (210)	86 **Rn** (222)
87 **Fr** (223)	88 **Ra** (226)	89-103 #	104 **Rf** (261)	105 **Db** (262)	106 **Sg** (266)	107 **Bh** (264)	108 **Hs** (277)	109 **Mt** (268)	110 **Ds** (281)	111 **Rg** (272)	112 **Uub** (285)	113 **Uut** (284)	114 **Uuq** (289)	115 **Uup** (288)	–	–	–

* Lanthanide series

57 **La** 138.91	58 **Ce** 140.12	59 **Pr** 140.91	60 **Nd** 144.24	61 **Pm** (145)	62 **Sm** 150.36	63 **Eu** 151.96	64 **Gd** 157.25	65 **Tb** 158.93	66 **Dy** 162.50	67 **Ho** 164.93	68 **Er** 167.26	69 **Tm** 168.93	70 **Yb** 173.04	71 **Lu** 174.97

Actinide series

89 **Ac** (227)	90 **Th** 232.04	91 **Pa** 231.04	92 **U** 238.03	93 **Np** (237)	94 **Pu** (244)	95 **Am** (243)	96 **Cm** (247)	97 **Bk** (247)	98 **Cf** (251)	99 **Es** (252)	100 **Fm** (257)	101 **Md** (258)	102 **No** (259)	103 **Lr** (262)

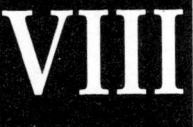
Abbreviations Used

acc.	accurately	m.p.	melting point
App.	appendix	ml	millilitre
Approx.	approximate	mm	millimetre
At. wt.	atomic weight	mu	millimicron = 10^{-8} millimetre
B.P.	British Pharmacopoeia	Mol. form.	Molecular formula
b.p.	boiling point	Mol. wt.	Molecular weight
B.P.C.	British Pharmaceutical Codex	μg	Microgramme
Chem. Form.	chemical formula	N	Normal (concentration)
cm	centimetre	p	page
conc.	concentrated	p.p.m.	Parts per million
° (temperature)	Degree centigrade	ppt	Precipitate
dil.	Dilute	s	see
f.p.	Freezing point	sp. gr.	Specific gravity
g	gramme	sol.	Solution
I.P.	Indian Pharmacopoeia	Syn.	Synonym
I.U.	International Unit	u	Unit
l	Litre	U.S.P.	United States Pharmacopoeia
LD 50	A dose lethal to 50 per cent of the organisms	v/v	Volume in volume
		w.r.t.	With reference to
M	Molar (concentration)	w/v	Weight in volume
min.	minutes	w/w	Weight in weight

Index